Textbook of
ELECTROTHERAPY

Textbook of ELECTROTHERAPY

Fourth Edition

Jagmohan Singh
Postdoctoral Fellow PhD
Ex-Postdoctoral Fellow
Department of Physical Therapy, University of Toronto, Canada
Ex-Dean, Faculty of Physiotherapy
Baba Farid University of Health Sciences
Faridkot, Punjab, India
Ex-Professor and Principal
Gian Sagar College of Physiotherapy
Rajpura, Patiala, Punjab, India
Ex-Professor and Principal
Adesh College of Physiotherapy
Bathinda and Muktsar, Punjab, India

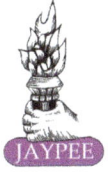

JAYPEE BROTHERS MEDICAL PUBLISHERS
The Health Sciences Publisher
New Delhi | London

Jaypee Brothers Medical Publishers (P) Ltd

Headquarters
Jaypee Brothers Medical Publishers (P) Ltd
EMCA House, 23/23-B
Ansari Road, Daryaganj
New Delhi 110 002, India
Landline: +91-11-23272143, +91-11-23272703
+91-11-23282021, +91-11-23245672
Email: jaypee@jaypeebrothers.com

Corporate Office
Jaypee Brothers Medical Publishers (P) Ltd
4838/24, Ansari Road, Daryaganj
New Delhi 110 002, India
Phone: +91-11-43574357
Fax: +91-11-43574314
Email: jaypee@jaypeebrothers.com

Overseas Office
J.P. Medical Ltd
83 Victoria Street, London
SW1H 0HW (UK)
Phone: +44 20 3170 8910
Fax: +44 (0)20 3008 6180
Email: info@jpmedpub.com

Website: www.jaypeebrothers.com
Website: www.jaypeedigital.com

© 2024, Jaypee Brothers Medical Publishers

The views and opinions expressed in this book are solely those of the original contributor(s)/author(s) and do not necessarily represent those of editor(s) and publisher of the book.

All rights reserved. No part of this publication may be reproduced, stored or transmitted in any form or by any means, electronic, mechanical, photocopying, recording or otherwise, without the prior permission in writing of the publishers.

All brand names and product names used in this book are trade names, service marks, trademarks or registered trademarks of their respective owners. The publisher is not associated with any product or vendor mentioned in this book.

Medical knowledge and practice change constantly. This book is designed to provide accurate, authoritative information about the subject matter in question. However, readers are advised to check the most current information available on procedures included and check information from the manufacturer of each product to be administered, to verify the recommended dose, formula, method and duration of administration, adverse effects and contraindications. It is the responsibility of the practitioner to take all appropriate safety precautions. Neither the publisher nor the author(s)/editor(s) assume any liability for any injury and/or damage to persons or property arising from or related to use of material in this book.

This book is sold on the understanding that the publisher is not engaged in providing professional medical services. If such advice or services are required, the services of a competent medical professional should be sought.

Every effort has been made where necessary to contact holders of copyright to obtain permission to reproduce copyright material. If any have been inadvertently overlooked, the publisher will be pleased to make the necessary arrangements at the first opportunity.

Inquiries for bulk sales may be solicited at: jaypee@jaypeebrothers.com

Textbook of Electrotherapy

First Edition: 2005
Second Edition: 2012
Third Edition: 2018
Fourth Edition: 2024

ISBN: 978-93-5696-388-7

Dedicated to

*My Parents, Teachers, Friends,
Students, Wife
and
My Daughters Jinia and Jinisha*

Preface to the Fourth Edition

Adding to the international experience in physiotherapy and after understanding the physiotherapy education, research and practice in a global scenario, this Fourth Edition of *Textbook of Electrotherapy* has been created.

A new chapter on Inflammation and Repair has been added.

It has been designed to cater to the long—pending needs of students of Bachelor of Physiotherapy (BPT) especially 1st and 2nd year and also of 3rd and 4th year. The book is also useful for professionals of physiotherapy, teachers, doctors, rehabilitation professionals, other paramedics and public in general.

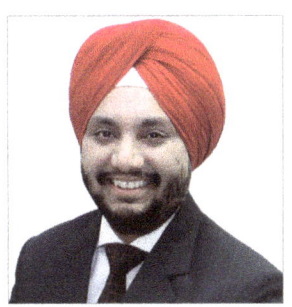

The book has been compiled and prepared as per the curriculum of electrotherapy for BPT degree courses devised by the following Universities: Baba Farid University of Health Sciences, Faridkot; The Tamil Nadu Dr MGR Medical University, Chennai, Tamil Nadu; Rajiv Gandhi University of Health Sciences (RGUHS), Bengaluru; Utkal University, Bhubaneswar, Odisha; Manipal Academy of Higher Education (MAHE), Manipal; NTR University of Health Sciences, Vijayawada, Andhra Pradesh; Guru Nanak Dev University, Amritsar, Punjab; Punjab University, Chandigarh; Punjabi University, Patiala; Postgraduate Institute of Medical Education and Research (PGIMER), Chandigarh; MM University, Mullana, Ambala; Choudhary Charan Singh (CCS) University, Meerut, Uttar Pradesh; HNB University, Srinagar, Garhwal, Uttaranchal; University of Allahabad; Dr Bhim Rao Ambedkar University, Agra; Guru Jambheshwar University, Hisar, Haryana; Kurukshetra University, Kurukshetra, Haryana; Nagpur University, Nagpur; University of Pune, Pune; Devi Ahilya University, Indore, Madhya Pradesh; University of Delhi; GGS Indraprastha University, New Delhi; Jamia Hamdard, New Delhi; Utkal University, Bhubaneswar, Odisha; University of Calcutta, Kolkata, West Bengal; Sri Ramachandra Medical Centre (SRMC), Chennai, Tamil Nadu; Alagappa University, Karaikudi, Tamil Nadu and many more other Indian and International Universities, etc.

Not many books on electrotherapy are available, especially the books which are written for the students studying physiotherapy. This subject is essential and is a basic subject of physiotherapy for the undergraduate as well as for the postgraduate courses. A limited number of textbooks are available in the market, which are suitable for the students. To avoid confusion in understanding each topic of the entire subject, *Textbook of Electrotherapy* has been written in a systematic manner in a very simple approach for the students, professionals of physiotherapy, teachers, doctors, rehabilitation professionals, other paramedics and public in general. Recently, lots of advances have taken place in the field of electrotherapy. Utmost efforts have been made to cover all the necessary aspects of electrotherapy. All chapters have been written in a very simple and lucid manner.

In ancient times, two modes of treatment—physical therapy and chemotherapy—were available to mankind, i.e., treatment by physical means and treatment by chemical means. Physical means included the use of sun, earth, air, water, electricity, etc. Chemical means included chemical agents which were therapeutically useful for clinical purposes. Electrotherapy is an ever-advancing field. Recent advances have made electrotherapy very interesting, and lots of new modalities have been found effective for the treatment of various ailments. Utmost efforts have been made to make the textbook up-to-date. Starting from the history of electrotherapy to the recent advances, all the aspects have been covered in detail.

I have tried to give a fairly complete coverage of the subject describing the most common modalities known to be employed by physiotherapists. The intention is to explain how these modalities work and their effects upon the patient. In the initial chapter, I have tried to lay the foundation of the principles of electrotherapy because a thorough understanding of these principles will ultimately lead to safer and more effective clinical practice. The nature, production, effects and uses on the body tissues of each modality are explained and illustrated.

Chapter One covers the Basics of Electricity, Light and Sound. Starting from the origin of Electricity, to the use in various experiments in sciences, to the conduction of electricity in nerves and contraction of muscles, all basic aspects have been covered in detail. Fundamental principles of electricity have been explained in detail, i.e., Ohm's law, Coulomb's law, law of conservation of energy, quantization of electricity, etc. Static electricity and current electricity have also been explained. Thermal and chemical effects of currents, magnetic effects of currents and electromagnetic waves have also been added. Physical principles of light and sound has been added in this edition.

Chapter Two covers Inflammation and Repair. Defining inflammation, causes of inflammation, acute and chronic inflammation. Pain: types and causes of pain. Acute, subacute and chronic conditions. The role of a physiotherapist and physical agents.

Chapter Three covers the Low Frequency Currents. Starting from faradic type current, modified faradic current, iontophoresis, commonly used ions and their indications for use, methods of treatment, safety and precautions have also been included. TENS, types of TENS, methods of treatment, indications for use, dangers and contraindications are also added. MENS has been added in this edition. Indications for the use of low frequency currents and physiological effects of low frequency currents have been explained in detail.

Methods of treatment are the special features of the book. Comprehensive proforma for the assessment of the patient's condition has been formulated for the convenience of the students. Methods of median nerve stimulation, ulnar nerve stimulation, radial nerve stimulation, Erb's paralysis, facial nerve stimulation, deltoid inhibition, quadriceps inhibition, lateral popliteal nerve stimulation, faradism under pressure and faradic foot bath have been explained in detail. Common motor points have also been demonstrated.

Chapter Four covers the Medium Frequency Currents. Interferential therapy, methods of treatment, advantages of interferential currents, physiological effects of interferential therapy have been explained in detail. Russian currents and Rebox-type currents are also explained.

Chapter Five covers the High Frequency Currents. Short wave diathermy, methods of applications, indications for use, physiological effects, therapeutic effects, dangers and contraindications are explained in detail.

Microwave diathermy, methods of applications, indications for use, physiological effects, therapeutic effects, dangers and contraindications are also explained in this chapter. Long-wave diathermy has been added in this edition.

Chapter Six covers the Radiation Therapy. Infrared therapy, ultraviolet radiation, types of generators, methods of applications, indications for use, physiological effects, therapeutic effects, dangers and contraindications have been explained in detail.

Chapter Seven covers the Laser Therapy. Production of lasers, types of lasers, methods of application, indications for use, physiological effects, therapeutic effects, dangers and contraindications have been explained in detail.

Chapter Eight covers the Superficial Heating Modalities. Its composition, methods of applications, indications for use, physiological effects, therapeutic effects, dangers and contraindications have been explained in detail. Hot packs, electric heating packs, whirlpool bath, contrast bath, heliotherapy and sauna bath have also been explained.

Chapter Nine covers the Ultrasonic Therapy. The production of ultrasound, thermal and mechanical effects of ultrasound, methods of applications, indications for use, physiological effects, therapeutic effects, dangers and contraindications have been explained in detail. Shockwave therapy is also added in this edition.

Chapter Ten covers the Cryotherapy. Methods of applications, indications for use, physiological effects, therapeutic effects, dangers and contraindications have been explained in detail.

Chapter Eleven covers the Biofeedback. Its instrumentation, types of biofeedback, effects and uses, indications for use have been explained in detail.

Chapter Twelve covers the Electromyography. Its instrumentation, uses, study of electromyograph, spontaneous potential, insertional activity, motor unit action potential and recruitment pattern, abnormal potentials, spontaneous activity, positive sharp waves, fasciculation potential, and repetitive discharges have been explained in detail.

Nerve conduction velocity, its instrumentation, sensory nerve conduction velocity, motor nerve conduction velocity, methods of stimulation and recording have also been included. The H reflex, F wave, and their clinical significance have also been explained. Kinesiological electromyography, surface and fine wire recording, placement of electrodes and its clinical importance have been explained.

Glossary of terms, Suggested Reading and Index are given at the end of this book.

Any suggestions from the teachers and students will be highly appreciated so that further improvements can be made in the subsequent edition in the light of the same.

Jagmohan Singh

Preface to the First Edition

The book titled *Textbook of Electrotherapy* has been designed to cater the long-pending needs of students of bachelor of physiotherapy especially 1st and 2nd year and also of 3rd and 4th year. The book is also useful for professionals of physiotherapy, teachers, doctors, rehabilitation professionals, other paramedics and public in general.

This book has been compiled and prepared as per the curriculum of electrotherapy for BPT degree courses devised by the following Universities: Baba Farid University of Health Sciences, Faridkot; The Tamil Nadu Dr MGR Medical University, Chennai; Rajiv Gandhi University of Health Sciences, Bengaluru; Manipal Academy of Higher Education, Manipal; NTR University of Health Sciences, Vijayawada; Guru Nanak Dev University, Amritsar; Punjab University, Chandigarh; Punjabi University, Patiala; PGIMER, Chandigarh; CCS University, Meerut; HNB Garhwal University, Srinagar, Garhwal (UA); University of Allahabad; Dr Bhim Rao Ambedkar University, Agra; Guru Jambheshwar University, Hisar (Haryana); Kurukshetra University, Kurukshetra (Haryana); Nagpur University, Nagpur; University of Pune, Pune; Devi Ahilya University, Indore (Madhya Pradesh); University of Delhi; GGS Indraprastha University, New Delhi; Jamia Hamdard, New Delhi; Utkal University, Bhubaneswar, Odisha; University of Calcutta; SRMC, Chennai; Alagappa University, Karaikudi, etc.

Not many books on electrotherapy are available in India, especially the book which is written for the students studying physiotherapy in India. This subject is essential and is a basic subject of physiotherapy for the undergraduate as well as for the postgraduate courses. Very few books by the Indian authors are available. A limited number of textbooks are available in the market, which are suitable for the students. To avoid confusion in understanding each topic of the entire subject, *Textbook of Electrotherapy* has been written in a systematic manner in a very simple approach for the students, professionals of physiotherapy, teachers, doctors, rehabilitation professionals, other paramedics and public in general. Recently, lots of advances have taken place in the field of electrotherapy. Utmost efforts have been made to cover all the necessary aspects of electrotherapy. All chapters have been written in a very simple and lucid manner.

In ancient times, two modes of treatments—physical therapy and chemotherapy were available to mankind, i.e., treatment by physical means and treatment by chemical means. Physical means included the use of sun, earth, air, water, electricity, etc. Chemical means included chemical agents which were therapeutically useful for clinical purposes. Electrotherapy is an ever-advancing field. Recent advances have made electrotherapy very interesting, and lots of new modalities have been found effective for the treatment of various ailments. Utmost efforts have been made to make this textbook up-to-date. Starting from the history of electrotherapy to the recent advances, all the aspects have been covered in detail.

I have tried to give a fairly complete coverage of the subject describing the most common modalities known to be employed by physiotherapists. The intention is to explain how these modalities work and their effects upon the patient. In the initial chapter, I have tried to lay the foundation of the principles of electrotherapy because a thorough understanding of these principles will ultimately lead to safer and more effective clinical practice. The nature, production, effects and uses on the body tissues of each modality are explained and illustrated.

Chapter One covers the Introduction of Electrotherapy. Starting from the origin of electricity, to the use in various experiments in sciences, to the conduction of electricity in nerves and contraction of muscles, all basic aspects have been covered in detail. Fundamental principles of electricity have been explained in detail, i.e., Ohm's law, Coulomb's law, law of conservation of energy, quantization of electricity, etc. Static electricity and current electricity have also been explained. Thermal and chemical effects of currents, magnetic effects of currents and electromagnetic waves have also been added.

Chapter Two covers the Low Frequency Currents. Starting from faradic type current, modified faradic current, electrotherapeutic currents including alternating, direct and pulsed currents, interrupted direct current, evenly alternating currents including sinusoidal currents and didynamic currents, interrupted Galvanic current to the electrical nerve stimulation, accommodation, effects of frequency of stimulation, strength of contraction, pathological changes in peripheral nerve, Seddon's classification of nerve injuries, process of denervation and regeneration of nerve. Different waveforms, waveform shape, pulse vs phases and direction of current flow, pulse amplitude, pulse charge, pulse rate of rise and decay time, asymmetric waveforms, exponential current, pulse duration, pulse frequency and current modulations have also been added in this chapter. Indications for the use of low frequency currents and physiological effects of low frequency currents have been explained in detail.

Methods of treatment are the special features of this book. Comprehensive proforma for the assessment of the patient's condition has been formulated for the convenience of the students. Methods of median nerve stimulation, ulnar nerve stimulation, radial nerve stimulation, Erb's paralysis, facial nerve stimulation, deltoid inhibition, quadriceps inhibition, lateral popliteal nerve stimulation, faradism under pressure and faradic foot bath have been explained in details. Common motor points have also been demonstrated.

Iontophoresis, commonly used ions and their indications for use, methods of treatment, safety and precautions have also been included. TENS, type of TENS, methods of treatment, indications for use, dangers and contraindications are also added.

Chapter Three covers the Middle Frequency Currents. Interferential therapy, methods of treatment, advantages of interferential currents, physiological effects of interferential therapy have been explained in details. Russian currents and Rebox-type currents are also explained.

Chapter Four covers the High Frequency Currents. Short wave diathermy, methods of application, indications for use, physiological effects, therapeutic effects, dangers and contraindications are explained in detail.

Microwave diathermy, methods of application, indications for use, physiological effects, therapeutic effects, dangers and contraindications are also explained in this chapter.

Chapter Five covers the Radiation Therapy. Infrared therapy, ultraviolet radiation, types of generators, methods of applications, indications for use, physiological effects, therapeutic effects, dangers and contraindications have been explained in detail.

Chapter Six covers the Laser Therapy. Production of lasers, types of lasers, methods of applications, indications for use, physiological effects, therapeutic effects, dangers and contraindications have been explained in detail.

Chapter Seven covers the Paraffin-wax Bath Therapy and Other Healing Modalities. Its composition, methods of applications, indications for use, physiological effects, therapeutic effects, dangers and contraindications have been explained in details. Hot packs, electric heating packs, whirlpool bath, contrast bath, heliotherapy and sauna bath have also been explained.

Chapter Eight covers the Ultrasonic Therapy. The production of ultrasound, thermal and mechanical effects of ultrasound, methods of applications, indications for use, physiological effects, therapeutic effects, dangers and contraindications have been explained in detail.

Chapter Nine covers the Cryotherapy. Methods of applications, indications for use, physiological effects, therapeutic effects, dangers and contraindications have been explained in detail.

Chapter Ten covers the Biofeedback. Its instrumentation, types of biofeedback, effects and uses, indications for use.

Chapter Eleven covers the EMG, NCV and Evoked Potentials. Its instrumentation, uses, study of electromyograph, spontaneous potential, insertional activity, motor unit action potential and recruitment pattern, abnormal potentials, spontaneous activity, positive sharp waves, fasciculation potential, and repetitive discharges have been explained in detail.

Nerve conduction velocity, its instrumentation, sensory nerve conduction velocity, motor nerve conduction velocity, methods of stimulation and recording has also been included. The H reflex, F wave, and their clinical significance have also been explained. Kinesiological electromyography, surface and fine wire recording, placement of electrodes and its clinical importance have been explained.

Glossary of terms, Suggested Reading and Index are also given at the end of this book.

Any suggestions from the teachers and students will be highly appreciated so that further improvements in the title can be made in the subsequent edition in the light of the same.

Jagmohan Singh

Acknowledgments

Textbook of Electrotherapy is a book that provides practical knowledge of the basic principles and techniques along with updated knowledge of the important aspects of electrotherapy.

I am indebted to my teachers Dr AG Dhandapani, Dr PP Mohanty, Dr Monalisa Pattnaik Mohanty, Dr Nanda and Dr C Misra who taught me the basics of physiotherapy.

I am indebted to my guide and mentor Dr Jaspal Singh Sandhu, Vice-Chancellor, Guru Nanak Dev University, Amritsar, Dr HS Gill, Chancellor, Adesh Group of Institutions, Bathinda, Dr MS Sohal, Ex-Professor and Head, Department of Physiotherapy and Sports Sciences, Punjabi University, Patiala and Dr Paramvir Singh, Associate Professor and Head, Department of Sports Sciences, Punjabi University, Patiala for encouraging me at every step of my life.

I am indebted to Dr Sukhwinder Singh, Vice-Chairman and Dr JP Singh, Director, Gian Sagar Educational and Charitable Trust and Dr Kamaljit Singh, Principal for encouraging me and providing me support for writing this book.

I am thankful to Dr Satwinder Kalra, Dr KEM Benzamin and Dr AG Sinha; their comments are of great value for elevating the profession of physiotherapy.

I am thankful to Dr Deepak Kumar, Dr Manish Arora, Dr Uma Shankar Mohanty, Dr Narkeesh Arumugham, Dr GD Singh, Dr Jitendra Sharma, Dr Harihara Prakash, Dr Lalit Arora, Dr Reena Arora, Dr Hemant Juneja, Dr Raju Sharma, Dr Pawas Jaiswal, Dr D Vijay Kumar, Dr Aruna Ravipati, Dr Sandeep Singh, Dr Sonia Singh, Dr Ramasubramania Raja, Dr Navkiran, Dr Sanjay, Dr Sabita, Dr Smarak Mishra, Dr Dayanand Kiran, Dr Anand Mishra, Dr Ram Prasad, Dr Deepali, Dr Navinder Singh, Dr Gagandeep Singh, Dr K Prabhu, Dr A Prabhu, Dr Rajni Arora, Dr AM Bhardwaj, Dr Surjit Chakrabarty, Dr Rati, Dr Jaspreet Vij and Dr Manu Goyal for their support.

In preparing the book, I have utilized the knowledge of a number of stalwarts in my profession and consulted many books and authors. I wish to express my appreciation and gratitude towards all of them. I especially thank my colleagues Dr M Neethi, Dr Janarthanan Reddy, Dr Anu Sharma, Dr Rajiv Sharma, Dr Amandeep Singh, Dr Bhanu, Dr Manpreet, Dr Shainy, Dr Sukhjinder Singh, and Dr Amit Gupta for their support and cooperation towards the successful completion of the book.

I especially thank Dr Ranbir Dhull, Shri Ashok Sharma and Mrs Lalita Aneja for their wholehearted support.

I am very grateful to the whole team of M/s Jaypee Brothers Medical Publishers (P) Ltd, New Delhi, India, who helped and guided me, especially Shri Jitendar P Vij (Group Chairman), Mr Ankit Vij (Managing Director), Mr MS Mani (Group President), Dr Madhu Choudhary (Director–Educational Publishing), Ms Pooja Bhandari [Director-Production (Books and Journals)], Ms Sunita Katla (Executive Assistant to Group Chairman and Publishing Manager), Mr Ajay Kumar Sharma (Deputy General Manager), Ms Samina Khan (Executive Assistant to Director–Educational Publishing), Dr Upma Tomar (Development Editor), Mr Rajesh Sharma (Production Coordinator), Ms Seema Dogra (Cover Visualizer) and Mr Laxmidhar Padhiary (Proofreader), Mr Kulwant Singh (Typesetter), Mr Nitesh Jain (Graphic Designer) and their team members, for all their support to work in this project and make it a success. Without their cooperation, I could not have completed this project.

My thanks also go to my students, viz. Dr Manpreet, Dr Gagandeep, Dr Gursharanjit, Dr Irvan, Dr Jasmeet, Dr Jasmeen, Dr Navjot, Dr Indermeet Singh, Dr Inderpal Singh, Dr Shallu, Dr Navpreet, Dr Sukhmeet, Dr Sachleen, Dr Aman Navneet, Dr Vishesh, Dr Iftikhar, Dr Neha, Dr Bavleen, Dr Pavneet, Dr Sakshi, Dr Bhanupriya, Dr Aakshi, Dr Prabhdeep, Dr Amanpreet, Dr Manjinder, Dr Shilpa and others for their enthusiasm for learning, which has inspired me a lot.

Special thanks to my daughters Jinia and Jinisha, who have always supported me while I was preparing this time. After all, their times with me goes into this book.

Last but not least, my thanks go to my wife Dr Harpreet Kaur for always having picked me up whenever I have needed and who endured five years of emotional stress, while I was deeply engrossed in preparing the book.

Contents

Chapter 1: Basics of Electricity, Light and Sound   1
- Structure of an Atom *3*
- Formation of Compounds *4*
- Types of Electricity *5*
- Static Electricity *5*
- Capacitance *9*
- Current Electricity *11*
- Thermal and Chemical Effects of Currents *18*
- Magnetic Effects of Electric Current *28*
- Magnets and Earth Magnetism *37*
- Electromagnetic Induction *44*
- Electric Shock *59*
- Physical Principles of Sound *67*

Chapter 2: Inflammation and Repair   71
- Inflammation *71*
- Acute Inflammation *72*
- Pain *74*
- The Role of a Physiotherapist and Physical Agents *75*

Chapter 3: Low Frequency Currents   76
- Faradic Type Current *76*
- Electrotherapeutic Currents *77*
- Nerve Transmission *83*
- Waveforms *86*
- Current Modulation *90*
- Indications for the Use of Low Frequency Currents *92*
- Physiological Effects of Low Frequency Currents *93*
- Treatment of Patient's Condition *94*
- Proforma for Patient's Assessment *95*
- Median Nerve Stimulation *99*
- Ulnar Nerve Stimulation *101*
- Radial Nerve Stimulation *104*
- Erb's Paralysis *107*
- Facial Nerve Stimulation *108*
- Deltoid Inhibition *111*
- Quadriceps Inhibition *112*
- Lateral Popliteal Nerve Injury *113*
- Faradism Under Pressure *115*
- Faradic Foot Bath *116*
- Strength Duration Curve *121*
- Iontophoresis *125*
- Transcutaneous Electrical Nerve Stimulation *127*
- Microcurrent Electrical Neuromuscular Stimulation *131*

Chapter 4: Medium Frequency Currents — 133
- Rebox-Type Currents *133*
- Russian Currents *133*
- Interferential Therapy *134*
- Treatment of Patient's Condition *137*
- Proforma for Patient's Assessment *137*
- Low Back Pain *141*
- Periarthritis Shoulder *143*
- Osteoarthritis Knee *144*
- Absorption of Exudates *145*
- Stress Incontinence *146*

Chapter 5: High Frequency Currents — 148
- Shortwave Diathermy *148*
- Microwave Diathermy *165*
- Longwave Diathermy *167*
- Treatment of the Patient's Condition *167*
- Proforma for Patient's Assessment *168*
- Cervical Spondylosis *170*
- Periarthritis Shoulder *172*
- Low Backache *173*
- Lumbar Spondylosis *176*
- Shortwave Diathermy to Hip Joint *177*
- Sciatica *178*
- Osteoarthritis of Knee *179*
- Secondary Osteoarthritis *180*
- Ligament Injuries *181*
- Plantar Fasciitis *185*
- Salpingitis (Pelvic Inflammatory Disease) *187*

Chapter 6: Radiation Therapy — 189
- Infrared Radiations *189*
- Dangers of Infrared Radiations *193*
- Treatment of Patient's Condition *194*
- Infrared Radiations Proforma for Patient's Assessment *194*
- Low Backache *196*
- Postimmobilization Stiffness *198*
- Absorption of Exudates or Edema *199*
- Production of Ultraviolet Radiations *201*
- Techniques of Application *203*
- Techniques of General Irradiation *204*
- Physiological Effects of Ultraviolet Radiations *204*
- Indications of Ultraviolet Irradiations *205*
- Contraindications *207*
- Treatment of Patient's Condition *207*
- Proforma for Patient's Assessment *207*
- Ulcers *209*
- Acne Vulgaris *211*
- Pressure Sores *212*
- Psoriasis *212*
- Rickets *214*
- General Debilitating Condition *214*
- Vitiligo *215*

- ❖ Alopecia *215*
- ❖ Sensitizers *215*

Chapter 7: Laser Therapy 217
- ❖ Historical Aspects *217*
- ❖ Properties of Laser *218*
- ❖ Production of Laser *218*
- ❖ Types of Laser *219*
- ❖ Techniques of Application *220*
- ❖ Dosage Parameters *220*
- ❖ Interaction of Laser with Body Tissues *221*
- ❖ Physiological Effects and Therapeutic Uses of Lasers *221*
- ❖ Dangers and Contraindications *222*
- ❖ Treatment of Patient's Condition *222*
- ❖ Proforma for Patient's Assessment *222*

Chapter 8: Superficial Heating Modalities 228
- ❖ Paraffin Wax Bath Therapy *228*
- ❖ Proforma for Patient's Assessment *230*
- ❖ Hot Packs/Hydrocollator Packs *230*
- ❖ Electric Heating Pads *232*
- ❖ Whirlpool Bath *233*
- ❖ Contrast Bath *234*
- ❖ Heliotherapy *234*
- ❖ Sauna Bath *235*

Chapter 9: Ultrasonic Therapy 236
- ❖ Frequency of Ultrasound *237*
- ❖ Properties of Waves *237*
- ❖ Production of Ultrasound *238*
- ❖ Techniques and Methods of Application *243*
- ❖ Dosage *246*
- ❖ Physiological Effects of Ultrasound *248*
- ❖ Therapeutic Uses of Ultrasound *250*
- ❖ Dangers of Ultrasound *250*
- ❖ Contraindications *251*
- ❖ Phonophoresis *251*
- ❖ Combination Therapy *254*
- ❖ Treatment of Patient's Condition *256*
- ❖ Proforma for Patient's Assessment *256*
- ❖ Tennis Elbow (Lateral Epicondylitis) *258*
- ❖ Golfer's Elbow (Medial Epicondylitis) *259*
- ❖ Supraspinatus Tendinitis *259*
- ❖ De Quervain's Disease (Tenosynovitis) *260*
- ❖ Bicipital Tendinitis *260*
- ❖ Subdeltoid Bursitis *260*
- ❖ Subacromial Bursitis *261*
- ❖ Metatarsalgia *261*

Chapter 10: Cryotherapy 262
- ❖ Techniques of Application *262*
- ❖ Basic Principles *264*
- ❖ Physiological Effects and Therapeutic Uses of Cold Therapy *264*
- ❖ Dangers and Contraindications *265*

- Proforma for Patient's Assessment *266*
- Ankle Sprain *267*
- Muscle Contusion/Hematoma *268*

Chapter 11: Biofeedback — **270**
- Biofeedback Instrumentation *270*
- General Principles *272*
- Biofeedback in Rehabilitation *272*
- Use of Electromyogram Biofeedback for Neuromuscular Re-education *273*
- Limitations of Biofeedback *273*
- Uses of Biofeedback *274*

Chapter 12: Electromyography — **275**
- Types of Electromyography *276*
- Motor Unit Action Potential *276*
- Components of Electromyography *276*
- The Electromyographic Examination *281*
- Kinesiological Electromyography *284*
- Nerve Conduction Velocity *284*
- Clinical Implications of Electromyography *290*

Glossary *293*

Suggested Reading *305*

Index *307*

CHAPTER 1

Basics of Electricity, Light and Sound

INTRODUCTION

Physiotherapy is the means of treating disorders by physical means. Electrotherapy is an integral part of physiotherapy. Electrotherapy is the treatment of diseases and disorders by using electrical modalities that apply electrical currents directly (such as low, medium and high frequency currents) and indirectly (such as ultrasound, hydrocollator, shock wave, cryotherapy, etc.) to the body for getting therapeutic effects.

Actinotherapy is the treatment of patient's conditions by visible or invisible radiations, such as infrared, ultraviolet and laser. Actinotherapy in its simplest form is the use of visible and invisible radiations for the treatment of patients. The word *Actis* is a Greek word which means "*a ray*" and treatment by using rays (such as lamp as a source of light) is called Actinotherapy.

The use of modalities for therapeutic use has a very old history. Hippocrates (430–380 BC) has used traction, manipulation, etc., which is evident from ancient medical literature. The use of electricity for therapeutic purposes has grown up in recent years and now includes a wide variety of apparatus and equipment. A large number of therapeutic modalities for treating several disorders are now in use.

❖ The evolution of electricity for therapeutic purposes starts way back in *1646* when *Thomas Rown* coined the term *Electricity*. After this period, there was a rapid development in the field of electricity. It became possible to store electricity for experiments. The important names during this period that contributed to these achievements included *Pieter Van Musschenbroek* of Leyden, *Benjamin Franklin* of Philadelphia and *Luigi Galvani* of Bologna (Cherington et al. 1994).

❖ *Benjamin Franklin* was a great thinker and statesman at the time of the American Revolution. In *1752*, he conducted famous kite experiment. *Franklin* charged his *Leyden jar* by using a kite during electrical storms. During that period, electricity has become a source of astonishment and amusement. *Franklin's* analysis of Leyden jar led to the discovery of the law of electrostatic induction. He postulated the two opposing forces of electricity, i.e., positive and negative charges.

❖ In *1780, Luigi Galvani,* a professor of Anatomy, proceeded his work on animal electricity. Galvani discovered that the nerves are a good conductor of electricity. He stimulated nerve of a frog with a knife during an experiment. This study revealed the relationship between electrical stimulation of nerve and contraction of its muscle.

- In *1826, George Simon Ohm* establishes the result which is now known as *Ohm's law*. He stated that the current flowing through a metallic conductor is proportional to the potential difference across its ends, provided the physical conditions remain constant.
- In *1833, Guillaume Duchenne* demonstrated that the muscle can be stimulated percutaneously. He was the first to systematically study the neuromuscular diseases and was first to study the muscular dystrophies. *Duchenne* was considered as the inventor of muscle nerve electricity or "localized faradizations" and also considered as *Father of Modern Electrotherapy*.
- In *1840*, England's first electrotherapy department was established at Guy's Hospital under *Dr Golding Bird*. The use of Galvanic currents was first documented there.
- In *1843, Emil Du Bois-Reymond* introduced the technique of stimulating nerve and muscle by means of a short duration (faradic) current from the modified induction coil. He was the first to demonstrate that there is change in polarity of nerve when it is stimulated. He is considered as *Father of Modern Electrophysiology*.
- In *1849, LeDuc* introduced interrupted direct current.
- In *1858, Remak* discovered that the points where the nerve enters into a muscle were easy to stimulate.
- In *1859, Baierlacher* reported that a paralyzed muscle responded to galvanic but not faradic current.
- In *1861, Erb* introduced the method of electrodiagnosis based on faradic and galvanic currents. Erb was the first to demonstrate increase electrical irritability of motor nerves in tetany which is known as *Erb's phenomenon*. He was also the first to electrically stimulate the brachial plexus. This is how evolution of electricity in the use of nerve muscle stimulation has taken place.
- In *1864, Keningsberg* reported the important role of duration of current in eliciting the muscle contraction. He developed a mechanical device which could rapidly interrupt the current; if the rate of interruption exceeded the limit, there was no muscle contraction.
- In *1891, Nicola Tesla* presented a paper in "Electrical Engineer" about Medical Application of High Frequency Currents. He observed when the body is transversed by alternating currents above a certain frequency, heat is perceived.
- In *1892, Arsene D'Arsonval* of France developed an apparatus capable of producing high-frequency currents; he was the first person to study the effects of high-frequency currents on humans. In a communication to Biological Society of France, he wrote that a current with frequency greater than 10,000 Hz can be passed through a body without producing any other sensation other than heat.
- In *1892, Weiss* first attempted to produce a rectangular pulse using ballistic rheotome.
- In *1907, Lapicque* defined rheobase as minimal continuous current intensity required for muscle excitation. He also defined chronaxie which is the minimal current duration required at an intensity twice the rheobase.
- In *1908, Nagel Schmidt* was the first person to coin the term "Diathermy". He performed several experiments independently over animal models and demonstrated the deep heating effects of diathermy.
- In *1910, Langevin* produced the first piezoelectric generator for emitting ultrasound.
- In *1916, Adrian* was the first to demonstrate strength duration curve. He noted that healthy muscles showed a fairly constant curve. There was a predictable shift of the curves during muscle degeneration as well as in different phases of recovery.

- In *1928, AW Hull* invented the magnetron.
- In *1946, Frank H Krusen* and his coworkers reported first clinical use of microwave diathermy.
- In *1965, Melzack* and *Wall* first postulated the pain gate theory.
- In *1972, Meyer* and *Fields* were the first to report the clinical use of TENS (transcutaneous electrical nerve stimulation) for relief of chronic pain.
- In *1982, Melzack* and *Wall* further modified their famous pain gate theory.
- In *1985, Cummings* performed several experiments on rat to see the effects of LASER (light amplification by the stimulated emission of radiation). His experiments suggested the use of LASER on wounds and ulcer healing.
- In *1991, Erwin Neher* and *Bert Sakmann* developed a technique that detects electrical currents in the membrane of the cell, establishing the existence of ion channels. They developed a device called Patch-clamp apparatus to record the small electrical potential of the cell. They were awarded *Nobel Prize in Physiology and Medicine* for their discoveries.

STRUCTURE OF AN ATOM

The structure of matter that shapes the world around us has been a subject of study since long. The first contribution came from *John Dalton (1808)*, who postulated that matter is composed of atoms. The structure of atom was first described by *JJ Thompson (1897)* and later modified by *Rutherford (1911)* and *Neil Bohr (1940)*. Historically, they were described as minute individual particles but the quantum physics has explained the existence of many subatomic particles.

An Atom

An atom can be described as the smallest particle of an element. It contains the central nucleus in which two particles protons and neutrons are held together by strong nuclear forces and are surrounded by negatively charged particles called electrons. The diameter of the atom is of the order of 10^{-10} m.

Nucleus

The whole mass of an atom is concentrated in the central part called the nucleus. Its diameter ranges from 10^{-15} m to 10^{-14} m. It consists of positively charged protons and neutral charged neutrons. The proton and neutron are regarded as two different charge state of same particle called *nucleon*. As the atom is electrically neutral, the number of electrons in the atom is equal to the number of protons inside the nucleus.

Proton

Protons were discovered by *Goldstein (1900)*. They are comparatively larger in size and bear a positive charge. It is the positive charge of proton which gives the nucleus of an atom an overall positive charge. Number of protons in the nucleus of an atom determines which element it is and is called the *atomic number*. For example, the atomic number of hydrogen is 1.

Neutron

Neutrons were discovered by *James Chadwick (1932)*. The neutrons possess no charge and are therefore electrically neutral. Usually, the number of neutrons approximately equals a number of protons but in larger elements there are more neutrons than protons. The sum of protons and neutrons in the nucleus gives rise to the *atomic mass*.

In certain elements, it is possible for different atoms to have different number of neutrons in their nuclei with the same number of protons. These are called *Isotopes* of an element. For example, carbon with atomic number 6 may have atomic masses 12, 13 or 14. So, an isotope is an atom of an element with same number of protons but different number of neutrons.

Electron

Electrons were discovered by *JJ Thomson (1897)*. Electrons are negatively charged particles found revolving around the nucleus in fixed orbits. Although electrons are very small (1/1,837 mass of a proton), they are responsible for various physical and chemical activities of an atom.

A force of attraction between nucleus and electron is very strong. Therefore, these electrons are tightly bound with the nucleus. These electrons lie close to nucleus and are called bound electrons. As the distance between the nucleus and electrons increases, force of attraction decreases. It means that there is an inverse relation between force of attraction and the distance between the two.

$$F \propto \frac{1}{d^2}$$

As the number of orbits increases, the force of attraction between nucleus and electron weakens and therefore, the last orbit electrons are bounded by weak force and as a result of which these electrons remain free and are known as free electrons. Transfer of these free electrons makes the body charged.

FORMATION OF COMPOUNDS

A compound is a substance formed by the union of two or more elements via the electrons of the atoms involved to form a molecule of the compound. Compounds may be either electrovalent or covalent.

- *Electrovalent compounds:* These are formed when an atom of one element gives an electron to the atom of another element. These atoms are then held together by their opposite electrical charges, e.g., NaCl.
- *Covalent compounds:* These are formed when the outer shells of atoms of the elements share a number of common or bonding electrons so that each atom has a complete outer shell, e.g., methane.

Conductors and Nonconductors of Electricity

Conductors: These are elements whose atoms have few electrons in their outer orbit. For example, copper has a single loosely held electron in its outer orbit. It is such conducting electrons which facilitate the passage of an electric current.

Nonconductors (insulators): These are materials made of atoms in which the electrons in the outer shell are firmly held in their orbits and do not leave the atom in order to conduct the current.

States of Matter

Matter can be solid, liquid or gaseous. The molecules of a substance are attracted by cohesive forces (force of attraction in molecules of same substance) and kinetic forces (force of movement of molecules).

In solids: There is a strong cohesive force which holds them in a rigid lattice formation so that shape remains same or constant. The kinetic force produces vibration of molecules about a mean position.

In liquids: When considerable amount of energy is applied to liquid, cohesive force decreases and kinetic force increases so that its structure collapses and liquid state is reached.

In gases: If even more heat is applied, there comes a point when, kinetic force is greater than cohesive force. Then molecules fly apart and form a gas. The molecules collide with each other and with the walls of the container, so that the pressure increases. As a result, temperature increases.

Latent heat: It is the energy required for (or released by) a change of state.
- Latent heat of fusion is the amount of heat required to convert 1 g of ice at 0°C to 1 g of water at 0°C (value is 336 J).
- Latent heat of vaporization is the amount of heat required to convert 1 g of water at 100°C to 1 g of steam at 100°C (value is 2268 J).

Transmission of Heat

Conduction: If one end of a solid metal rod is heated, the energy added causes an increased vibration of molecules. This is transmitted and thus, heat is conducted from area of high temperature to area of low temperature, e.g., metals.

Convection: If one part of a fluid is heated, the kinetic energy of the molecules in that part is increased, they move further apart and this part becomes less dense. As a result it rises, displacing the more dense fluid above which descends to take its place. The current produced is called convection current. For example, it takes place in fluids.

Radiation: As a substance is heated, it causes the electron to move to the higher-energy shell. As it returns to its normal shell, the energy is released as a pulse of infrared electromagnetic energy. For example, heat may be transmitted by infrared electromagnetic radiation.

TYPES OF ELECTRICITY

- *Static electricity:* When the charges on a body do not flow, then it is called *static electricity.*
- *Current electricity:* When charges flow through a conductor, it is known as *current electricity.*
- *Charges:* There are two types of charges—positive and negative.

STATIC ELECTRICITY

The simplest way of producing a static electric charge is to rub two materials together. If the materials involved are insulators, the charges are held on the surfaces of objects and spread themselves evenly over the surfaces unless there are points or corners, at which charges tend to concentrate.

Experiments to prove the existence of charge:

Experiment 1: Take a glass rod and a silk cloth. Rub glass rod on silk cloth. After rubbing hang it with the help of nonmetallic string. Take another ebonite rod and repeat this experiment. Bring it close to hanged rod; we see force of repulsion between them.

Experiment 2: Take ebonite rod and a woolen cloth. Rub the rod on woolen cloth and hang it with the help of nonmetallic string. Take another ebonite rod and repeat the above process. Bring it close to first hang rod; we observe the property of force of repulsion.

Experiment 3: Take a glass rod and a silk cloth. Rub the rod on the silk cloth. Hang it with the help of a nonmetallic string. Now take an ebonite rod and a woolen cloth. Rub these with each other and bring this rod close to the glass rod; we observe the property of force of attraction.

Conclusion: On the basis of these experiments, we conclude that charge is produced on glass rod. Later, American scientist *Benjamin Franklin* (1706–1790) confirms these charges as positive and negative charges. When glass rod is rubbed with silk, charge produced on glass rod is known as positive charge. When ebonite rod is rubbed on woolen cloth, charge produced on ebonite rod is known as negative charge.

We may conclude that like charges repel each other but unlike charges attract each other.

Other Methods of Producing Electricity

According to the *law of conservation of energy*, energy can neither be created nor be destroyed, but can be converted from one form to another. When it is produced by friction, mechanical energy is converted into electrical energy. When it is produced in dry cells, chemical energy is converted into electrical energy, etc.

Quantization of Electric Charge

The quantization of electric charge is the property by virtue of which any charge exists only in discrete lumps or packets or bundles of certain minimum charge ±e, where −e is the charge of an electron and +e is the charge of a proton. The least charge found on any body is equal to the charge of electron or proton.

$$e = 1.6 \times 10^{-19} \text{ coulomb}$$

Also, charge on any body can only be the integral multiple of the charge of electron, i.e.:

$$q = \pm ne$$

where *n* is an integer 1, 2, 3,....

Coulomb's Law

According to this law, *the force of interaction between any two point charges is directly proportional to the product of charges and inversely proportional to the square of distance between them.*

Suppose two bodies having charges q1 and q2 are separated in vacuum by a distance r. Let their linear dimensions be much smaller than the distance r so that they act as point charges.

According to Coulomb's law

$$F \propto q1\ q2/r^2$$
$$F = K\ q1\ q2/r^2$$

Where, K is electrostatic force constant.

Coulomb's law of electrostatic force between two charges corresponds to the Newton's Law of Gravitational force between two masses, i.e.:

$$F = G\ m1\ m2/r^2$$

A unit charge is that much charge which when placed in vacuum at a distance of 1 meter from an equal and similar charge would repel it with a force of 9×10^9 Newton.

Electric Field Intensity due to a Group of Charges

The electric field intensity at any point due to a group of point charges is equal to the vector sum of the electrical field intensities due to the individual charges at the same point.

$$\vec{E} = \vec{E}1 + \vec{E}2 + \vec{E}2 + \ldots \ldots \vec{E}n$$

Electric Lines of Forces

Michael Faraday invented the idea of electric lines of force. They give us partial qualitative information about *an electric field. We may define an electric line of force as a path, straight or curved, such that tangent to it at any point gives the direction of electric field intensity at that point.* In fact, it is the path along which a unit positive charge actually moves in the electrostatic field, if free to do so.

In **Figure 1.1**, AB is an electrostatic line of force. The tangent to the line at any point P gives us the direction of electric intensity $\vec{E}p$ at P. Similarly, tangent to AB at Q gives us the direction of $\vec{E}q$

It is important to note here that the lines of force do not actually exist, but what they represent is a reality.

Figure 1.2 shows some lines of force due to single positive point charge. These are directed radially outward. The lines of force extend to infinity.

On the contrary, lines of force due to singly negative point charge are directed radially inward, **Figure 1.3**.

Figure 1.4 shows lines of force due to a pair of equal and opposite charges. The lines of force due to two equal positive point charges of different strength are shown in **Figures 1.5 and 1.6**.

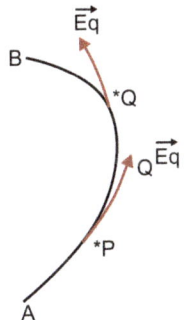

Fig. 1.1: Electric lines of forces.

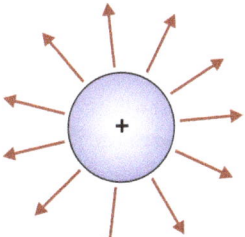

Fig. 1.2: Lines of force due to positive charge.

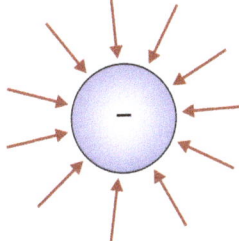

Fig. 1.3: Lines of force due to negative charge.

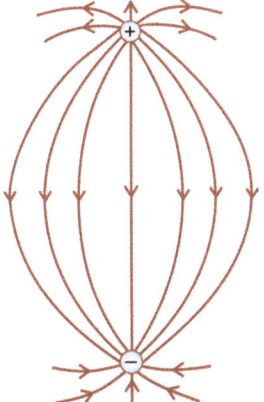

Fig. 1.4: Lines of force due to pair of equal and opposite charges.

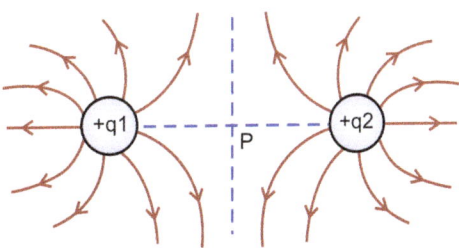

Fig. 1.5: Lines of force due to pair of equal charges.

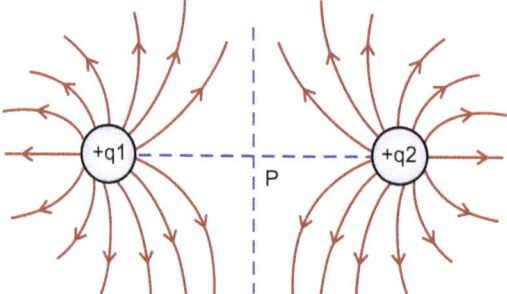
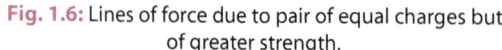
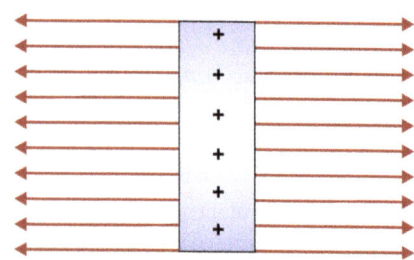

Fig. 1.6: Lines of force due to pair of equal charges but of greater strength.

Fig. 1.7: Lines of force due to large sheet.

When the charges are equal, P lies at the center of the line joining the charges. However, when the charges are unequal, the neutral point P is closer to the smaller charge. **Figure 1.7** shows lines of force for a section of an infinitely large sheet of positive charge.

Properties of Electric Lines of Forces

Electric lines of force are *discontinuous curves*. They start from a positively charged body and end at a negatively charged body. No electric lines of force exit inside the charged body.
* Tangent to the line of force at any point gives the *direction* of electric intensity at that point.
* No two electric lines of force can intersect each other. This is because at the point of intersection P, we can draw two tangents PA and PB to the two lines of force **(Fig. 1.8)**. This would mean two directions of electric intensity at the same point, which is not possible. Hence, no two lines of force can cross each other.
* The electric lines of force are always normal to the surface of a conductor, both while starting and ending on the conductor. Therefore, there is no component of electric field intensity parallel to the surface of the conductor.
* The electric lines of force contract longitudinally, on account of attraction between unlike changes.
* The electric lines of force exert a lateral pressure on account of repulsion between like charges.

Electric dipole: An electric dipole consists of a pair of equal and opposite point charges separated by a very small distance. Atoms or molecules of ammonia, water, alcohol, carbon dioxide, HCl, etc., are some of the examples of electric dipoles, because in their cases, the centers of positive and negative charge distributions are separated by some small distance. **Figure 1.9** shows an electric dipole consisting of two equal and opposite point charges (±q) separated by a small distance "2a".

Dipole moment: Dipole moment ($\vec{p}$) is a measure of the strength of electric dipole. It is a vector quantity whose magnitude is equal to product to the magnitude of either charge or the distance between them, i.e.:

$$\vec{p} = q\,(2\vec{a})$$
$$\text{or} \quad |\vec{p}| = q\,(2a)$$

The direction of $\vec{p}$ is from negative charge to positive charge. The SI unit of dipole moment is Coulomb-meter (C/m).

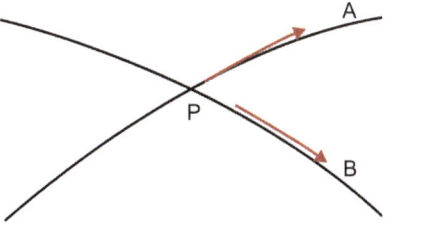

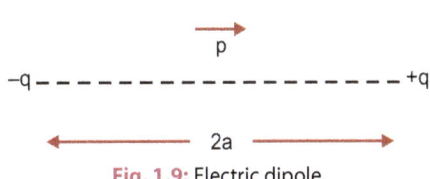

Fig. 1.8: Tangents to two lines of force.

Fig. 1.9: Electric dipole.

If charge q gets larger; and the distance 2a gets smaller and smaller, keeping the product |p| = q × 2a = constant, we get what is called an ideal dipole. Thus, an ideal dipole is the smallest dipole having almost no size.

Dipole field: The dipole field is the electric field produced by an electric dipole. It is the space around the dipole in which the electric effect of the dipole can be experienced. To calculate dipole field intensity at any point, we imagine a unit positive charge held at that point. We calculate force on this charge due to each charge of the dipole and take vector sum of the two forces. This gives us dipole field intensity at that point.

CAPACITANCE

The capacitance of an object is the ability of the body to hold an electrical charge. The unit of capacitance is farad.

A farad is the capacity of an object which is charged to a potential of 1 volt by 1 coulomb of electricity.

In practice, microfarad is used most commonly (1 microfarad = 1/1,000,000 farad).

At any stage, if q is the charge of the conductor and V is the potential of the conductor, then

$$q \propto V$$
$$q = CV$$

Where, C is a constant of proportionality and is called capacity or *capacitance* of the conductor. The value of C depends on the shape and size of the conductor and also on the nature of the medium in which the capacitance is located.

Factors affecting capacity of a conductor:
- *Area of conductor:* It is inversely related to capacity.
- *Presence of any conductor nearby:* In this case, potential decreases, so capacity increases.
- *Medium around conductor:* The capacity increases when any other medium is placed around conductor.

Parallel plate capacitor is the capacitor which is used most commonly. It consists of two thin conducting plates of area A, held parallel to each other, suitable distance "d" apart. The plates are separated by an insulating medium such as air, paper, mica, glass, etc., or dielectric constant k **(Fig. 1.10)**.

Spherical capacitor consists of a hollow conducting sphere A of radius Ra surrounded by another concentric conducting spherical shell B of radius Rb **(Fig. 1.11)**.

Variable capacitor consists of two sets of plates interleaving with one another, constructed in such a way that one set of plates can be moved relative to the other, thus varying the surface area of the plates facing each other. When all the surfaces of both the sets of plates are fully

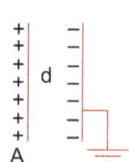
Fig. 1.10: Parallel plate capacitor.

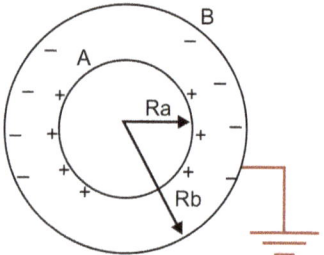
Fig. 1.11: Spherical capacitor.

interleaved, the capacitance is maximum. Variable sets are found in radio sets and shortwave diathermy machine.

Grouping of Capacitors

In many electrical circuits, capacitors are to be grouped suitably to obtain the desired capacitance. Two most commonly used modes of grouping of capacitors are: *Series and parallel.*
1. *Capacitors in series:* A voltage applied across four capacitors in series induces charges of +Q and –Q on the plates of each. As we know:

$$1/C = V/Q$$

The potential difference across the row is the sum of the potentials across each capacitor and so, the single capacitance C equivalent to the three capacitors C1, C2, C3 is given by as in **Figure 1.12**.

$$\begin{aligned} 1/C &= (V1 + V2 + V3 + V4)/Q \\ &= V1/Q + V2/Q + V3/Q + V4/Q \\ &= 1/C1 + 1/C2 + 1/C3 + 1/C4 \end{aligned}$$

2. *Capacitors in parallel:* If capacitors are connected in parallel, the total charge developed on them is the sum of the charges on each of them. The effective capacitance is given by as in **Figure 1.13**.

$$C = Q/V$$

where
$$Q = Q1 + Q2 + Q3 + Q4$$
and so,
$$\begin{aligned} C &= Q1/V + Q2/V + Q3/V + Q4/V \\ &= C1 + C2 + C3 + C4 \end{aligned}$$

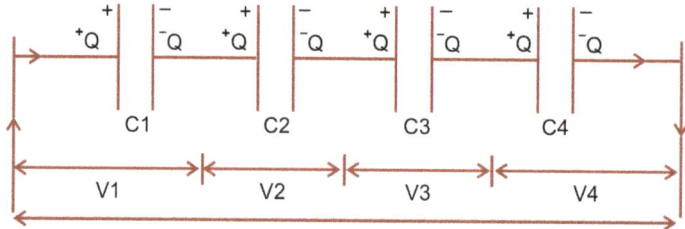
Fig. 1.12: Capacitors in series.

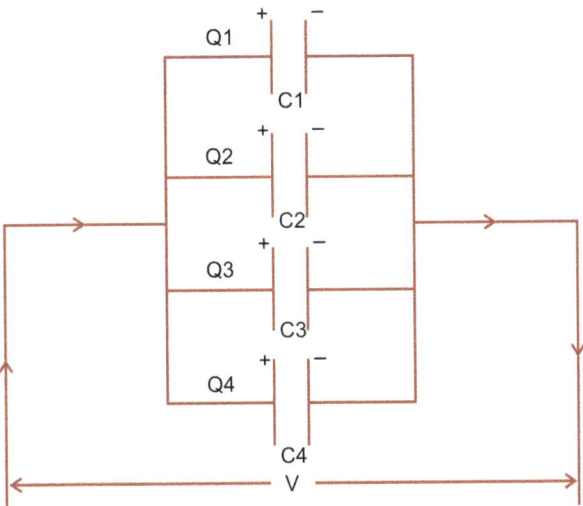

Fig. 1.13: Capacitors in parallel.

CURRENT ELECTRICITY

When charges flow through a conductor, the study of this is known as current electricity.

Electric Current

The flow of charge in a conductor is known as electric current. The essentials for the production of electric current are:
- Potential difference
- Pathway along which current can move.

Electric potential: The electric potential of a body is the condition of that body when compared to the neutral potential of the Earth. Its unit is the *volt*.

One Volt is that electromotive force (emf) which when applied to a conductor with a resistance of 1 ohm produces a current of 1 ampere. In simple words, it is the repelling power between the charges.

Potential gradient: The rate of change of potential with respect to distance is called potential gradient. It is directed from an area of low potential to an area of high potential. It is a vector quantity.

$$E = v/d$$

Where,
  E = Potential gradient
  v = Potential of that point
  d = Distance

From this equation, we conclude that potential gradient can be increased by bringing two plates together.

Current Carriers

The charged particles whose flow in a definite direction constitutes the electric current are called *current carriers*.

Current carriers in solid conductors: In solid conductors like metals, the valence electrons of the atoms do not remain attached to individual atoms but are free to move throughout the volume of the conductor. Under the effect of an external electric field, the valence electrons move in a definite direction causing electric current in the conductors. Thus, valence electrons are the current carriers in solid conductors.

Current carriers in liquids: In an electrolyte like $CuSO_4$, NaCl, etc., there are positively and negatively charged ions (such as Cu^{++}, SO^{--}, Na^+, Cl^-). These are forced to move in definite directions under the effect of an external electric field, causing electric current. Thus, current carriers in liquids are positive and negative charged ions.

Current carriers in gases: Ordinarily, the gases are insulators of electricity. But they can be ionized by applying a high potential difference at low pressures or by their exposures to X-rays, etc. The ionized gas contains positive ions and electrons. Thus, positive ions and electrons are the current carriers in gases.

Electromotive Force

It is the force producing the flow of electrons from the more negative to the less negative body, if similar bodies are charged with different quantities of electricity.

If a pathway is provided, the emf produces a flow of electrons, but if there is no pathway, so that no current can pass, the force still exists. The greater the potential difference, the greater is the emf, and both are measured in the same unit, i.e., the volt.

A volt is that emf which when applied to a conductor with a resistance of one Ohm produces a current of one Ampere.

Electrons move only so long as a potential difference exists between the ends of the pathway, i.e., so long as the emf is maintained. A potential difference can be produced by friction, but when a pathway is completed the charges quickly neutralize each other and current ceases to flow. Other methods of producing a potential difference, and so an emf, are by the chemical action in cells, by electromagnetic induction (EMI) in dynamo, by heat in a thermocouple and from radiant energy in a photoelectric cell. With all these methods the potential difference is maintained in spite of the electron flow.

As fast as electrons move away from the negative end of the conductor, they are replaced by others from the generator, while those which reach the positive end are drawn away by the generator. Thus, the potential difference is maintained and current continues to flow.

Electric current: The flow of charge in a definite direction constitutes the electric current and the time rate of flow of charge through any cross section of a conductor is the measure of electric current, i.e.:

$$\text{Electric current} = \frac{\text{Total charge flowing}}{\text{Time taken}}$$

$$I = q/t$$

Unit of electric current: SI unit of electric current is *Ampere*.

$$1 \text{ Ampere} = \frac{1 \text{ coulomb}}{1 \text{ sec}}$$

Thus, the current through a wire is said to be 1 ampere, if 1 coulomb charge is flowing per second through a section of the wire.

Direction of electric current: As a matter of convention, the direction of flow of positive charge gives the direction of current. This is called conventional current. The direction of flow of electrons gives the direction of electronic current. The direction of flow of conventional current is opposite to that of electronic current **(Fig. 1.14)**.

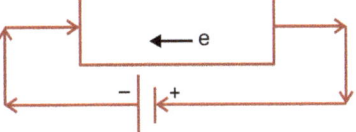

Fig. 1.14: Direction of electric current.

Current density: Current density at a point is defined as the amount of current flowing per unit are of the conductor around that point provided the area is held in a direction normal to the current.

Resistance

It is the obstruction to the flow of electrons in a conductor. The unit of electrical resistance is the *ohm*. It is the resistance offered to current flow by a column of mercury 1.063 m long and 1 mm square in cross section at 0°C.

Cause of resistance of a conductor: Resistance of a given conducting wire is due to the collisions of free electrons with the ions or atoms of the conductor while drifting toward the positive end of the conductor which in turn depends upon the arrangement of atoms in the conducting material (silver, copper, etc.) as well as on the length and thickness of the conducting wire.

Resistance is directly proportional to length and inversely proportional to area of cross section, temperature and number of free electrons in a unit volume.

Ohm's Law

It was given by a German scientist *George Simon Ohm*, in the year 1828. It states that:

The current flowing through a metallic conductor is proportional to the potential difference across its ends, provided that all physical conditions remain constant.

$$V \propto I$$

If V = Potential difference and I = current then,

$$V = IR$$

Where R is resistance and is the constant of proportionality.

Also,
$$R = V/I$$

So, 1 ohm is defined as the resistance of a body such that 1 volt potential difference across the body results in a current of 1 ampere through it.

Limitations of Ohm's Law

- Temperature of the conductor should remain constant.
- The conducting body should not be deformed.
- It takes place in metallic conductors only.

Resistance in Series

If the components of a circuit are connected in series, there is only one possible pathway for the current, i.e., the components carry the same current. The total resistance equals the sum of individual resistances **(Fig. 1.15)**.

If R1, R2, R3 = resistance and V1, V2, V3 = potential difference,

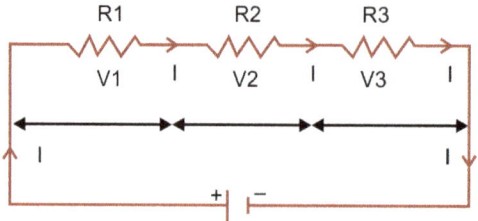

Fig. 1.15: Resistance in series.

Then from Ohm's law, we have,
$$V_1 = IR_1$$
$$V_2 = IR_2$$
$$V_3 = IR_3$$

If potential difference between A and B is V,

Then,
$$V = V_1 + V_2 + V_3$$

So,
$$V = IR_1 + IR_2 + IR_3$$
$$V = I(R_1 + R_2 + R_3)$$
$$R = R_1 + R_2 + R_3$$

So, in series combination, equivalent resistance is equal to sum of individual resistances.

Resistance in Parallel

In this case, there are a number of alternative routes offered to the current. However, potential difference remains the same. It has been found by the application of Ohm's law that the largest resistance carries the smallest current and vice versa.

If three resistances R_1, R_2, R_3 are connected in parallel across points A and B. At point A current I gets divided into I_1, I_2, and I_3 **(Fig. 1.16)**.

Potential difference across A and B is V.

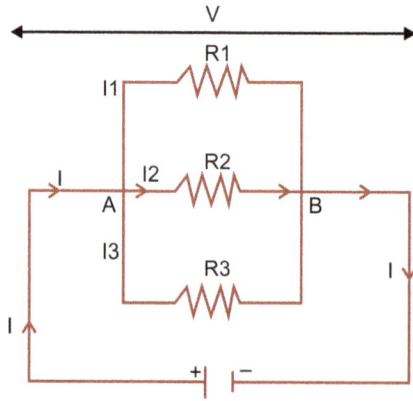

Fig. 1.16: Resistance in parallel.

Then from Ohm's law,

I = V/R1 + V/R2 + V/R3
I = V (1/R1 + 1/R2 + 1/R3)
V/R = V (1/R1 + 1/R2 + 1/R3)
1/R = 1/R1 + 1/R2 + 1/R3

Hence, in a parallel combination, the reciprocal of equivalent resistance is equal to the sum of reciprocals of individual resistances.

Electric conductivity: The inverse of resistivity of a conductor is called its conductivity.

Rheostat

Rheostat is a device used to regulate current by altering either the resistance of the current or potential in the part of the circuit. It consists of a coil of high resistance wire wound onto an insulating block with each turn insulated from adjacent turns.

Types

There are two types of rheostat:
1. *Series rheostat:* In this, the rheostat is wired in series with the apparatus. If all the wires in the rheostat are included in the circuit, resistance is at its maximum and current at its lowest. In the physiotherapy department, it is found in the apparatus where an effect on the degree of heating is required. For example, for wax baths. It is also known as variable rheostat.
2. *Shunt rheostat:* It is wired across a source of potential difference and any other circuit has to be taken off in parallel to it. This apparatus has a current regulating mechanism in which an electric current is applied directly to the patient, as the current intensity can be increased gradually from zero up to maximum. It is also known as potentiometer rheostat.

Non-Ohmic Conductors

Those conductors which do not obey the Ohm's law are called the non-Ohmic conductors. For example, vacuum tubes, semiconductor diode, liquid electrolyte, transistor, etc.

The relation V/I = R is valid for Ohmic and non-Ohmic conductors. The value of R is constant for Ohmic conductors but not so for non-Ohmic conductors.

Thermistors

A thermistor is a heat sensitive device whose resistivity changes very rapidly with the change of temperature. The thermistors are usually prepared from the oxides of nickel, copper, iron, cobalt, etc. These are generally in the form of beads, disks or rods. Pair of platinum leads is attached at the two ends of the electric connections. This arrangement is sealed in a small glass bulb. A thermistor can have a resistance in the range of 0.1 Ohm to 10^7 Ohm, depending upon its composition. A thermistor can be used over a wide range of temperatures.

Important applications of thermistors:
- Thermistors can be used to detect small temperature changes. A typical thermistor can easily measure a change in temperature of $10^{-3}°C$.
- Thermistors are used to safeguard the filament of the picture tube of a television set against the variation of electric current.
- Thermistors are used in temperature control units of industry.

- Thermistors are used for voltage stabilization.
- Thermistors are used in the protection of windings of generators, transformers and motors.

Semiconductors

Semiconductors are elements whose conductivity is between conductors and insulators. Elements, such as germanium, silicon and carbon are insulators of electricity. But when impurities are added to it, they become semiconductors. Semiconductors are insulators at low temperature. The resistance of semiconductors decreases when the temperature increases.

The process of deliberate addition of impurities to a pure semiconductor to enhance conductivity is called *doping*. The impurity atoms are called *dopants*.

The semiconductors are thus called n-type or p-type. The n-type is with excess of electrons and p-type is with deficient electron.

Types of Semiconductors

Semiconductors are of two types*:*
1. Intrinsic semiconductors
2. Extrinsic semiconductors.

Intrinsic semiconductors: A pure semiconductor which is free of every impurity is called *intrinsic semiconductor*. Germanium and silicon are important examples of intrinsic semiconductors which are widely used in electronics industry.

Extrinsic semiconductors: A doped semiconductor or a semiconductor with suitable impurity atoms added to it is called *extrinsic semiconductor*.

Extrinsic semiconductor is of two types*:*
1. N-type semiconductor
2. P-type semiconductor.

N-type semiconductor: When a pure semiconductor of silicon (Si), in which each Si atom has four valence electrons, is doped with a controlled amount of pentavalent atoms, say arsenic or phosphorus or antimony or bismuth, which have five valence electrons, the impurity atoms will replace the silicon atoms. The four of the five valence electrons of the impurity atoms will form covalent bonds by sharing the electrons with the adjoining four atoms of silicon, while the fifth electron is very loosely bound with the parent impurity atom and is comparatively free to move **(Fig. 1.17)**.

Thus, each impurity atom added donates one free electron to the crystal structure. These impurity atoms which donate free electrons for the conduction are called *donor atoms*. Since the conduction of electricity is due to the motion of electrons, i.e., negative charges or n-type carriers, therefore, the resulting semiconductor is called *donor-type or n-type semiconductor*. On giving up their fifth electron, the donor atoms become positively charged. However, the matter remains electrically neutral as a whole.

P-type semiconductor: When a pure semiconductor of silicon (Si) in which atom has four valence electrons is doped with a controlled amount of trivalent atoms, say indium (In) or boron (B) or aluminum (Al), which have three valence electrons, the impurity atoms will replace the silicon atoms **(Fig. 1.18)**.

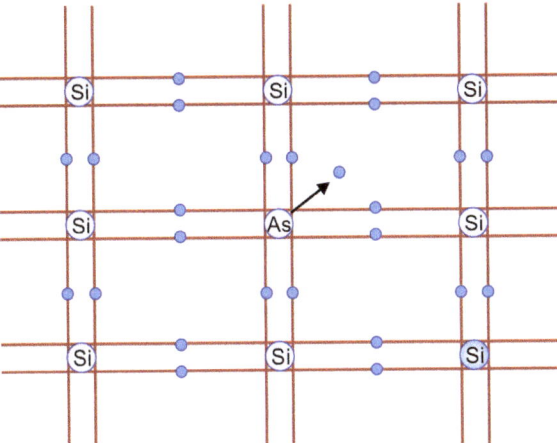

Fig. 1.17: N-type semiconductor.

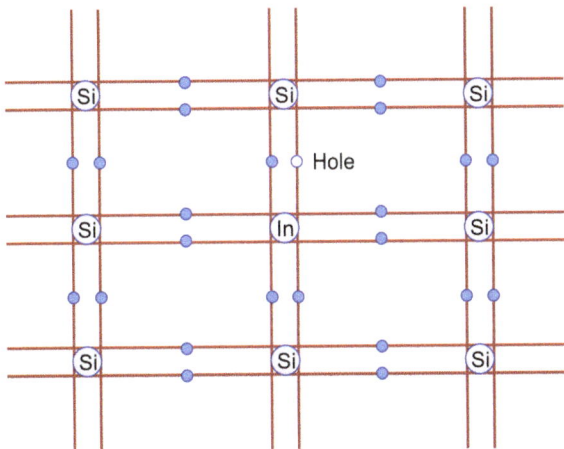

Fig. 1.18: P-type semiconductor.

The three valence electrons of the impurity atom will form covalent bonds by sharing the electrons of the adjoining three atoms of silicon, while there will be one incomplete covalent bond with the neighboring Si atom, due to the deficiency of an electron. This deficiency is completed by taking an electron from one of the Si-Si bonds, thus completing the In-Si bond. This makes Indium ionized (negatively charged) and creates a hole. An electron moving from a Si-Si bond to fill a hole, leaves a hole behind. That is how, holes move in the semiconductor structure. The trivalent atoms are called acceptor atoms and the conduction of electricity due to motion of holes, i.e., positive charges or p-type carriers. That is why, the resulting semiconductor is called acceptor type or p-type semiconductor.

Superconductivity

Professor K Onnes in 1911 discovered that certain metals and alloys at very low temperature lose their resistance considerably. This phenomenon is known as *superconductivity*. As the temperature decreases, the resistance of the material also decreases, but when the temperature reaches a certain critical value (called critical temperature or transition temperature), the resistance of the material completely disappears, i.e., it becomes zero. Then the material behaves as if it is a superconductor and there will be flow of electrons without any resistance what so ever. The critical temperature is different for different materials. It has been found that mercury at critical temperature 4.2 K, lead at 7.25 K and niobium at critical temperature 9.2 K become superconductors.

The cause of superconductivity is that the free electrons in superconductor are no longer independent but are mutually dependent and coherent when the critical temperature is reached. The ionic vibrations which could deflect free electrons in metals are unable to deflect this coherent or cooperative cloud of electrons in superconductors. It means that coherent cloud of electrons makes no collisions with ions of the superconductor and, as such, there is no resistance offered by the superconductor to the flow of electrons.

Applications of Superconductor

- Superconductors are used for making very strong electromagnets.
- Superconductivity is used to produce very high speed computers.
- Superconductors are used for the transmission of electric power.

THERMAL AND CHEMICAL EFFECTS OF CURRENTS

Thermal Effects of the Electric Current

The thermal effect was discovered by *James Prescott Joule*, a British scientist in the year 1841. He established the law called Joule's law.

When current is passed through a conductor, some of its energy is converted into thermal energy. The amount of heat produced can be calculated using Joule's law which states that:

The amount of heat produced in a conductor is directly proportional to the square of current, the resistance, and the time for which the current flows.

This is given by:

$$Q = I^2 Rt$$

Where, I = current in amperes
R = resistance in Ohms
t = time in seconds.

This equation is known as Joule's law of heating.

Cause of heating effect of current: When a potential difference is applied across the ends of a conductor, an electric field is set up across its ends and the electric current flows through it. The large number of free electrons present in the conductor gets accelerated toward the positive end, i.e., in a direction opposite to the electric field developed, and acquires kinetic energy in addition to their own kinetic energy due to their thermal motion. Due to which an electric current flows through the conductor. These accelerated electrons on their way suffer frequent collisions with the ions or atoms of the lattice and transfer their gained kinetic energy to them. As a result of this, the average kinetic energy of vibration of the ions or atoms of the conductors, rises and consequently the temperature of the conductor rises. Thus, the conductor gets heated due to flow of electric current through it. Obviously, the electrical energy supplied by the source of emf is converted to this heat energy.

Electrical Energy and Power

Energy: Energy is the ability to do work.

According to the Law of conservation of energy, energy can neither be created nor can be destroyed. It only be converted from one form to another.

The amount of work done is given by:

$$W = E \times C$$

Where, W = work done in joules
E = emf in volts
C = quantity of electricity in coulombs.

Or   Electric energy = Power × time

$$W = P \times t$$
$$W = VI \times t$$

SI unit of electric energy is Joule, where:

1 Joule = 1 volt × 1 ampere × 1 sec
1 Joule = 1 watt × 1 sec

The commercial unit of electric energy is called a kilowatt-hour (kWh).

1 kWh = 1 kilowatt × 1 hour
1 kWh = 1,000 watts × 1 hour

Thus, 1 kilowatt-hour is the total electric energy consumed when an electrical appliance of power 1 kilowatt works for 1 hour.

1 kWh = 1,000 watt hour
1 kWh = 1,000 watt × 60 × 60 sec
1 kWh = 3.6 × 10^6 Joules

Number of units of electricity consumed:

= Number of kilowatt hour
= watt × hour/1,000

Power: It is the rate of doing work.

Electric power: The rate at which work is done by the source of emf in maintaining the current in electric circuit is called the electric power of the circuit.

It is given by:

Power (P) = emf (E) × Current (I)
= I^2 R (as, V = IR)

Also,   Power (P) = work/time

Its unit is the watt.

If an emf of 1 volt moves 1 coulomb of electrons in 1 second then the power of system is said to be 1 watt.

Bigger units of power are kilowatt (10^3 watts) and megawatt (10^6 watts).

Commercial unit of power is *horsepower*.

1 horsepower = 746 watts.

Some Aspects of Heating Effects of Currents

❖ The wire supplying current to an electric lamp is not practically heated while that of the filament of the lamp becomes white hot. We know that, the heat produce due to a current in a conductor is proportional to its resistance. The lamp and the supply wires are in series. The resistance of the wires supplying the current to the lamp is very small as compared to that of the filament of the lamp. Therefore, there is more heating effect in the filament of the lamp than that in the supply wires. Due to it, the filament of the lamp becomes white hot where the wires remain practically unheated.

- Electric iron, electric heater and heating rod are some of the important household electric appliances whose working is based on the heating effect of the electric current. In all such appliances, the heating element used is of a nichrome (an alloy of nickel and chromium) wire. The wire of nichrome is used because:
  - It has high melting point and high value of specific resistance
  - It can be easily drawn into wires
  - It is not oxidized easily when heated in air.

  Electric iron, electric heater and heating rod are of high power instruments. As, electric power, $P = VI$. Therefore, for the given voltage V, $P \propto I$. Thus, the higher is the power of the electrical appliance, the larger is the current drawn by it. Since the heat produced, $H \propto I^2$, hence the heat produced due to current, is high in both of them.

  It should be noted that electric power, $P = V^2/R$. Therefore, for the given voltage V, $P \propto 1/R$. This shows that the resistance of high electric power instrument is smaller than that of low power. The heater wire must be of high resistivity and of high melting point. Heat produced, $H = V^2 t/R = V^2 At/\rho l$. The resistivity is kept high so that the length l, used for the given area of cross section of the wire and heat to be produced, may be small. Nichrome wire is used in heater due to its high resistivity as compared to platinum, tungsten and copper.

- *Incandescent electric lamp:* It consists of metal filament of fine wire (generally of tungsten) enclosed in a glass bulb with some inert gas at suitable pressure. The metal filament must be of very high melting point. When voltage is applied across the bulb, the current is passed through the filament. The filament gets heated to a very high temperature. It then becomes white hot *(incandescent state)* and then starts emitting white light at once.

- *Fuse wire:* A fuse wire is generally prepared from tin-lead alloy (63% tin + 37% lead). It should have high resistance and low melting point. It is used in series with the electrical installations and protects them from the strong currents. All of a sudden, if strong current flows, the fuse wire melt away, causing the breakage in the circuit, thereby saving the main installations from being damaged. Thus, very cheap fuse wire is capable of saving very costly appliances.

- *Efficiency of an electric device (η):* Efficiency of an electric device is defined as the ratio of its output power to the input power, i.e.:

$$\eta = \frac{\text{Output power}}{\text{Input power}}$$

In case of an electric motor,

$$\text{Efficiency} = \frac{\text{Output mechanical power}}{\text{Input electric power}}$$

Here, Input electric power = Output mechanical power + Power lost in heat.

Efficiency of a battery or cell is maximum when its internal resistance is equal to external resistance of the circuit.

Chemical Effects of the Electric Current

When we pass current through a solid conductor, it gets heated and also a magnetic field is produced around the conductor. It shows that there is a heating effect as well as magnetic effect of current, but there is no chemical effect in a solid conductor. On the other hand if current is passed through a liquid, it may or may not allow the current to pass through it. On the basis of electric behavior, the liquids can be classified into three categories:
1. *Insulators:* These are those liquids which do not allow current to pass through them. For example, vegetable oil, distilled water, etc.
2. *Good conductors:* These are those liquids which allow the current to pass through them but do not dissociate into ions. For example, mercury (a liquid metal at ordinary temperature).
3. *Electrolytes:* The liquids which allow current to pass through them and also dissociate into ions or passing through them are called electrolytes. For example, the solution of salts, acids and bases in water, alcohol, etc.

Therefore, when current is passed through an electrolyte, it dissociates into positive and negative ions. This is called chemical effect of electric current and was studied in detail by *Michael Faraday* in *1933*.

Commonly used Terms

Electrolysis: The process of decomposition of electrolyte solution into ions on passing the current through is called *electrolysis.*

Electrolyte: The substance which decomposes into positive and negative ions on passing current through is called *electrolyte*. For example, acids, basis, salts, dissolved in water, alcohol, etc., are common electrolytes. Pure salt like NaCl, KCl are electrolyte, in their molten state.

Electrodes: These are the two metal plates which are partially dipped in the electrolyte for passing the current through the electrolyte.

Anode: The electrode connected to the positive terminal of the battery, i.e., the electrode at higher potential is called *anode.*

Cathode: The electrode connected to the negative terminal of the battery, i.e., the electrode at lower potential is called is *cathode.*

The current flows through the electrolyte from anode to cathode.

Ions: The charged constituents of the electrolyte which are liberated on passing current are called *ions.*

Anions: The ions which carry negative charge and moves toward the anode during electrolysis are called *anions*. The ions formed when chemical reaction involves addition of electrons (i.e., reduction) are called anions.

Cations: The ions which carry positive charge and move toward the cathode during electrolysis are called *cations*. The ions formed when chemical reaction involves removal of electrons (i.e., oxidation) are called *cations.*

Voltameter: The vessel in which the electrolysis is carried is called a *voltameter.* It contains two electrodes and a solution electrolyte. It is also known as electrolytic cell.

Faraday's Laws of Electrolysis

Faraday, from his experimental study, arrived at the two laws of electrolysis which are given next.

First law: The mass of the substance liberated or deposited at an electrode during electrolysis is directly proportional to the quantity of charge passed through the electrolyte.

If m is the mass of a substance deposited or liberated at an electrode during electrolysis when a charge q passes through the electrolyte, then according to Faraday's First Law of electrolysis:

$$m \propto q$$
$$\text{Or } m = zq$$

Where z is a constant of proportionality and is called *electrochemical equivalent* (ECE) of the substance.

If an electric current I flows for a time t to pass the charge q through the electrolyte, then:

$$q = It$$
$$m = zIt, \text{ when } q = 1, \text{ then } m = z \times 1 = z$$

Hence, ECE of a substance is defined as the mass of the substance liberated or deposited on an electrode during electrolysis, when one Coulomb of charge (or 1 ampere current for 1 second) is passed through the electrolyte.

Generally, ECE of a substance is expressed in gram/Coulomb (g/C). The value of ECE of copper and hydrogen are 0.0003294 g/C and 0.0000105 g/C, respectively.

Second law: When the same amount of charge is made to pass through any number of electrolytes, the masses of the substances liberated or deposited at the electrodes are proportional to their chemical equivalents.

If m1 and m2 are masses of the substances liberated or deposited on various electrodes, when same current is passed for the same time through their electrolytes.

E1 and E2 are the chemical equivalents of the substances liberated or deposited. Then according to the Faraday's Second Law of electrolysis:

$$m1/m2 = E1/E2$$

Faraday's Second Law of electrolysis also states that the ECE of a substance is directly proportional to its chemical equivalent.

If E1 and E2 are the chemical equivalents of the two substances and z1 and z2 are ECE of those two substances, then according to Faraday's Second Law of electrolysis:

$$z1/z2 = E1/E2$$

Faraday's constant: From Faraday's Second Law of electrolysis:

$$z \propto E$$
$$\text{or } E \propto z$$
$$E = Fz$$

Where, F is Faraday's constant
Thus, Faraday's constant is:

$$F = E/z$$
$$F = E/m/q = qE/m \ (m = zq)$$

If m = E, then F = q

Hence, Faraday's constant is equal to the amount of charge required to liberate the mass of a substance at an electrode during electrolysis, equal to its chemical equivalent (in grams).

Practical application of electrolysis:
- *Electroplating:* It is a process of depositing a thin layer of one metal over another metal by the method of electrolysis. The articles of cheaper metals are coated with precious metals like silver and gold to make their looks more attractive. The article to be electroplated is made the cathode and the metal to be deposited is made the anode. A soluble salt of the precious metal is taken as the electrolyte. When current is passed, a thin layer of the metal (made anode) is deposited on the article made (made cathode).
- *Extraction of metals from ores:* Certain metals like aluminum, copper, zinc, magnesium, etc., are extracted from their ores by the method of electrolysis.
- *Purification of metals:* Impure metals are purified by electrolysis. Blister copper is purified by this method.
- *Anodizing:* It is the process of coating aluminum with its oxide electrochemically to protect it against corrosion. It dilute sulfuric acid as electrolyte, the aluminum article is made the anode. To give surface of articles beautiful colors, dyes are mixed in the electrolyte.
- *Medical applications:* Similar principles of electrolysis are also used in nerve stimulation. Also, similar principles are used for removing unwanted hairs from the body.

Cell

In current electricity, cell means an electrochemical cell. Cell is a device by which chemical energy is converted into electrical energy. Electrochemical cells are of two types:
1. The primary cells
2. The secondary cells.

The primary cells are those in which electrical energy is produced due to chemical energy. The chemical reaction in the primary cell is irreversible. The examples of primary cells are Voltaic cell, Daniel cell, Leclanché cell, Dry cell, etc.

The secondary cells are those in which the electrical energy is first stored up as the chemical energy. When current is required to drawn from the secondary cell, then the chemical energy is reconverted into the electrical energy. The chemical reaction in the secondary cell is reversible. The examples of secondary cells are Lead-acid accumulators, alkali accumulators or Edison cell.

The initial cost of a primary cell is low as compared to the secondary cell. But, the running cost of a secondary cell is low as compared to the primary cell.

Primary Cells

Voltaic cell: Voltaic cell was invented by *Allexandro de Volta* in *1800*. It consists of two rods (called electrodes) one of copper and another of zinc, partly immersed in dilute sulfuric acid (called electrolyte) contained in a glass vessel **(Fig. 1.19)**. The copper rod acts as positive electrode and zinc rod acts as negative electrode.

When the electrodes are connected to an external resistor, the circuit is completed. There will be flow of electrons from the negatively charged zinc rod to the positively charged copper rod through the external resistor. Now, the conventional electric current is said to flow from copper to zinc.

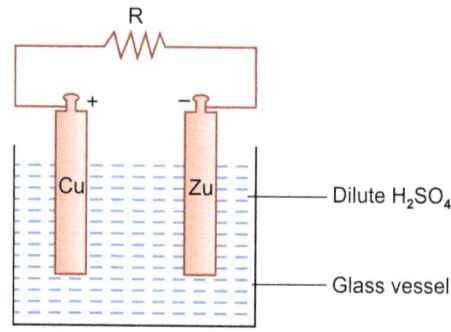

Fig. 1.19: Voltaic cell.

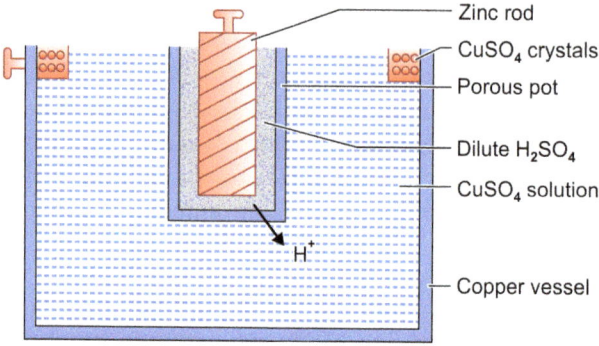

Fig. 1.20: Daniel cell.

Daniel cell: It consists of a copper vessel containing saturated copper sulfate solution. The copper vessel itself acts as the positive electrode or anode. A porous pot containing 10% dilute sulfuric acid (called electrolyte) and amalgamated zinc rod (called cathode), is placed in the copper vessel and is partly immersed in a copper sulfate solution. The porous pot prevents the solution from mixing, but allows the hydrogen ions to pass through it. A perforated shelf containing the copper sulfate crystal is placed at the top of the vessel in order to keep the concentration of the copper sulfate solution same **(Fig. 1.20)**.

In this cell, as the reaction continues, the concentration of copper sulfate solution decreases. Some $CuSO_4$ crystals get dissolved immediately from the perforated shelf into $CuSO_4$ solution. Thus, the concentration of $CuSO_4$ is maintained. As the concentration of the copper sulfate solution remains constant, when Daniel cell is in use, therefore, its emf remains constant.

Leclanché cell: A Leclanché cell consists of a vessel of glass containing strong solution of ammonium chloride which acts as electrolyte. An amalgamated zinc rod dipping in ammonium chloride acts as negative electrode or cathode. A porous pot is placed inside the glass vessel. The carbon rod placed inside the porous pot acts as positive electrode or anode. The space in the porous pot is filled with manganese dioxide (MnO_2) and charcoal powder **(Fig. 1.21)**. The charcoal powder makes the manganese dioxide electrically, conducting and manganese dioxide acts as depolarizer. The inner side of glass vessel near the open end is coated with black paint which works as reflector for the ammonium chloride crystals as they have the tendency to creep

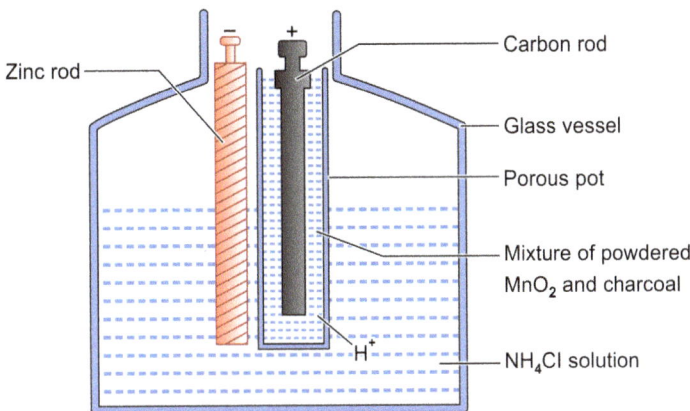

Fig. 1.21: Leclanché cell.

along the glass wall. This helps in maintaining the proper concentration of ammonium chloride solution. The electrons released are collected by zinc rod, making it as negative potential with respect to electrolyte. The ammonia gas so produced escapes. The hydrogen ions diffuse through the porous pot and interact with manganese dioxide.

The positive charge is transferred to the carbon rod which attains the positive potential with respect to electrolyte. The depolarizer (MnO_2) in Leclanché cell is in solid form and is slow in action. Therefore, when the current is drawn from the Leclanché cell, the hydrogen is liberated quickly than MnO_2 can use it up. So, after some time, a partial polarization sets due to accumulation of hydrogen on anode and thereby, the current falls off. When the circuit is switched off, the hydrogen gas escapes. The cell regains its original emf and is again ready for use.

Thus, Leclanché cell is useful in those experiments where intermittent supply of current is needed.

The emf of Leclanché cell is 1.45 V and its internal resistance can vary from 0.1 Ohm to 10 Ohm.

Dry cell: A dry cell is a portable form of Leclanché cell. It consists of zinc vessel which acts as a negative electrode or cathode. The vessel contains a moist paste of sawdust saturated with a solution of ammonium chloride and zinc chloride. The ammonium chloride acts as an electrolyte and the purpose of zinc chloride is to maintain the moistness of the paste being highly hygroscopic. The carbon rod covered with the brass cap is placed in the middle of the vessel. It acts as positive electrode or anode. It is surrounded by a closely packed mixture of charcoal and manganese dioxide in a muslin bag. Here MnO_2 acts as a depolarizer. The zinc vessel is sealed at the top with pitch or shellac. A small hole is provided in it to allow the gases formed by the chemical action to escape **(Fig. 1.22)**.

The emf of dry cell is 1.5 V. If this cell is used continuously, the polarization defect may develop in this cell but it regains its emf, if allowed to rest for a while.

Secondary Cell

A secondary cell is that cell in which the electrical energy is first stored up as a chemical energy and when the outside circuit is closed to draw the current from the cell, the chemical energy is reconverted into electrical energy. The chemical reactions are reversible in this cell.

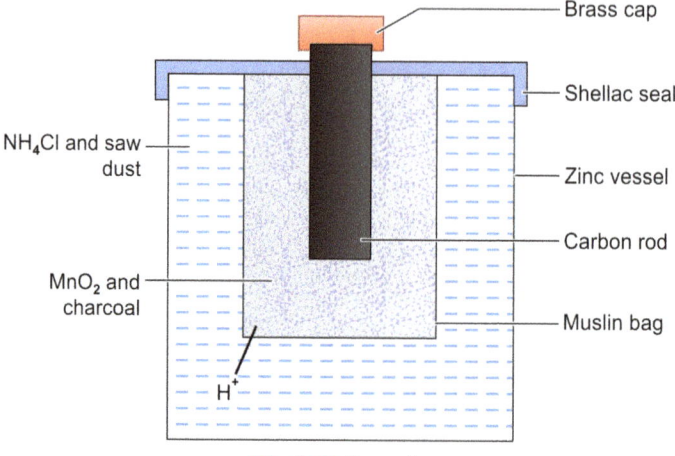

Fig. 1.22: Dry cell.

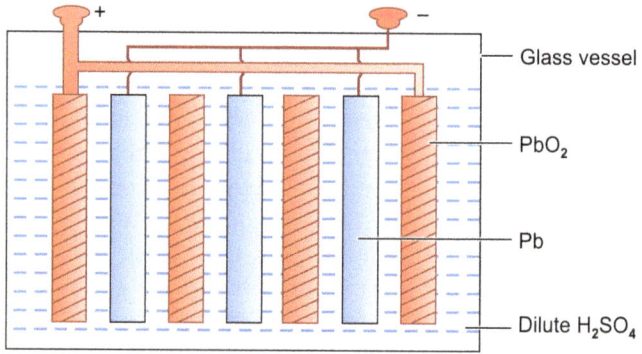

Fig. 1.23: Secondary cell (lead-acid accumulator).

The secondary cells are also called storage cells or accumulators because they act in such a way as if they were reservoir of electricity, i.e., the current can be drawn from them whenever required and when they are discharged, they can be recharged. The commonly used secondary cells are lead-acid accumulator and Edison cell.

Lead-acid accumulator: It consists of a glass or hard rubber vessel containing dilute sulfuric acid (20% conc.), which acts as electrolyte. There are two sets of perforated lead plates arranged alternately parallel to each other inside the vessel **(Fig. 1.23)**. These plates are held apart by strips of wood or celluloid. Alternate plates are soldered together to one lead rod forming one electrode while remaining once soldered to another common lead rod forming another electrode. The holes or perforations in the lead plates are filled with red lead or lead oxide (PbO_2).

Charging: Charging means storing of electrical energy. To charge this accumulator a source of steady current or battery charger is connected across the two terminals of two electrodes. The electrode which is connected to positive terminal of external source serves as anode and the other electrode serves as cathode. The dissociation of H_2SO_4 gives the H^+ and SO_4^{2-}. When current is passed through the cell by the help of external source, hydrogen ions move to the negative electrode (called cathode) and the sulfate ions go to positive electrode (called anode).

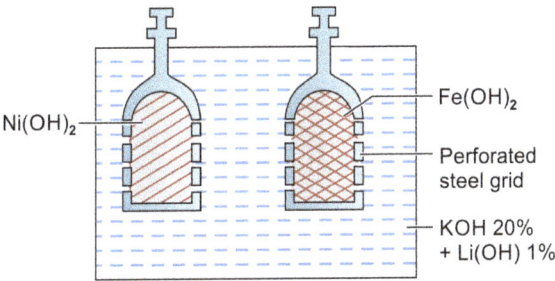

Fig. 1.24: Alkali accumulator or Edison cell.

During charging electron moves from the anode to cathode, thus raising the potential difference between the electrodes. In charging process, water is consumed and sulfuric acid is formed. When the specific gravity of sulfuric acid solution becomes 1.25, the cell is fully charged. The emf of the cell at this stage is 2.2 volts.

Discharging: If the cell is connected to the external circuit, the current is drawn from the cell. The sulfuric acid dissociates into hydrogen ions and sulfate ions. After giving their charges, they react with the electrodes and reduce the active material of each plate to lead sulfate.

In discharging process, the electrons moves from the cathode to anode, thus lowering the potential difference between electrodes. Hence, the emf of cell falls. In this process, sulfuric acid is consumed and water is formed. Therefore, the specific gravity of sulfuric acid also falls. If the specific gravity of sulfuric acid falls below 1.18, the cell requires recharging.

Alkali accumulator (Ni-Fe) or Edison cell: It is also known as alkaline secondary cell or Edison cell. It consists of a steel vessel containing 20% solution of KOH in distilled water (as electrolyte) and 1% lithium hydroxide to make it conducting. Here anode is a perforated steel plate in the form of a grid. Its holes are packed with nickel hydrochloride and trace of nickel to make it conducting. The cathode is also made of a steel grid. Its holes are packed with an iron hydrochloride and trace of mercury oxide for lowering its internal resistance **(Fig. 1.24)**.

Working: Potassium hydroxide solution breaks up into positive potassium ions and negative hydroxyl ions due to ionization.

Charging: On passing the current from an external source, the anode attracts negative hydroxyl ions and cathode attracts positive potassium ions. These ions on reaching the respective electrodes lose their charge and react with them. Thus, when accumulator is charged $Ni(OH)_4$ is formed on the anode and a spongy Fe on the cathode. In this process, electrons moves from anode to cathode, raising the potential difference between the two electrodes of cell. When this potential difference becomes 1.36 V, the cell is fully charged.

Discharging: When the two electrodes of the cell are connected together through a resistor, there is discharging of the cell, i.e., the cell is giving the current. Now the anode attracts the potassium ions and cathode attracts hydroxyl ions. These ions on reaching the respective electrodes give their charges and react with them. The electrons moves from cathode to anode, thus lowering the potential difference between two electrodes, due to which emf of the cell falls. When the emf becomes less than 1.1 V, then the cell requires recharging.

The emf of Ni-Fe cell is 1.36 V. Its internal resistance is low but is higher than net storage cell.

Advantages

- It can withstand rough handling.
- It is lighter, stronger and more durable than the lead accumulator.
- It is not damaged or over recharged.
- It is not spoiled even if left uncharged for a long time.

Disadvantages

- Its initial cost is high.
- Its emf is smaller and internal resistance is greater than that of lead accumulator. Therefore, it cannot give us very strong currents.
- It absorbs carbon dioxide when exposed to atmosphere and thus its capacity is considerably reduced.

MAGNETIC EFFECTS OF ELECTRIC CURRENT

Oersted (1820) showed that the electric current through the wire deflects the magnetic needle below the wire. The direction of deflection of the magnetic needle is reversed if the deflection of current in the wire is reversed.

An electric current is equivalent to the charges (or electrons) in motion. Such charges produce magnetic interaction. The magnetic field produce by the conductor carrying current thus interacts with the magnetic needle and deflects it **(Fig. 1.25)**.

As a rule, if we imagine a man swimming along the wire in the direction of current with his face always turned toward the needle, so that the current enters at his feet and leaves at his head, then the North pole of the magnetic needle will be deflected toward his left hand. This rule can be recollected with the help of the word SNOW. It means current from South to North, in a wire over the magnetic needle, the North pole of the needle is deflected toward West.

A magnetic field is the space around a magnet or a space around a conductor carrying current in which magnetic influence can be experienced. In the latter case, the magnetic field disappears as soon as the current is switched off. It suggests that motion of electrons in the wire produces a magnetic field. In general, a moving charge is a source of magnetic field.

Due to the interaction between the magnetic field produced due to a moving charge, i.e., current and the magnetic field applied, the charge q then experiences a force, which depends upon the following factors **(Fig. 1.26)**:

- The magnitude of the force F experienced is directly proportional to the magnitude of the charge, i.e."

$$F \propto q$$

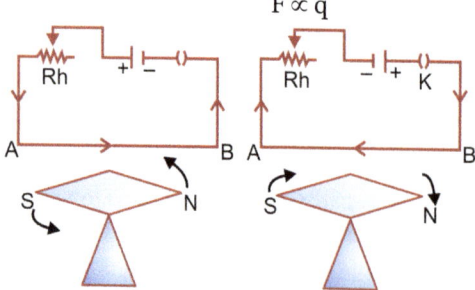

Fig. 1.25: Magnetic effects of electric current.

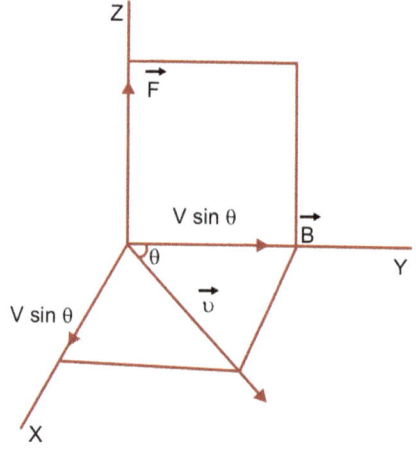

Fig. 1.26: Effects on magnitude of force.

- The magnitude of the force F is directly proportional to the component of velocity acting perpendicular to the direction of magnetic field, i.e.:
$$F \propto v \sin \theta$$
- The magnitude of the force F is directly proportional to the magnitude of the magnetic field applied, i.e.:
$$F \propto B$$

Thus, combing the above factors, we get:
$$F \propto q v \sin \theta B$$
$$F = k q v \sin \theta B$$

Where, k is the constant of proportionality and its value is found to be 1.
$$F = q v \sin \theta B$$
or
$$|\vec{F}| = q |\vec{v} \times \vec{B}|$$
or
$$\vec{F} = q |\vec{v} \times \vec{B}|$$

It is the equation of a magnetic Lorentz force experienced by a charged particle moving in the magnetic field.

If $v = 1, q = 1$ and $\sin \theta = 1$
or $\theta = 90°$, then $F = 1 \times 1 \times B \times 1 = B$

Thus, the magnetic field induction at any point in the field is equal to the force acting on a unit charge moving with a unit velocity perpendicular to the direction of magnetic field at that point. In cases where,

1. $\theta = 0°$ or $180°$, then $\sin \theta = 0$
   $F = q v \sin \theta B = 0$
   Thus, a charged particle moving parallel to the direction of magnetic field does not experience any force.
2. If $v = 0$, then
   $F = q v \sin \theta B = 0$
   It means that if a charged particle is at rest in a magnetic field, it experiences no force.
3. If $\theta = 90°$, then $\sin \theta = 1$
   $F = q v (1) B = q v B$
   It means that if a charge particle is moving along a line perpendicular to the direction of a magnetic field, it experiences a maximum force.

The direction of this force is determined by *Fleming's left hand rule*.

Fleming's left hand rule states that, if we stretch the first finger, the central finger and the thumb of left hand mutually perpendicular to each other such that the first finger points to the direction of magnetic field, the central finger points to the direction of electric current (motion of the positive charge) then the thumb represents the direction of force experienced by the charge particle.

If v is along X-axis and B along Y-axis, then F will be along Z-axis **(Fig. 1.27)**.

Unit of B in SI units is Tesla (T)
$$B = F/q v \sin \theta$$

If $q = 1$ C, $v = 1$ m/s, $\theta = 90°$
or $\sin \theta = 1$ and $F = 1$ N
Then, $B = 1/1 \times 1 \times 1 = 1$ T

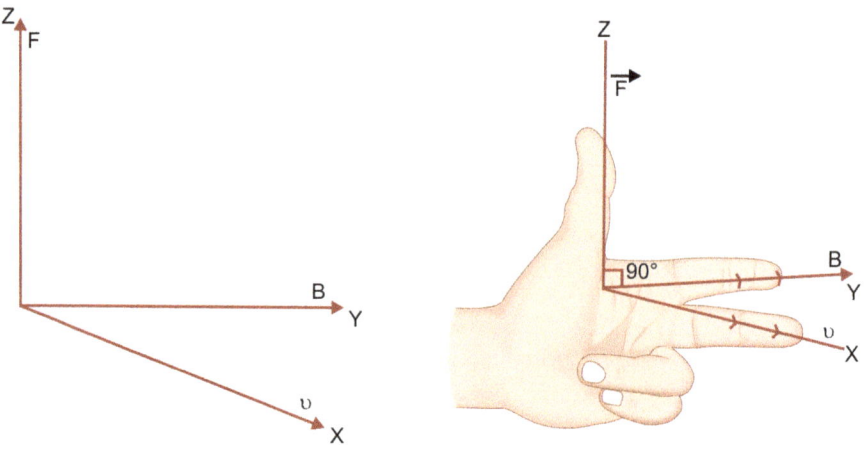

Fig. 1.27: Fleming's left hand rule.

Thus, the magnetic field induction at a point is said to be one Tesla, if a charge of one coulomb while moving at right angle to a magnetic field, with the velocity of one m/s experiences a force of one N, at that point.

Biot–Savart's Law

Biot–Savart's law is an experimental law predicted by *Biot* and *Savart* in the year *1820*. This law deals with the magnetic field induction at a point due to a small current element (a part of any conductor carrying current).

Let AB is a small element of length dl of the conductor XY which is carrying I. Let r be the position vector of the point P from the current element dl (the current element dl is a vector which is tangent to the element and is in the direction of current flow in the conductor) and be the angle dl and r **(Fig. 1.28)**.

According to Biot-Savart's law, the magnetic field induction dB (also called magnetic flux density) at a point P due to current element depends on the factors as stated next:
- $dB \propto I$
- $dB \propto dl$
- $dB \propto \sin \theta$
- $dB \propto 1/r^2$

On combining these factors, we get:
$$dB \propto I \, dl \sin \theta / r^2$$
$$dB = K I \, dl \sin \theta / r^2$$
Where, K is the constant of proportionality.

Important Features of Biot–Savart's Law

- This law is applicable only to very small length conductor carrying current.
- This law cannot be easily verified experimentally as the conductor of very small length cannot be obtained practically.
- This law is analogous to Coulomb's law in electrostatics.
- $\vec{dB}$ is perpendicular to both $\vec{dl}$ and $\vec{r}$.

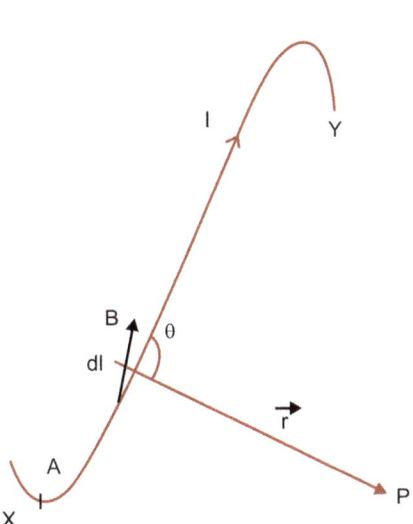

Fig. 1.28: Explanation of Biot–Savart's law.

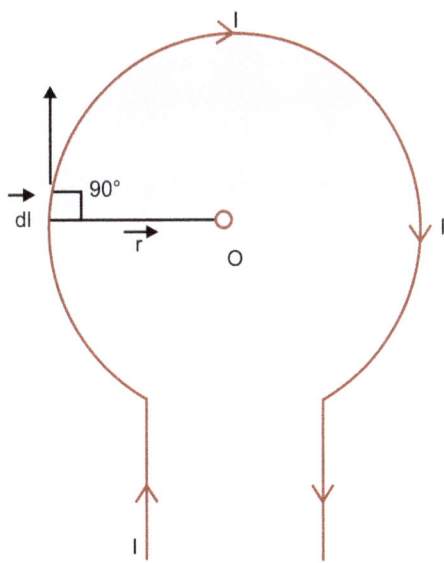

Fig. 1.29: Magnetic field at the center of circular coil carrying current.

- If $\theta = 0°$, i.e., the point P lies on the conductor itself, then $dB = K I l \sin \theta / r^2$
- $dB = 0$ ($\sin \theta = 0$). Thus, there is no magnetic field induction at any point on the conductor.
- If $\theta = 90°$ dB is maximum. Then, $dB = K I l \sin \theta / r^2$.

A magnetic field at the center of the circular coil carrying current: Consider a circular coil of radius r with center O, lying with its plane in the plane of paper. Let I be the current flowing in the circular coil in a particular direction **(Fig. 1.29)**. Suppose the circular coil is made up of a large number of current elements each of length dl.

According to Biot-Savart's law, the magnetic field at the center of the circular coil due to the current element dl is given by:

$$d\vec{B} = KI \frac{(\vec{dl} \times \vec{r})}{r^3}$$

$$K = \frac{\mu_o}{4\pi}$$

Where $\vec{r}$ is the position vector of point O from the current element.

The magnetic lines of force due to circular coil carrying current are perpendicular to the plane of the wire loop and are circular near the wire and practically straight near the center of the wire loop. If the radius of the current loop is very large, the magnetic field near the center of the current loop is almost uniform **(Fig. 1.30)**. The magnetic field at the center of circular current loop is given by right hand palm rule.

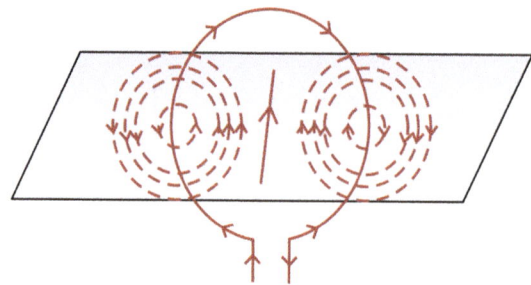

Fig. 1.30: Magnetic field near the center of current loop of larger radius.

Right hand palm rule: According to this rule, if we hold the thumb of right hand mutually perpendicular to the grip of the fingers such that the curvature of the finger represents the direction of current in the wire loop, then the thumb of the right hand will point in a direction of magnetic field near the center of the current loop.

Magnetic field due to a straight conductor carrying current: Consider a long straight conductor XY lying in a plane of paper carrying current I in the direction X to Y **(Fig. 1.31)**.

Let P be a point at a perpendicular distance from the straight conductor. Clearly, PC = a. Consider a small current element of length dl of the straight conductor at O. Let $\vec{r}$ be the position vector of P with respect to current element and θ be the angle between $\vec{dl}$ and $\vec{r}$ and CO = l.

According to Biot-Savart's law, the magnetic field induction, i.e., magnetic flux density at a point P due to current element dl is given by:

$$dB = KI\,(dl \times r/r^3)$$

$$\text{or } dB = \frac{\mu_0 I}{4\pi}\,(dl \times \sin\theta/r^2)$$

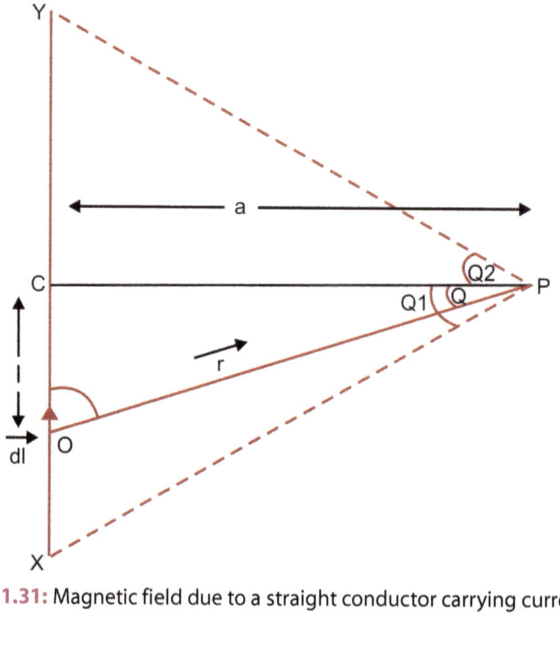

Fig. 1.31: Magnetic field due to a straight conductor carrying current.

In right angled triangle POC, $\theta + \varphi = 90°$

$$dB = \frac{\mu_0 I}{4\pi a} \cos\varphi \, d\varphi$$

The direction of dB, according to right hand thumb rule, will be perpendicular to the plane of paper and directed inward. As all the current elements of the conductor will also produce magnetic field in the same direction, therefore, the total magnetic field at point P due to current through the whole straight conductor XY can be obtained.

$$dB = \frac{\mu_0 I}{4\pi a} (\sin\theta_1 + \sin\theta_2)$$

Direction of magnetic field: The magnetic lines of force due to straight conductor carrying current are in the form of concentric circles with the conductor as center, lying in a plane perpendicular to the straight conductor. The direction of magnetic lines of force is anticlockwise, if the current flows from A to B in the straight conductor and is clockwise if the current flows from B to A in the straight conductor **(Fig. 1.32)**.

The direction of magnetic lines of force can be given by right hand thumb rule or Maxwell's cork screw rule.

Right hand thumb rule: According to this rule, if we imagine the linear conductor to be held in the grip of the right hand so that the thumb points in the direction of current, then the curvature of the fingers around the conductor will represent the direction of magnetic lines of force **(Fig. 1.33)**.

Maxwell's cork screw rule: According to this rule, if we imagine a right-handed screw placed along the current carrying linear conductor, be rotated such that the screw moves in a direction of flow of current, then the direction of rotation of the thumb gives the direction of magnetic lines of force **(Fig. 1.34)**.

Ampere's circuital law: Ampere's circuital law states that the line integral of magnetic field induction $\vec{B}$ around any closed path in vacuum is equal to μ_0 times the total current threading the closed path, i.e.:

$$\oint \vec{B} \cdot \vec{dl} = \mu_0 I$$

This is independent of the size and shape of the closed curve enclosing a current.

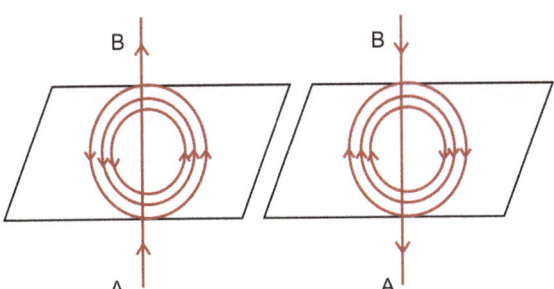

Fig. 1.32: Direction of magnetic lines of force.

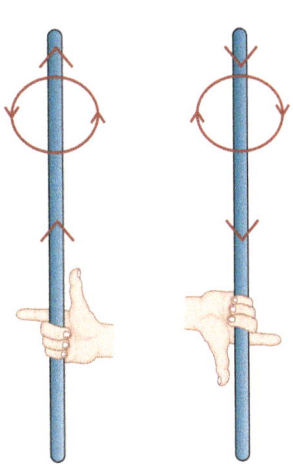

Fig. 1.33: Right hand thumb rule.

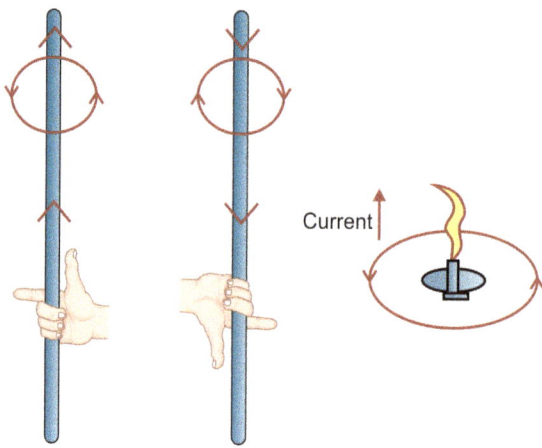

Fig. 1.34: Maxwell's cork screw rule.

Lorentz force: The force experienced by a charged particle moving in space where both electric and magnetic fields exist is called Lorentz force.

Force due to electric field: When a charged particle carrying charge +q is subjected to an electric field of strength E, it experiences a force given by:

$$\vec{F} = q\vec{E}$$

Whose direction is the same as that of $\vec{E}$.

Force due to magnetic field: If the charged particle is moving in a magnetic field B, with a velocity v it experiences a force given by:

$$\vec{F}m = q\,(\vec{v} \times \vec{B})$$

The direction of this force is in the direction of $\vec{v} \times \vec{B}$, i.e., perpendicular to the plane containing v and B and is directed as given by right hand screw rule.

Due to both the electric and magnetic fields, the total force experienced by the charged particle will be given by:

$$\vec{F} = \vec{F}e + \vec{F}m = q\vec{E} + q\,(\vec{v} \times \vec{B})$$
$$= q\,(\vec{E} + \vec{v} \times \vec{B})$$

This is called Lorentz force.

Moving Coil Galvanometer

Moving coil galvanometer is an instrument used for detection and measurement of small electric currents **(Fig. 1.35)**.

Principle: Its working is based on the fact that when a current carrying coil is placed in a magnetic field, it experiences a torque. It means the deflection produced is proportional to the current flowing through the galvanometer.

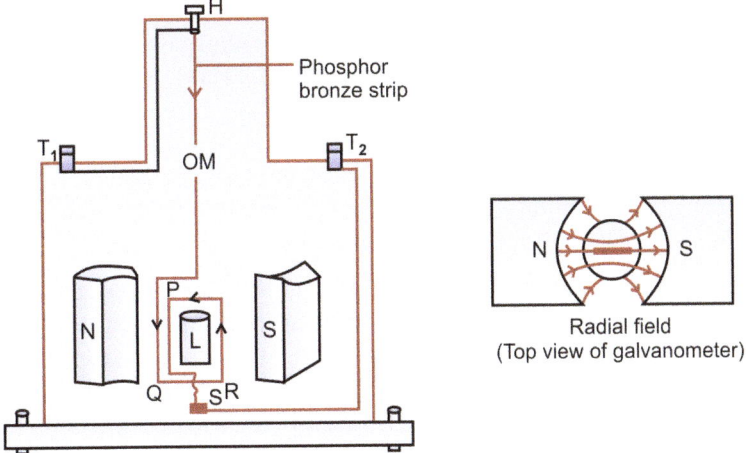

Fig. 1.35: Moving coil galvanometer.

Current sensitivity of a galvanometer is defined as the deflection produced in the galvanometer, when a unit current flows through it.

Voltage sensitivity of a galvanometer is defined as the deflection produced in the galvanometer when a unit voltage is applied across the two terminals of the galvanometer.

Conditions for a Sensitive Galvanometer

A galvanometer is said to be very sensitive if it shows large deflection even when a small current is passed through it.

From the theory of galvanometer:
$$\theta = nBAI/k$$

For a given value of I, θ will be large if nBA/k is large. It is so if:
1. n is large
2. B is large
3. A is large
4. k is small.

1. The value of n cannot be increased beyond a certain limit because it results in an increase of the resistance of the galvanometer and also makes the galvanometer bulky. This tends to decrease the sensitivity. Hence, n cannot be increased beyond a certain limit.
2. The value of B can be increased by using a strong horseshoe magnet.
3. The value of A cannot be increased beyond a certain limit because in that case the coil will not be in a uniform magnetic field. Moreover, it will make the galvanometer bulky and unmanageable.
4. The value of k can be decreased. The value of k depends upon the nature of the material used as suspension strip. The value of k is very small for quartz or phosphor bronze. That is why, in sensitive galvanometer, quartz or phosphor bronze is used as a suspension strip.

Shunt: Shunt is a low resistance connected in parallel with the galvanometer or ammeter. It protects the galvanometer or ammeter from the strong currents.

If the current flowing in a circuit is strong, a galvanometer or ammeter cannot be put directly in it because the instrument may be damaged. To overcome this difficulty, a low resistance (i.e., shunt) is connected in parallel with the instrument. Then a major portion of the current passes through this low resistance (i.e., shunt) and only a small portion passes through the instrument. Due to it the galvanometer or ammeter remains same **(Fig. 1.36)**.

Uses of Shunt

- A shunt is used to protect the galvanometer from the strong currents.
- A shunt is used for converting a galvanometer into an ammeter.
- A shunt may be used for increasing the range of ammeter.

Ammeter: An ammeter is a low resistance galvanometer. It is used to measure the current in a circuit in amperes. A galvanometer can be converted into an ammeter by using a low resistance wire in parallel with the galvanometer **(Fig. 1.37)**. The resistance of the wire (called the shunt wire) depends upon the range of the ammeter. As the shunt resistance is small, the combined resistance of the galvanometer and the shunt is very low and hence ammeter has a much lower resistance than galvanometer. An ideal ammeter has zero resistance.

Voltmeter: A voltmeter is a high resistance galvanometer. It is used to measure the potential difference between two points of a circuit in volt. A galvanometer can be converted into a voltmeter by using a high resistance in series with the galvanometer. The value of the resistance depends upon the range of the voltmeter. For voltmeter, a high resistance R is connected in series with the galvanometer, therefore, the resistance of voltmeter is very large as compared to that of galvanometer. The resistance of an ideal voltmeter is infinity **(Fig. 1.38)**.

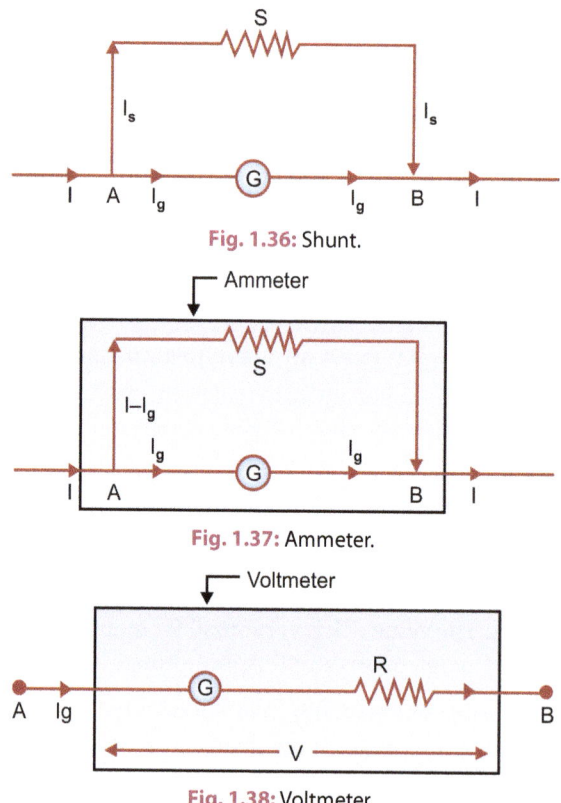

Fig. 1.36: Shunt.

Fig. 1.37: Ammeter.

Fig. 1.38: Voltmeter.

MAGNETS AND EARTH MAGNETISM

A Greek philosopher, *Thales* of Miletus, had observed as long back as 600 BC that a naturally occurring ore of iron attracted small pieces of iron toward it. This ore was found in the district of Magnesia in Asia Minor in Greece. Hence, the ore was named magnetite. The phenomenon of attraction of small bits of iron, steel, cobalt, nickel, etc., toward the ore was called *magnetism*. The iron ore showing this effect was called a *natural magnet*.

The Chinese discovered that a piece of magnetite, when suspended freely, always points out roughly in the North-South direction. Thus, a natural magnet has attractive and directive properties. A magnetic compass based on directive property of magnets was used by navigators to find their way in steering the ships.

That is why, magnetite was called the "load stone" in the sense of leading stone.

The natural magnets have often irregular shape and they are weak. It is found that a piece of iron or steel can acquire magnetic properties, on rubbing with a magnet. Such magnets made out of iron and steel are called artificial magnets. Artificial magnets can have desired shape and desired strength. A bar magnet, a horseshoe magnet, magnetic needle, compass needle, etc., all are artificial magnets.

Basic Properties of Magnets

Following are some basic properties of magnets:

* A magnet attracts magnetic substances like iron, steel, cobalt and nickel toward it. When a magnet is put in a heap of iron fillings, they cling to the magnet. The attraction appears to be maximum at the ends of the magnet **(Fig. 1.39)**. These ends are called *poles* of the magnet.
* When a magnet is suspended freely with the help of an unspun thread, it comes to rest along the North-South direction. If it is turned from this direction and left, it again returns to this direction. The pole which points toward the geographic north is called North pole and the pole which points toward geographic south is called South pole **(Fig. 1.40)**.

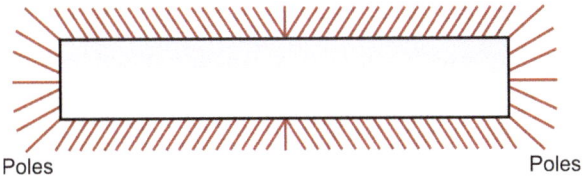

Fig. 1.39: Attraction by the magnet (maximum at poles).

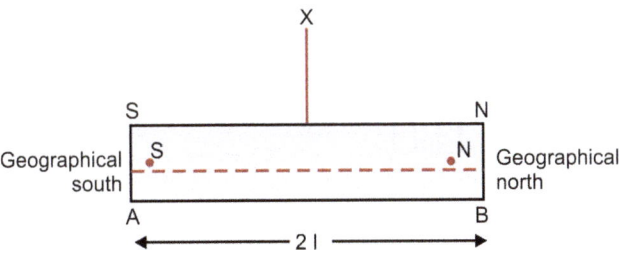

Fig. 1.40: A suspended magnet.

It should be clearly understood that poles exist always in pairs; two poles of a magnet are always of equal strength. Further, poles North and South are situated a little inward from the geometrical ends A and B of the magnet. The magnetic length (North-South) of magnet is roughly 6/7 of its geometric length (AB). We represent North-South by 2l (and not l); this is done for simplification of calculations.

The straight line passing through North-and-South poles of a magnet is called axial line of the magnet. The line passing through center of a magnet in a direction perpendicular to the length of the magnet is called equatorial line of the magnet.

The straight line joining North-and-South poles of a freely suspended magnet represents magnetic North-South direction. A vertical plane passing through North-South line of a freely suspended magnet is called magnetic meridian.

- Like poles repel each other and unlike poles attract each other. To show this, we suspend a bar magnet with the help of a thread. When we bring North pole of another magnet near the North pole of suspended magnet, we observe repulsion. Similarly, South pole of one magnet repels South pole of the other. However, when South pole of one is brought near North pole of suspended magnet, there is attraction **(Fig. 1.41)**.

- The force of attraction or repulsion F between two magnetic poles of strengths m1 and m2 separated by a distance r is directly proportional to the product of pole strengths and inversely proportional to the square of the distance between their centers, i.e.:

$$F \propto m_1 m_2 / r^2$$
$$F = K m_1 m_2 / r^2$$

Where K is magnetic force constant:

$$\text{In SI units, } K = \mu_0/4\pi$$
$$= 10^{-7} \text{ Wb A}^{-1} \text{ m}^{-1}$$

Where μ_0 is absolute magnetic permeability of free space (air/vacuum).

$$F = \frac{\mu_0 m_1 m_2}{4\pi r^2}$$

This is called Coulomb's law of magnetic force. However in CGS (centimeter-gram-second) system, the value of K = 1.

- The magnetic poles always exist in pairs, i.e., magnetic monopoles do not exist. In an attempt to separate the magnetic poles, if we break a magnet, we find new poles formed at the broken ends. If the two pieces are broken again, we find the broken ends contain new poles. Thus

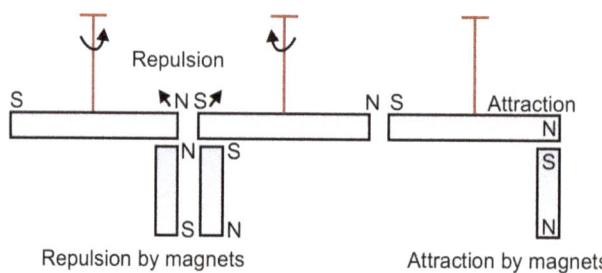

Fig. 1.41: Repulsion and attraction by magnets.

each piece, howsoever small, is a complete magnet in itself. Even if a magnet is broken into molecules, each molecule shall be a complete magnet. Note that pole strength (m) of each piece broken lengthwise, remains unchanged, although dipole moment M = m × 2l goes on decreasing, with decreasing length.

Atomic/Molecular Theory of Magnetism

The molecular theory of magnetism was given by *Weber* and modified later by Ewing. According to this theory:

- Every molecule of a magnetic substance (whether magnetized or not) is a complete in itself, having a North pole and a South pole of equal strength.
- In an unmagnetized substance, the molecular magnets are randomly oriented such that they form closed chains **(Fig. 1.42)**. The North pole of one molecular magnet cancels the effect of South pole of the other so that the resultant magnetism of the unmagnetized specimen is zero.
- On magnetizing the substance, the molecular magnets are realigned so that North-poles of all molecular magnets point in one direction and South poles of all molecular magnets point in opposite direction **(Fig. 1.43)**.

  The extent of magnetization of the specimen is the extent of realignment of the molecular magnets.
- When all the molecular magnets are fully aligned, the substance is said to be saturated with magnetism.
- At all stages, the strengths of the two poles developed will always be equal.
- On heating the magnetized specimen, molecular magnets acquire some kinetic energy. Some of the molecules may get back to the closed chain arrangement. That is why magnetism of the specimen would reduce on heating.

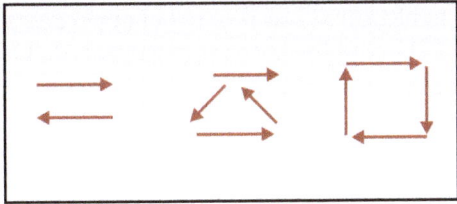

Fig. 1.42: Unmagnetized magnet.

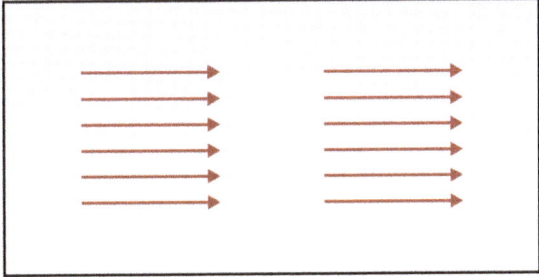

Fig. 1.43: Magnetized magnet.

Magnetic Lines of Force

The concept of magnetic lines of force or simply the field lines was developed to visualize the effect of the magnetic field. The magnetic field lines represent the magnetic field in the same way as the electric field lines represent an electric field.

The magnetic lines of force do not exist in reality. They are only hypothetical lines, which enable us to understand certain phenomena in magnetism. To draw these lines, we have to take a test object which is a magnetic dipole, such as a small compass needle.

If we imagine a number of small compass needles around a magnet, each compass needle experiences a torque due to the field of the magnet. The torque acting on a compass needle aligns it in the direction of the magnetic field. The path along which the compass needles are aligned is known as magnetic lines of force. It should be clearly understood that tangent to a field line at any point P gives the direction of magnetic field B at that point **(Fig. 1.44)**.

Properties of magnetic lines: Following are some of the important properties of the magnetic lines of force:

- Magnetic lines of force are closed continuous curves; we may imagine them to be extending through the body of the magnet.
- Outside the body of the magnet, the direction of magnetic lines of force is from North pole to South pole **(Fig. 1.45)**.
- The tangent to magnetic lines of force at any point gives the direction of magnetic field at that point.
- No two magnetic lines of force can intersect each other **(Fig. 1.46)**.
- Magnetic lines of force contract longitudinally and they dilate laterally.
- Crowding of magnetic lines of force represents stronger magnetic field and vice versa **(Fig. 1.47)**.

It should be clearly understood that there is one fundamental difference between electricity and magnetism. Whereas in electricity, an isolated charge can exist, and in magnetism, an isolated pole does not exist. The simplest magnetic structure that can exist is only a magnetic dipole, characterized by magnetic dipole moment $\vec{M}$. Thus for mapping magnetic field, the

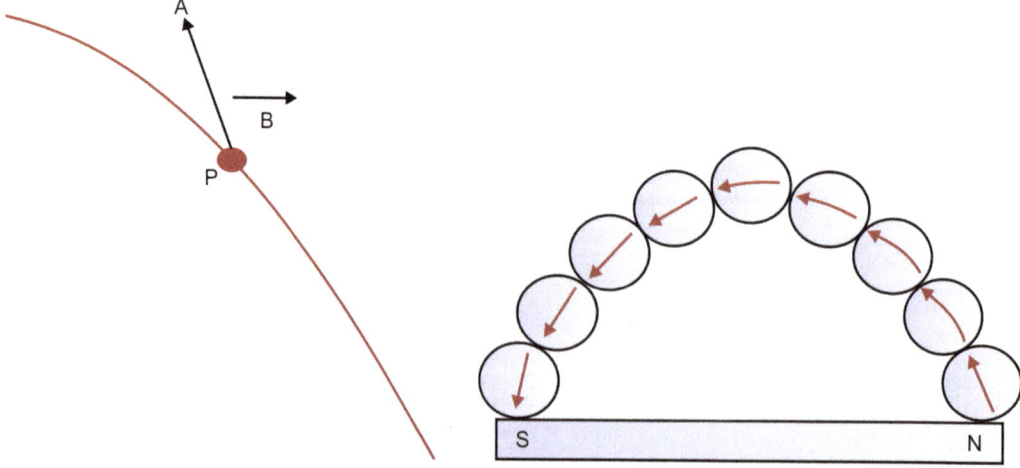

Fig. 1.44: Tangent to a magnetic line of force.   **Fig. 1.45:** Magnetic line of force.

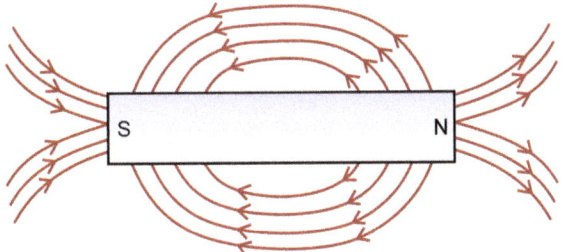

Fig. 1.46: Direction of magnetic lines of force.

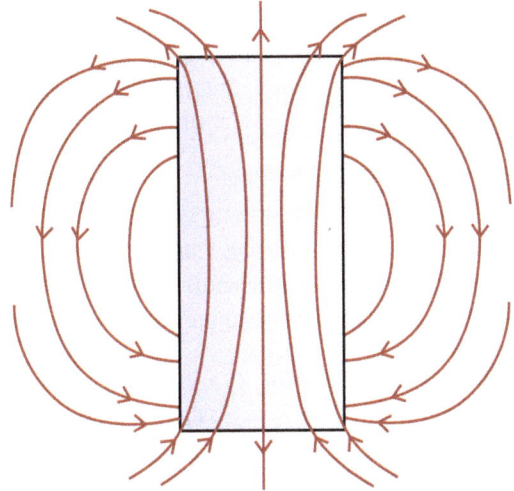

Fig. 1.47: Crowding of magnetic lines of force.

simplest test object is a dipole. That is why in the definition of $\vec{B}$ above, we have used the word "hypothetical" isolated North pole. However, this definition of $\vec{B}$ (corresponding to definition of $\vec{B}$) enables us to simplify some calculations.

Thus, magnetic dipole is characterized by a vector $\vec{M}$ in place of a scalar charge q in electricity. We shall show that in an external magnetic field, the dipole experiences a torque (unlike the force experienced by charge q in electric field). The effect of torque is to align the dipole along the external magnetic field. The directive property of a magnet is attributed to the torque acting on the magnetic dipole due to earth's magnetic field.

Each electric line of force starts from a positive charge and ends at a negative charge. It should be clearly understood that the electric lines are discontinuous only in the sense that no such lines exist inside a charged body. However, from a positively charged body to a negatively charged body, there is no discontinuity in the electric lines of force. In magnetism, as there are no monopoles, therefore, the magnetic field lines will be along closed loops with no starting or ending. The magnetic lines of force would pass through body of the magnet. At very far off points, the field lines due to an electric dipole and a magnetic dipole will appear identical.

Remember that electric lines of force are discontinuous, whereas magnetic lines of force are closed continuous curves.

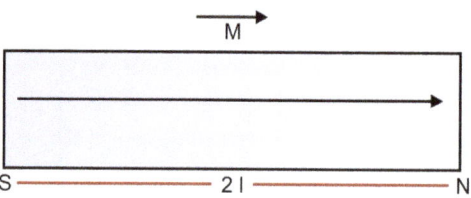
Fig. 1.48: Magnetic dipole.

Magnetic Dipole

A magnetic dipole consists of two unlike poles of equal strength and separated by a small distance. For example, a bar magnet, a compass needle, etc., are magnetic dipoles. An atom of a magnetic material behaves as a dipole due to electrons revolving around the nucleus. Magnetic dipole moment is defined as the product of pole strength and the distance between the two poles. This distance between the poles is called magnetic length and is represented by 2l. If m is the strength of each pole, then magnetic dipole moment (M) is:

$$M = m\,(2l)$$

Magnetic dipole moment is a vector quantity directed from South-to-North-pole. The SI units of M are joule/tesla and ampere-meter^2 **(Fig. 1.48)**.

The direction of magnetic moment (M) is from south to north. This corresponds to the electric dipole moment (p) of an electric dipole from negative charge to positive charge.

Gauss's Theorem (or Gauss's Law) on Magnetism

According to Gauss's theorem, the surface integral of electrostatic field E over a closed surface S is equal to $1/\varepsilon_o$ times the total charge q inside the surface, where ε_o is absolute electrical permittivity of free space, i.e.:

$$\oint \vec{E} \cdot \vec{ds} = q/\varepsilon_o$$

If an electric dipole was enclosed by the surface, equal and opposite charges in the dipole add up to zero. Therefore, surface integral of electric field of a dipole over a closed surface enclosing an electric dipole is zero, i.e.:

$$\oint \vec{E} \cdot \vec{ds} = 0$$

Whereas, electric field can be produced by isolated charge, the magnetic field is produced only by a magnetic dipole. This is because isolated magnetic poles do not exist. Hence, magnetic analog equation is as follows:

$$\oint \vec{B} \cdot \vec{ds} = 0$$

That is surface integral of magnetic field over a surface (closed or open) is always zero, i.e., the net magnetic flux (ψ_B) through any surface S is always zero. This is called *Gauss's law in magnetism*. In terms of magnetic field lines, the law means that there are as many lines entering S, as are leaving it **(Fig. 1.49)**.

Magnetic Field of Earth

Sir William Gilbert was the first to suggest in the year 1600, that earth itself is a huge magnet. His statement was based on the following evidence:

* A magnet suspended from a thread and free to rotate in a horizontal plane comes to rest along the North-South direction. On disturbing, the magnet returns quickly to its

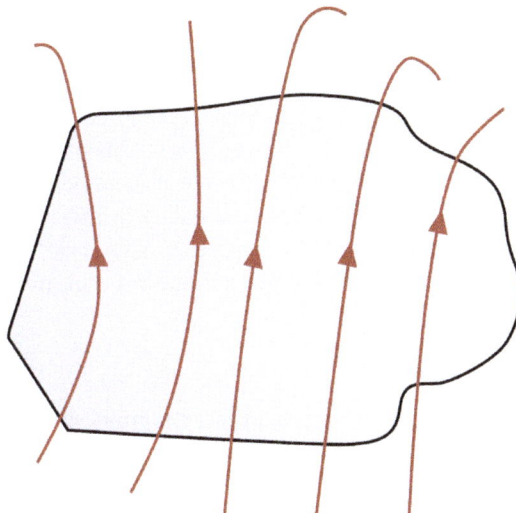

Fig. 1.49: Magnetic field lines.

North-South direction again this is as if huge bar magnet lies along the diameter of the earth. The North pole of this fictitious magnet must be toward geographic south so as to attract South pole of the suspended magnet and vice versa.

* When a soft iron piece is buried under the surface of earth in the North-South direction, it is found to acquire the properties of a magnet after some time.
* When we draw field lines of a magnet, we come across neutral points. At these points, magnetic field due to the magnet is neutralized or cancelled exactly by the magnetic field of earth. If earth had no magnetism of its own, we would never observe neutral points.

The branch of physics which deals with the study of magnetism of earth is called terrestrial magnetism or geomagnetism.

It has been established that earth's magnetic field is fairly uniform. The strength of this field is approximately 10^{-4} tesla or 1 gauss. The field is not confined only to earth's surface. It extends up to a height nearly 5 times the radius of the earth.

Cause of Earth's Magnetism

The exact cause of earth's magnetism is not yet known. However, some important postulates in this respect are as follows:

* The earth's magnetism may be due to molten charged metallic fluid in the core of earth. The radius of this core is about 3,500 km with the rotation of earth; the fluid also rotates resulting in the development of currents in the core of earth. These currents magnetize the earth.
* According to *Professor Brackett*, earth's magnetism may be due to rotation of earth about its axis. This is because every substance is made of charged particles (protons and electrons). Therefore, a substance rotating about an axis is equivalent to circulating currents, which are responsible for its magnetization.
* In the outer layers of earth's atmosphere, gases are in the ionized state, primarily on account of cosmic rays. As earth rotates, strong electric currents are set up due to movement of (charged) ions. These currents might be magnetizing the earth.

ELECTROMAGNETIC INDUCTION

Michael Faraday in UK and *Joseph Henry* in USA observed that an emf is produced across the ends of a conductor when the number of magnetic lines of force associated with the conductor changes. The emf lasts so long as this change continues. This phenomenon of generating an emf by changing the number of magnetic lines of force associated with the conductor is called *electromagnetic induction*. The emf so developed is called induced emf. If the conductor is in the form of a closed circuit, a current flows in the circuit. This is called *induced current*.

The phenomenon of EMI is the basis of power generators, dynamos, transformers, etc., and hence it is important.

Magnetic Flux

The magnetic flux (Φ) through any surface held in a magnetic field is measured by the total number of magnetic lines of force crossing the surface. The unit of magnetic flux is *weber* (*Wb*). One weber is the amount of magnetic flux over an area of 1 m² held uniform to a uniform magnetic field of one tesla. Also, magnetic flux is a scalar quantity.

Faraday's Experiments

Experiment 1: **Figure 1.50** shows a circular insulated wire of one or more turns connected to a sensitive galvanometer G. North-South is a bar magnet which can be moved with respect to the coil. Faraday observed the following:

- Whenever there is a relative motion between the coil and the magnet, the galvanometer shows a sudden deflection. This deflection indicates that current is induced in the coil.
- The deflection is temporary. It lasts so long as relative motion between the coil and the magnet continues.
- The deflection is more when the magnet is moved faster and less when the magnet is moved slowly.
- The direction of deflection is reversed when same pole of magnet is moved in the opposite direction or opposite pole of magnet is moved in the same direction.

The motion of the magnet implies that the number of magnetic lines of force threading the coil is changing.

Experiment 2: **Figure 1.51** shows the experimental set up. Coil 1 is connected to a battery, a rheostat and a key K. Coil 2 is connected to a sensitive galvanometer G and is held close to coil 1.

When we press K, galvanometer G in coil 2 shows a sudden temporary deflection. This indicates that current is induced in coil 2. This is because current in coil 1 increases from zero to a certain steady value increasing the magnetic field of coil 1 and hence the number of magnetic lines of force entering coil 2. Their direction is shown in **Figure 1.51**.

On releasing K, galvanometer shows a sudden temporary deflection in the opposite direction. This is because on releasing K, current in coil 1 decreases from maximum to zero value, decreasing thereby the magnetic field of coil 1 and hence the number of magnetic lines of force entering coil 2.

Thus, the results of the two experiments are identical.

Note: In both the experiments discussed, we find that induced emf appears in a coil whenever the amount of magnetic flux linked with the coil changes. Hence, we conclude that the cause

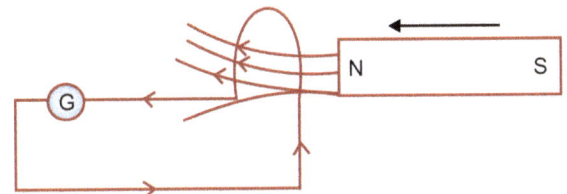

Fig. 1.50: Electromotive force induced in a coil due to moving magnet.

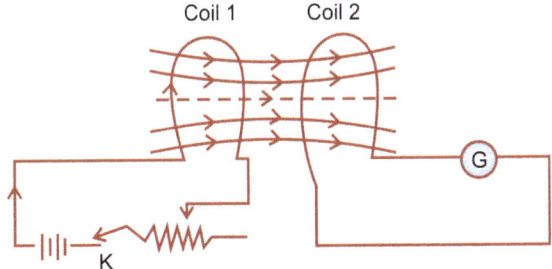

Fig. 1.51: Electromyography induced in a coil due to current carrying coil.

of emf induced in a coil is change in magnetic flux linked with the coil. It should be clearly understood that mere presence of magnetic flux is not enough. The amount of magnetic flux linked with a coil must change in order to produce any induced emf in the coil.

Faraday's Laws of Electromagnetic Induction

Following are the laws of EMI as given by Faraday. Both the laws follow from Faraday's experiments discussed earlier.

First law: Whenever the amount of magnetic flux linked with a circuit changes, an emf is induced in the circuit. The induced emf lasts so long as the change in magnetic flux continues.

Second law: The magnitude of emf induced in a circuit is directly proportional to the rate of change of magnetic flux linked with a circuit.

Explanation

First law: In Faraday's experiment, when magnet is moved toward the coil, number of magnetic lines of force linked with the coil increases, i.e., magnetic flux increases. When the magnet is moved away, the magnetic flux linked with the coil decreases. In both the cases, galvanometer shows deflection indicating that emf is induced in the coil.

When there is no relative motion between the magnet and the coil, magnetic flux linked with the coil remains constant. That is why galvanometer shows no deflection. Thus, induced emf is produced when magnetic flux changes and induced emf continues so long as the change in magnetic flux continues. This is first law. The same results follow from Faraday's second experiment.

Second law: In Faraday's experiment, when magnet is moved faster, the magnetic flux linked with the coil changes at a faster. Therefore, galvanometer deflection is more. However, when the magnet is moved slowly, rate of change of magnetic flux is smaller. Therefore, galvanometer deflection is smaller. Hence magnitude of emf induced varies directly as the rate of change of magnetic flux linked with the coil. This is second law.

If it is amount of magnetic flux linked with the coil at any time and is the magnetic flux linked with the coil after t second then:

Rate of change of magnetic flux = According to Faraday's second law, induced emf

$$e \propto \frac{\phi_2 - \phi_1}{t}$$

$$\text{or } e = \frac{K(\phi_2 - \phi_1)}{t}$$

Where, K is a constant of proportionality. As K = 1 (in all systems of units)

$$E = \frac{\phi_2 - \phi_1}{t}$$

If d is small change in magnetic flux in a small time dt, then:

$$E = \frac{-d\phi}{dt}$$

Negative sign is taken because induced emf always opposes any change in magnetic flux associated with the circuit.

Lenz's Law

This law gives us the direction of current in a circuit. According to this law, the induced current will appear in such a direction that it opposes the change (in magnetic flux) responsible for its production.

The law refers to induced currents, which means that it applies only to closed circuits. When we push the magnet toward the coil (or the loop toward the magnet), an induced current appears. In terms of Lenz's law, induced current will oppose the push when face of the loop toward the magnet becomes a North pole. Therefore, induced current will be anticlockwise, as we see along the magnet toward the loop.

If we pull the magnet away from the coil, the induced current will oppose the pull by creating a South pole on the face of the loop toward the magnet. Therefore, induced current will be clockwise.

The agent that moves the magnet, either toward the coil or away from it, will always experience a resisting force and will thus be required to do the work.

Experimental Verification of Lenz's Law (Fig. 1.52)

A coil of a few turns is connected to a cell C and a sensitive galvanometer G through a two way key 1, 2, and 3.

Put in the plug of key between 1 and 2. Cell sends current through the coil. At the upper face of the coil, the current is anticlockwise, which would produce North pole on this face. Suppose the galvanometer deflection is to the right. Obviously, if galvanometer deflection were to the left, current would be clockwise at the upper face, which would behave as South pole.

Chapter 1: Basics of Electricity, Light and Sound

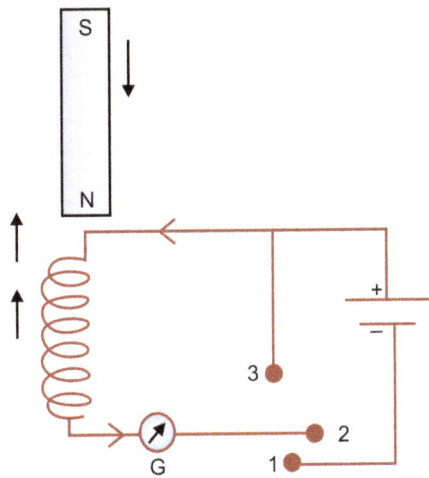

Fig. 1.52: Experimental set-up for verifying Lenz's law.

Remove the plug of key from 1 and 2. Insert the plug of key between 2 and 3. Now, move North pole of a bar magnet toward the coil. The galvanometer shows a sudden deflection to the right indicating that current induced in the coil is anticlockwise and upper end of the coil behaves as north. It opposes the inward motion of North pole of the bar magnet, which is the cause of induced current.

Similarly, when North pole of the bar magnet is moved away from the coil, the galvanometer shows a sudden deflection to the left, indicating that current induced in the coil is clockwise and upper end of the coil behaves as south. It opposes the outward motion of North pole of the bar magnet, i.e., cause of induced emf is opposed.

Exactly similar results follow when South pole of magnet is moved instead of North pole.

Hence, induced current always opposes the change which produces it. This verifies Lenz's law.

Lenz's Law and Energy Conservation

Lenz's law is in accordance with the law of conservation of energy.

For example, in the experimental verification of Lenz's law, when North pole of magnet is moved toward the coil, the upper face of the coil acquires north polarity. Therefore, work has to be done against the force of repulsion, in bringing the magnet closer to the coil. Similarly, when North pole of magnet is moved away, south polarity develops on the upper face of the coil. Therefore, work has to be done against the force of attraction, in taking the magnet away from the coil.

It is this mechanical work done in moving the magnet with respect to the coil that changes into electrical energy producing induced current. Thus, energy is being transformed only.

When we do not move the magnet, work done is zero. Therefore, induced current is also not produced.

Hence, Lenz's law obeys the principle of energy conservation.

Conversely, Lenz's law can be treated as a consequence of the principle of energy conservation.

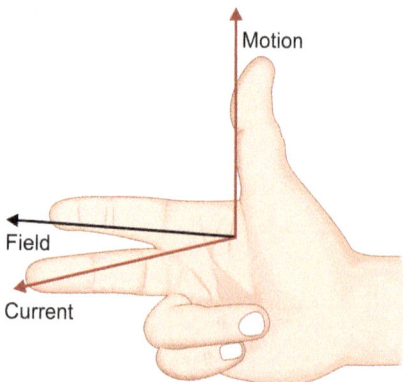

Fig. 1.53: Fleming's right hand rule.

Fleming's Right Hand Rule

Fleming's right hand rule also gives the direction of induced emf/current, in a conductor moving in a magnetic field. According to this rule, if we stretch the first finger, central finger and thumb of our right hand in mutually perpendicular directions such that first finger points along the direction of the field and thumb is along the direction of motion of the conductor, then the central finger would give us the direction of induced current **(Fig. 1.53)**.

The direction of induced current given by Lenz's law and Fleming's right hand rule is the same.

Eddy Currents

Eddy currents are the currents induced in the body of the conductor when the amount of magnetic flux linked with the conductor changes. These were discovered by *Foucault* in the year *1895* and hence they are also called *Foucault currents*.

The magnitude of eddy current is:

$$i = \text{induced emf/resistance} = e/R$$
$$\text{but} \quad e = -d\varphi/dt$$
$$i = \frac{-d\varphi/dt}{R}$$

The direction of eddy currents is given by Lenz's law or Fleming's right hand rule.

Note: Eddy currents are basically the currents induced in the body of a conductor due to change in magnetic flux linked with the conductor.

Experimental Demonstration

Experiment 1: Hold a light metallic disk D atop the cross section of an electromagnet connected to a source of AC **(Fig. 1.54)**. When AC is switched on, the disk is thrown up into the air.

This is due to eddy currents developed in the disk. As current through the solenoid increases, the magnetic flux along the axis of the solenoid increases. Therefore, magnetic flux linked with the disk increases. Induced currents or eddy currents develop in the disk and magnetize it. If upper end of solenoid initially acquires north polarity, the lower face of disk also acquires north polarity in accordance with the Lenz's law. The force of repulsion between the two throws the disk up in the air.

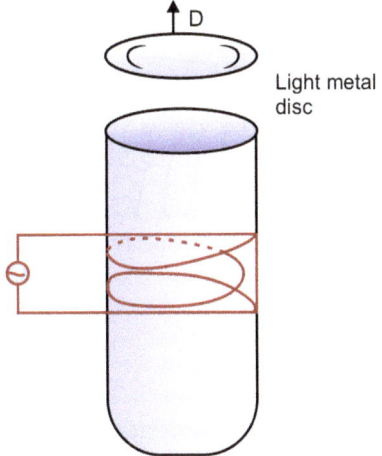

Fig. 1.54: Eddy currents on a disk.

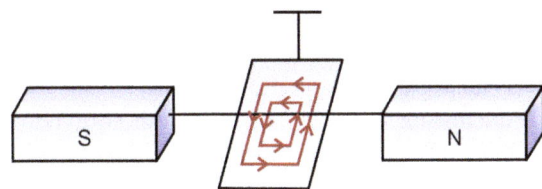

Fig. 1.55: Eddy currents on a flat metallic plate.

Experiment 2: Suspend a flat metallic plate between pole pieces N and S of an electromagnet (**Fig. 1.55**).

When the magnetic field is off, the metallic plate disturbed once from its equilibrium position and left, oscillates freely for a longer time. But when the electromagnet is switched on, the vibrations of the plate are damped. This is because of eddy currents developed in the vibrating plate.

In the normal position of rest of the plate, magnetic flux linked with the plate is maximum. When it is displaced toward any one extreme position, area of plate in the field decreases. Therefore, magnetic flux through the plate decreases. Eddy currents develop in the plate which, according to Lenz's law, opposes the motion of the plate toward extreme position. Similarly, when plate returns from extreme position to mean position, area of plate in the field increases, magnetic flux linked with the plate increases. Eddy currents are developed which oppose the motion of the plate toward the mean position.

In either case, vibrations of the plate are damped.

Figure 1.56 shows the same metallic plate with slots cut in it. When such a plate is made to oscillate in the magnetic field, the damping effect is there, but it is much smaller compared to the case when no slots were cut.

This means eddy currents are reduced. This is because closed loop of a given area now has a much longer path. As longer path means more resistance, eddy currents will reduce. We can only minimize eddy currents but cannot reduce such currents to zero.

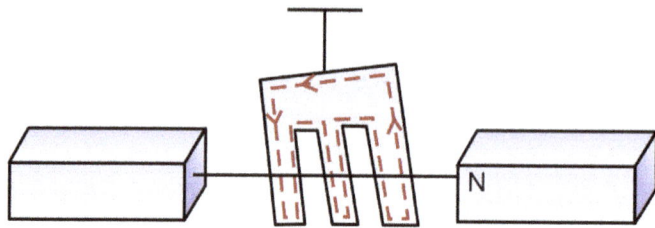

Fig. 1.56: Eddy currents on metallic plate with slots.

Applications of Eddy Currents

Eddy currents are useful in many ways.
Some of the applications of eddy currents are:
- *Electromagnetic damping:* This is used in designing dead beat galvanometers. When a steady current is passed through the coil of a galvanometer, it is deflected. Normally, the coil oscillates about its equilibrium position for some time before coming to rest.
  To avoid delay due to these oscillations, the coil is wound over a metallic frame. As the coil is deflected, eddy currents set up in the metallic frame oppose its motion.
  Therefore, the coil attains its equilibrium position almost instantly. Thus, the motion of coil is damped. This is called electromagnetic damping.
- *Induction furnace:* It makes use of the heating effect of eddy currents. The substance to be heated/melted is placed in a high frequency magnetic field. The large eddy currents developed in the substance produce so much heat that it melts. Such an arrangement is called induction furnace. It is used for extracting a metal from its ore and also in the preparation of certain alloys.
- *Electromagnetic brakes:* They are used in controlling the speed of electric trains. A strong magnetic field is applied to a metallic drum rotating with the axle connecting the wheels. Large eddy currents set up in the rotating drum oppose the motion of the drum and tend to stop the train.
- *Induction motor:* An induction motor or AC motor is another important application of eddy currents. A rotating magnetic field produces strong eddy currents in a rotor, which starts rotating in the direction of the rotating magnetic field.
- *Speedometers:* In speedometers of automobiles and energy meters.
- *Eddy currents in diathermy:* They are also used in diathermy, i.e., in deep heat treatment of the human body.

Some of the *undesirable effects* of eddy currents are:
- They oppose the relative motion.
- They involve loss of energy in the form of heat.
- The excessive heating may break the insulation in the appliances and reduce their life.

To minimize the eddy currents, the metal core to be used in an appliance like dynamo, transformer, choke coil, etc., is taken in the form of thin sheets. Each sheet is electrically insulated from the other by insulating varnish. Such a core is called a laminated core. The planes of these sheets are arranged parallel to the magnetic flux.

Large resistance between the thin sheets confines the eddy currents to the individual sheets. Hence, the eddy currents are reduced to a large extent.

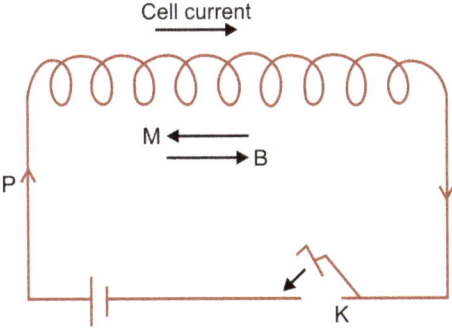

Fig. 1.57: Self-induction.

Self-induction

Self-induction is the property of a coil by virtue of which, the coil opposes any change in the strength of current flowing through it by inducing an emf in itself. For this reason, self-induction is also called the *inertia of electricity*.

Suppose there is a coil connected to a cell through a tap key K **(Fig. 1.57)**.

On pressing K, current through the coil increases from zero to a certain maximum value. It takes some time. During this time (of make M), current through the coil is increasing, magnetic flux linked with the coil is increasing. Therefore, a current is induced in the coil. According to Lenz's law, the induced current at make will oppose the growth of current in the coil, by flowing in a direction opposite to the direction of the cell current.

On releasing K, current through the coil decreases from maximum to zero value. It takes some time. During the time (of break B), current through the coil is decreasing. Therefore, magnetic flux linked with the coil is decreasing. A current is induced in the coil. According to Lenz's law, the induced current at break will oppose the decay of current in the coil, by flowing in the direction of the cell current, so as to prolong it.

Coefficient of self-induction (L) of a coil is equal to the emf induced in the coil when rate of change of current through the coil is unity.

The SI unit of L is *henry*. Self-inductance of a coil is said to be 1 henry, when a current change at the rate of 1 ampere/sec through the coil induces an emf of 1 volt in the coil.

Mutual Induction

Mutual induction is the property of two coils by virtue of which each opposes any change in the strength of current flowing through the other by developing an induced emf.

Suppose there are two coils P and S which are held closely. P is connected to a cell through a key K. S is connected to a sensitive galvanometer G **(Fig. 1.58)**.

On pressing or releasing K, galvanometer shows a temporary deflection. This is due to mutual induction as detailed next.

On pressing K, current in P increases from zero to maximum value. It takes some time. During this time (of make M), current in P is increasing. Therefore, magnetic flux linked with P is increasing. As S is close by, magnetic flux associated with S also increases. An emf is induced in S, according to Lenz's law, the induced current in S would oppose increase in current in P by flowing in a direction opposite to the cell current in P.

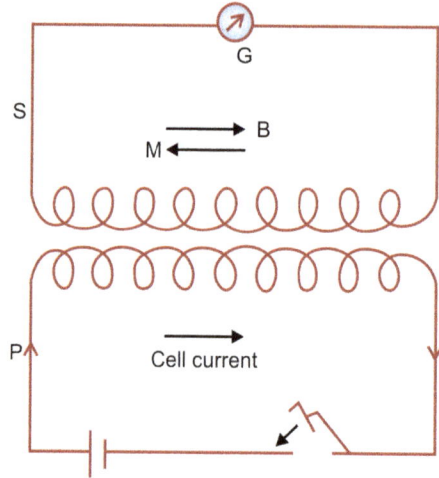

Fig. 1.58: Mutual induction.

On releasing K, current in P decreases from maximum to zero value. It takes some time. During this time (of break B), current in P is decreasing. Therefore, magnetic flux linked with P is decreasing. As S is close by, magnetic flux associated with S also decreases. An emf is induced in S. According to Lenz's law, the induced current in S during break flows in the direction of the cell current in P so as to oppose the decrease in current in P, i.e., it prolongs the decay of current.

Coefficient of mutual inductance of two coils is numerically equal to the amount of magnetic flux linked with one coil when unit current flows through the neighboring coil.

Coefficient of mutual induction (M) of two coils is equal to the emf induced in one coil when rate of change of current through the other coil is unity.

The SI unit of *M* is *henry*. Coefficient of mutual inductance of two coils is said to be 1 henry, when a current change at the rate of 1 ampere/sec in one coil induces an emf of 1 volt in the other coil.

The mutual inductance of two coils depends on:
- Geometry of two coils, i.e., size of coils, their shape, number of turns, nature of material on which two coils are wound
- Distance between two coils
- Relative placement of two coils (i.e., orientation of the coils).

Note: In self-induction, change in strength of current in a coil is opposed by the coil itself by inducing an emf in itself. However, in mutual induction, one coil opposes any change in the strength of current in the neighboring coil. It should be clearly understood that mutual induction is over and the self-induction of each coil, due to change in magnetic flux in both.

AC Generator/Dynamo

An AC generator or dynamo is a machine which produces alternating current energy from mechanical energy. It is one of the most important applications of the phenomenon of EMI. The generator was designed by Yugoslav scientist, *Nikola Tesla*. It is an alternator converting one form of energy into another.

Principle: An AC generator or dynamo is based on the phenomenon of EMI, i.e., whenever amount of magnetic flux linked with the coil changes, an emf is induced in the coil. It lasts so long as the magnetic flux through the coil continues. The direction of current induced is given by Fleming's right hand rule.

Multiphase AC Generator

- *Two-phase AC generator*: In this generator, there are two armature coils held at 90º to each other. Each coil has its own pair of slip rings and brushes. When this pair of coils is rotated in magnetic field, emf is induced in each coil. When emf induced in one coil is maximum, it is minimum in the other coil and vice versa. Thus, the emf's induced in the two coils differ in phase by 90º. This is called two-phase AC **(Fig. 1.59)**.
- *Three-phase AC generator*: In this generator, there are three armature coils equally inclined to one another at 60º. Each coil has its own pair of slip rings and brushes. When this arrangement of coils is rotated in magnetic field, emf is induced in each coil. Thus we obtain three alternating emf's differing in phase from one another by 60º. This is called three-phase AC **(Fig. 1.60)**.
- *In general*: When there are a number of separate coils, each having its own pair of slip rings and brushes, the generator is called polyphase generator. The current produced is called polyphase alternating current.

In actual practice one end of each coil is brought to a common point through shaft of the generator. The line wire from this line is called neutral line. Separate slip rings are provided for other ends of different coils. The line wires from these rings (through these brushes) are called phase lines.

It should be clearly understood that the principle of generator discussed here applies to all the practical devices for the purpose ranging from portable generator to giant hydroelectric and thermal power generators and even nuclear power generators.

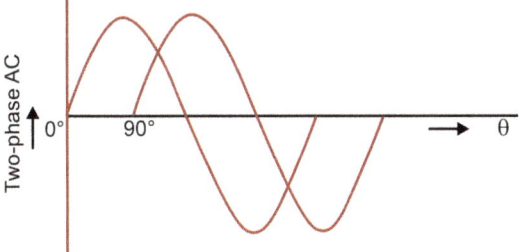

Fig. 1.59: Two-phase AC.

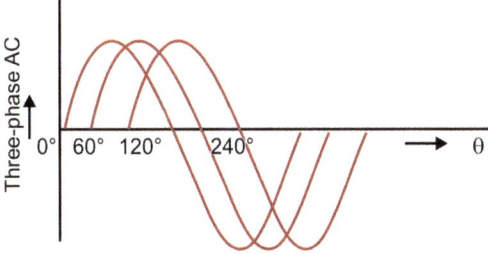

Fig. 1.60: Three-phase AC.

In a hydroelectric power station, water is stored to a great height in a dam, from where it falls on to giant turbines (popularly known as water wheels). These turbines are connected to loops of wires in AC generator. Thus, kinetic energy of falling water is converted into rotational energy of turbines, which leads to the production of electric energy by the generator.

In a thermal power station, superheated steam is produced by boiling water using coal or oil as fuel. The superheated steam pushes past the turbines and rotates them. This leads to the production of electrical energy by the generator.

DC Generator/Dynamo

A DC generator or dynamo is device which is used for producing direct current energy from mechanical energy.

The principle of DC generator is the same as that of AC generator.

Motor starter: A starter is a device which is used for starting a DC motor safely. Its function is to introduce a suitable resistance in the circuit at the time of starting of the motor. This resistance decreases gradually and reduces to zero when the motor runs at full speed.

In fact, resistance of armature of DC motor is kept low (to reduce the copper losses) and when armature is stationary, there is no back emf. Therefore, when operating voltage is applied, the current through armature coil may become so large ($I = V/R$) that the motor may burn. A starter is needed to avoid this.

Transformer

A transformer is an electric device which is used for changing the AC voltages.

A transformer which increases the AC voltages is called a step-up transformer. A transformer which decreases the AC voltages is called a step-down transformer.

Principle: A transformer is based on the principle of mutual induction, i.e., whenever the amount of magnetic flux linked with the coil changes, an emf is induced in the neighboring coil.

Construction: The transformer consists of two coils of insulated wire wound onto a laminated soft-iron frame. The two coils may be wound on top of one another or on opposite sides of the frame.

Working: An alternating current is passed through the primary coil and this sets up a varying magnetic field which cuts the secondary coil. By EMI, an EMF is induced into the secondary circuit.

Step-up transformer: In this, the number of turns in the primary coil is less than that in the secondary coil **(Fig. 1.61)**.

The primary coil is made up of thick insulated copper wire, with less number of turns, while the secondary coil is made up of thin insulated copper wire, with large number of turns. It converts a low voltage at high current into high voltage at low current.

Step-down transformer: In this, the number of turns in the primary coil is more than that in the secondary coil **(Fig. 1.62)**.

The primary coil is made up of thin insulated copper wire with larger number of turns, while the secondary coil is made up of thick copper wire with less number of turns. It converts a high voltage at low current into low voltage at high current.

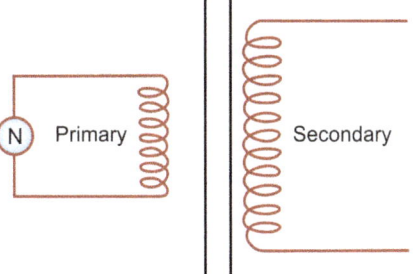

Fig. 1.61: Step-up transformer.

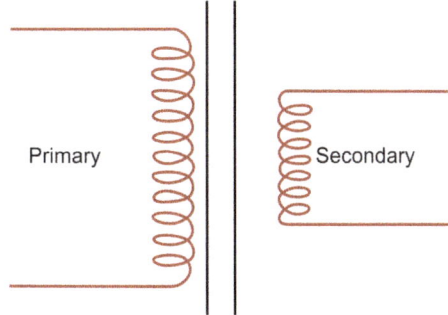

Fig. 1.62: Step-down transformer.

Types of Transformers

- *Static transformer*: It has been described earlier.
- *Variable transformer*: This consists of a primary and a secondary coil and is made so that one of them can be altered in length. The primary coil has a number of tappings and a movable contact can be placed on any one of these by turning a knobs. There is a step-up voltage in the secondary coil. In this way, a very crude control of voltage is obtained.
- *The autotransformer*: It consists of a single coil of wire with four contact points coming from it. It works on the principles of EMI, but it has the disadvantage that it allows only a small step up and does not render the current earth free.

Energy Losses in a Transformer

Following are the major sources of energy loss in a transformer:
- *Copper loss*: It is the energy loss in the form of heat in the copper coils of the transformer. This is due to Joule heating of conducting wires.
- *Iron loss*: It is the energy loss in the form of heat in the iron core of the transformer. This is due to formation of eddy currents in iron core. It is minimized by taking laminated cores.
- *Leakage of magnetic flux*: It occurs in spite of best insulations. Therefore, rate of change of magnetic flux linked with each turn of $S_1 S_2$ is less than the rate of change of magnetic flux linked with each turn of $P_1 P_2$.
- *Hysteresis loss*: This is the loss of energy due to repeated magnetization and demagnetization of the iron core when AC is fed to it.
- *Magnetostriction*: That is humming noise of a transformer.
  Therefore, output power in a transformer is roughly 90% of the input power.

Uses of Transformer

A transformer is used in almost all AC operations, e.g.:
1. In voltage regulators of TV, refrigerator, computer, air conditioner, etc.
2. In the induction furnaces
3. A step-down transformer is used for welding purposes
4. In the transmission of AC over long distances.

Electromagnetic Waves

History of Electromagnetic Waves

Faraday from his experimental study of EMI concluded that a magnetic field changing with time at a point produces an electric field at that point. Maxwell in 1865 from his theoretical study pointed out "there is a great symmetry in nature", i.e., an electric field changing with time at a point produces a magnetic field there. It means a change in either field (electric or magnetic) with time produces the other field. This idea led Maxwell to conclude that the variation in electric and magnetic field vectors perpendicular to each other leads to the production of electromagnetic disturbances in space. These disturbances have the properties of wave and can travel in space even without any material medium. These waves are called electromagnetic waves.

According to Maxwell, the electromagnetic waves are those waves in which there are sinusoidal variation of electric and magnetic field vectors at right angles to each other as well as at right angles to the direction of wave propagation. Both these fields vary with time and space and have the same frequency.

In **Figure 1.63**, the electric field vector (E) and magnetic field (B) are vibrating along Y and Z directions and propagation of electromagnetic wave is shown in X-direction.

Maxwell also found that the electromagnetic wave should travel in free space (or vacuum) also.

Maxwell also concluded that electromagnetic wave is transverse in nature and light is electromagnetic wave.

Examples of electromagnetic waves are radio waves, microwaves, infrared rays, light waves, ultraviolet rays, X-rays and ϒ-rays.

In 1888, *Hertz* confirmed experimentally the existence of electromagnetic waves. With the help of his experiment, Hertz produced electromagnetic waves of wavelength about 6 m.

In 1894, an Indian Physicist *Jagdish Chander Bose* was able to produce electromagnetic waves of wavelength = 5–25 mm but his experiment was confined to laboratory only.

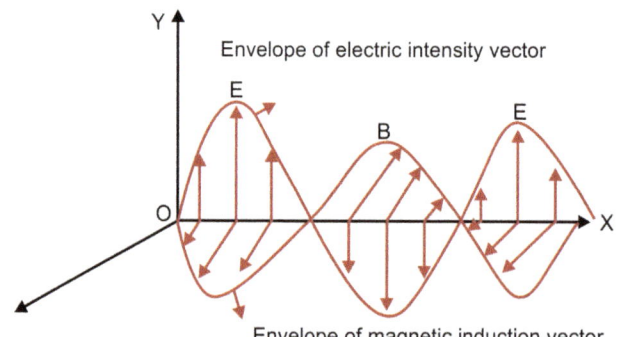

Fig. 1.63: Electromagnetic waves.

In 1899, *Guglielmo Marconi* was the first to transmit electromagnetic waves up to a few kilometers and established a wireless communication across the English channel, a distance of about 50 km.

Production of Electromagnetic Waves

We know that an electric charge at rest has electric field in the region around it, but no magnetic field. A moving charge produces both the electric and magnetic fields. If a charge is moving with a constant velocity (i.e., if current is not changing with time), the electric and magnetic fields will not change with time; hence, no electromagnetic wave can be produced. But if the charge is moving with a non-zero acceleration (i.e., charge is accelerated) both the magnetic field and electric fields will change with space and time, it then produces electromagnetic wave. This shows that an accelerated charge emits electromagnetic waves.

In an atom, an electron while orbiting around the nucleus in a stable orbit, although accelerating, does not emit electromagnetic waves. Electromagnetic waves are emitted only when it falls from higher energy orbit to lower energy orbit.

Electromagnetic waves (i.e., X-rays) are also produced when fast moving electrons are suddenly stopped by the metal target of high atomic number.

Important Facts about the Electromagnetic Waves

- The electromagnetic waves are produced by accelerated or oscillated charge.
- These waves do not require any material medium for propagation.
- These waves travel in free space with a speed 3×10^8 m/s (i.e., speed of light).
- The sinusoidal variation in both electric and magnetic field vectors (E and B) occurs simultaneously. As a result, they attain the maxima and minima at the same place and at the same time.
- The directions of variation of electric and magnetic field vectors are perpendicular to each other as well as perpendicular to the direction of propagation of waves. Therefore, electromagnetic waves are transverse in nature like light waves.
- The velocity of electromagnetic waves depends entirely on the electric and magnetic properties of the medium in which these waves travel and is independent of the amplitude of the field vectors.
- The velocity of electromagnetic waves in dielectric is less than 3×10^8 m/s.
- The energy in electromagnetic waves is equally divided between electric and magnetic vectors.
- The electric vector is responsible for the optical effects of an electromagnetic wave and is called the light vector.
- The electromagnetic waves being uncharged are not deflected by electric and magnetic fields.

Electromagnetic Spectrum

Maxwell in 1865 predicted electromagnetic waves from theoretical considerations and their existence was confirmed experimentally by *Hertz* in 1888.

Hertz experiment was based on the fact that an oscillating electric charge radiates electromagnetic waves and these waves carry energy which is being supplied at the cost of kinetic energy of the oscillating charge. The detailed study revealed that the electromagnetic radiation is significant only if the distance to which the charge oscillates is comparable to the wavelength of radiation.

After the experimental discovery of electromagnetic waves by Hertz, many other electromagnetic waves were discovered by different ways of excitation.

The orderly distribution of electromagnetic radiations according to their wavelength or frequency is called electromagnetic spectrum.

The electromagnetic spectrum has much wider range with wavelength variation of $\sim 10^{-14}$ m to 6×10^{6} m.

The whole electromagnetic spectrum has been classified into different parts or subparts in order of increasing wavelength, according to their type of excitation. There is overlapping in certain parts of the spectrum, showing that the corresponding radiations can be produced by two methods. It may be noted that the physical properties of electromagnetic waves are decided by their wavelengths and not by the method of their excitation.

Table 1.1 shows the various parts of the electromagnetic spectrum with wavelength range, frequency range and the names of the sources of the various electromagnetic radiations.

Uses of Electromagnetic Spectrum

The following are some of the uses of electromagnetic spectrum:
- Radio and microwave radiations are used in radio and TV communication system.
- Infrared radiations are used:
    - In revealing the secret writings on the ancient walls
    - In green houses to keep the plants warm
    - In war fare, for looking through haze, fog or mist as these radiations can pass through them
    - In electrotherapy for the heating of soft tissues.
- Ultraviolet radiations are used in the detection of invisible writing, forged documents, finger prints in forensic laboratory and to preserve the food stuffs. Ultraviolet radiations are used in electrotherapy for the treatment of various skin conditions.

Table 1.1: Various parts of the electromagnetic spectrum.

S. No.	Name	Wavelength range (m)	Frequency range (Hz)	Source
1.	Gamma rays	6×10^{-14} to 1×10^{-11}	5×10^{22} to 3×10^{19}	Nuclear origin
2.	X-rays	1×10^{-11} to 3×10^{-8}	3×10^{19} to 1×10^{16}	Sudden declaration of high energy electrons
3.	Ultraviolet rays	6×10^{-10} to 4×10^{-7}	5×10^{17} to 8×10^{14}	Excitation of atom, spark and arc lamp
4.	Visible light	4×10^{-7} to 8×10^{-7}	8×10^{14} to 4×10^{14}	Excitation of valence electrons
5.	Infrared	8×10^{-7} to 3×10^{-5}	4×10^{14} to 1×10^{13}	Excitation of atoms and molecules
6.	Heat radiations	10^{-5} to 10^{-1}	3×10^{13} to 3×10^{9}	Hot bodies
7.	Microwaves	10^{-3} to 0.3	3×10^{11} to 1×10^{9}	Oscillating current in special vacuum tube
8.	Ultra high frequency	1×10^{-1} to 1	3×10^{9} to 3×10^{8}	Oscillating circuit
9.	Very high radio frequency	1 to 10	3×10^{8} to 3×10^{7}	Oscillating circuit
10.	Radio frequencies	10 to 10^{4}	3×10^{7} to 3×10^{4}	Oscillating circuit
11.	Power frequencies	5×10^{6} to 6×10^{6}	60 to 50	Weak radiations from AC circuits

- X-rays can pass through soft tissues but not through bones. This property of X-rays is used in medical diagnosis, after X-ray films are made.
- Electromagnetic waves of suitable frequencies are used in medical science for the treatment of various diseases.
- Super-high frequency electromagnetic waves are used in radar and satellite communication.

ELECTRIC SHOCK

Shock: Shock is a stage of unconsciousness which could be due to so many causes. Examples are: hypovolemic, neurogenic, psychogenic and electric shock, etc.

Electric shock: Electric shock is a painful stimulation of sensory nerves caused by:
- Sudden flow of current
- Cessation or pause of flow of current
- Variation of the current passing through the body.

Causes of Electric Shock
- Poorly designed electromedical apparatus
- Improper insulation of equipment
- Improper insulation of wires
- Badly serviced medical equipment
- Mishandling of apparatus
- Improper guidance to the patient
- Lack of proper safety measures.

Severity of Electric Shock
- In accordance with the Ohm's law, resistance is inversely proportional to current. Hence, lower the resistance of the skin, the greater the current which passes through the body. Therefore, if exposed part of the circuit is touched with wet hands, the shock is more likely to be severe than if the hands are dry.
- The greater the current passing through the body, the more severe is the shock.
- The severity also depends upon the path taken by the current. A strong current through the head, neck or heart proves to be more fatal.
- The severity also depends upon the type of current which passes through the body. Individuals can be electrocuted by using appliances of as little as 40 V direct current in industry.

Types of Electric Shock
According to the severity of the shock, it could be of following types:
- Minor electric shock
- Major or severe electric shock.

Effects of Electric Shock
- *Minor electric shock*: In minor electric shock, the victim gets frightened and distressed. In this type of shock, there is no loss of consciousness.

- *Major or severe electric shock*: In major or severe electric shock, there is a fall of blood pressure and patient may become unconscious. There could be cessation of respiration, followed by ventricular fibrillations and cardiac arrest. These could be diagnosed by seeing absence of pulse in the carotid artery and with fully dilated pupils.

Treatment of Electric Shock
- The current should be switched off immediately.
- The victim to be disconnected from the source of supply.
- If there is no switch in the circuit, the victim must be removed from contact with the conductor, but rescuer must take care not to receive a shock himself from touching the affected person, contact with whom should be made only through a thick layer of insulating material.
- Following a minor shock, the patient is to be reassured that everything is alright and allowed to rest.
- Water may be given to drink, but hot drinks should be avoided as they may cause vasodilatation.
- Tight clothing should be loosened and plenty of air allowed.
- If respiration has ceased, the airway must be cleared and artificial respiration is to be commenced immediately by the mouth-to-mouth or mouth-to-nose method.
- Cardiopulmonary resuscitation may also be given.
- Oxygen therapy may also be administered if required.
- Patient must be shifted to the hospital after the primary care.

Precautions to Avoid Electric Shock
- All apparatus should be tested before use.
- Connections to be checked before application.
- Controls should be checked to ensure that they are at zero before switching on.
- Adequate warming up time should be allowed.
- The current intensity should be increased with care.
- Patients should never be allowed to touch electrical equipment.
- All apparatus should be serviced regularly by a competent person.
- Machine should be properly insulated.
- Mishandling of apparatus by unqualified person should be avoided.
- All safety measures should be taken before application to the patient.

Earth shock: When a shock is due to a connection between the live wire of the main and the earth it is called an earth shock.

Earth circuit: Electric power is transmitted by one live cable and one neutral cable which are connected to earth. The earth forms part of the conducting pathway and any connection between the live wire of the main and earth completes a circuit through which current passes. If some person forms part of this circuit he receives an earth shock. Thus an earth shock is liable to occur if any person makes contact with the live wire of the main while connected to earth.

Causes of Earth Shock
Earth shock may be caused by the following two reasons:
1. Connection to the live wire
2. Connection to the earth.

Connection to the Live Wire
* When wire is not properly insulated.
* When the switch is put in the neutral wire, the neutral wire is disconnected and live wire is not disconnected.
* Live wire is touched to metal casing.
* Live wire is touched to any wet thing.

Connection to the Earth
* If the floor is made up of stone.
* If the conductor is touching any wire which is connected to the earth, such as gas pipe or water pipes.
* If the conductor is touched to any radiated metal casing or metal wire.

Precautions
* Proper arrangement of the physiotherapy department.
* Proper flooring should be done with rexine.
* Insulation should be proper.
* While treatment patient should not touch any of the machine part.
* The metal casing of all apparatus must be connected to the earth.
* The floor should be kept dry.
* While using water containers, containing water, should be kept on an insulating material, e.g., a wooden table.
* Leaky bathtub should not be used.
* The bathtub should not have fixed taps or water pipes.

Examples
Simultaneous connection to the live wire and earth can occur in a variety of ways:
* A patient who is receiving treatment with a current that is not earth-free may rest her hand on a water pipe.
* A physiotherapist holding an electrode that is connected to the live wire may touch the earthed apparatus casing.
* If someone standing on a damp stone floor touches the casing of apparatus which is not connected to earth and with which the live wire is in contact, he too will receive an earth shock.

Physical Principles of Light
Multicolored rainbows, blue skies, green forests, etc., can be enjoyed by those who have eyes with which to see them. By studying the branch of physics called *optics,* which deals with the behavior of light and other electromagnetic waves, we can reach deeper appreciation of the visible world. A knowledge of the properties of light allows us to understand the colors of the rainbow and designs of the optical devices, such as telescopes, microscopes, cameras, eyeglasses and the human eyes. The same basic principles of light also lie at the heart of the some modern equipments like laser, optical fibers, holograms, optical computers and new techniques in medical imaging.

In this part of the chapter, we will study the laws of reflection and refraction and concepts of dispersion, polarization and scattering of light. Also we will compare the various possible description of light in terms of particles, rays or waves and how mirrors and lenses work in cameras, telescopes or microscopes.

Until the time of *Sir Isaac Newton* (1642–1727), most scientists thought that light consisted of streams of particles (called corpuscles) emitted by light sources. Galileo and others tried to measure speed of light. Around 1665, it was evident that light has wave properties. In 1873, *James Clark Maxwell* predicted the existence of electromagnetic waves and calculated its speed of propagation. This development along with the work of *Heinrich Hertz* in 1887 showed conclusively that light is indeed an electromagnetic wave.

The wave picture of light does not reveal the whole story. Several effects associated with emission and absorption of light concludes a particle aspect, in that the energy carried by light waves is packed in discrete bundles called *photons or quanta*. These apparently contradictory wave and particle properties have been reconciled in 1930s with development of quanta electrodynamics which is a comprehensive theory that includes both wave and particle properties. The propagation of light is best described by a wave model and the understanding of emission and absorption requires a particle approach.

The fundamental sources of all electromagnetic radiation are electric charges in accelerated motion. All bodies emit electromagnetic radiation as a result of thermal motion of their molecules. This radiation called thermal radiation is a mixture of different wavelengths. At sufficiently high temperatures, all matter emits enough visible light to become luminous. Thus, hot matter in any form is a source of light. Familiar examples are incandescent lamp, flame of a candle, coils in an electric heater, etc.

Light is also produced during electrical discharges through ionized gases. The bluish light of mercury arc lamp, the orange-yellow light of sodium vapor lamp and various colors of neon sign boards are common examples. A variation of the mercury arc lamp is a fluorescent lamp. This light source uses a material called a phosphor to convert the ultraviolet radiation from a mercury arc into a visible light. This conversion makes fluorescent lamps more efficient than the incandescent lamps in converting electrical energy into light.

A light source that has attained prominence in recent years is *LASER*. It is an acronym of Light Amplification of Stimulated Emission of Radiation. In most light sources, light is emitted independently by different atoms within the source. In a laser, by contrast, atoms are induced to emit light in a cooperative, coherent fashion. The result is a very narrow beam of radiation that can be enormously intense and that is monochromatic, i.e., having single frequency than light from any other source. Laser nowadays is used by physiotherapists for treatment purposes.

Reflection and Refraction

The ray model of light explains two of the most important aspects of light propagation: (i) reflection and (ii) refraction. In a homogeneous medium, light travels along a straight path. When a light wave strikes a smooth interface separating two transparent materials (such as air and glass or water and glass), the wave is generally partly reflected and partly refracted (transmitted) into the second material **(Fig. 1.64)**. The phenomenon of change in path of light as it goes from one medium to another is called refraction.

Laws of Reflection and Refraction

- The incident, reflected and refracted rays and the normal to the surface all lie in the same plane **(Fig. 1.65)**. The plane of the three rays is perpendicular to the plane of the boundary surface between the two materials.

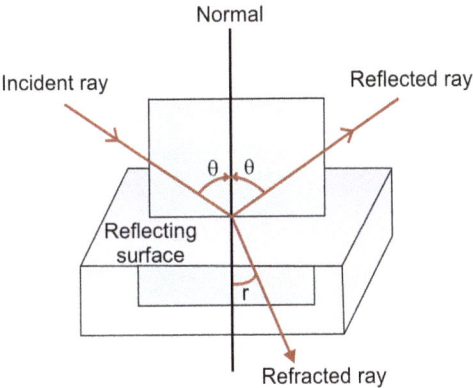

Fig. 1.64: Refraction and reflection of light.

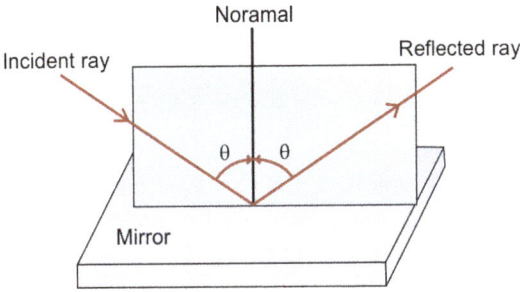

Fig. 1.65: The incident ray, reflected ray and the normal to the reflecting surface lie in the same plane.

- The angle of reflection is equal to the angle of incidence for all wavelengths and any pair of materials. This relation, together with the observation that the incident and reflected rays and the normal all lie in the same plane is called the law of reflection.
- For monochromatic light and for a given pair of materials, a and b, on opposite sides of the interface, the ratio of the sines of the angles where both angles are measured from the normal to the surface, is equal to the inverse ratio of the two indexes of refraction.

This experimental result, together with the observation that the incident and refracted rays and the normal all lie in the same plane, is called the *law of refraction or Snell's law,* after the Dutch scientist Willebrord Snell.

Characteristic of the image formed by a plane mirror:
- Image is as far as behind the mirror, as the object is in front of the mirror
- The size of the image is same as that of the object
- The image formed is virtual in nature
- The image formed is erect in nature
- The image formed is laterally inverted. The lateral inversion means that the right side of the object appears as the left side of the image and vice versa.

The portion of a reflecting surface, which forms part of a sphere, is called a spherical mirror. The spherical mirrors are of two types:
1. *Concave spherical mirror*: A spherical mirror whose reflecting surface is toward the center of the sphere of which mirror forms a part is called concave spherical mirror.

2. *Convex spherical mirror*: A spherical mirror whose reflecting surface is away from the center of the sphere of which mirror forms a part is called convex spherical mirror.

Pole: The center of spherical mirror is called its pole.

Principal axis: The line joining the pole and the center of curvature of the mirror is called the principal axis of the mirror.

Center of curvature: The center of sphere of which mirror forms a part is called the center of curvature of the mirror.

Radius of curvature: The radius of sphere of which mirror forms a part is called the radius of curvature of the mirror.

Aperture: The diameter of the mirror is called aperture of the mirror.

Principal focus: The point at which a narrow beam of light incident on the mirror parallel to its principal axis after reflection from the mirror meets or appears to come from is called principal focus of the mirror.

Focal length: The distance between the pole and the principal focus of the mirror is called the focal length of the mirror.

Applications of plane or curved mirrors:
- Concave mirrors are used for dressing up or used as make up mirrors. It is because a person keeps his body or face between pole and focus of the concave mirror, a highly magnified image of his body or face is formed.
- Concave mirrors are used by dental surgeons for examining dental cavities.
- Concave mirrors are used by ophthalmologists for examining the eye.
- Concave mirrors are used as reflectors in cinema projectors, magic lanterns, etc.
- Concave mirrors are used to make reflecting type astronomical telescope of large aperture.
- Concave parabolic mirrors are used in search lights.
- Convex mirrors are used in vehicles as drivers' mirror. The driver of the vehicle can get a clear and much wider field of view of the objects behind him.
- Convex mirrors are used as a safety feature at sharp turns or dangerous corners of the road. These are also used to prevent shop lifting activities in the market.

Dispersion

Ordinary white light is a superposition of waves with wavelengths extending throughout the visible spectrum. The speed of light *in vacuum* is the same for all wavelengths, but the speed in a material substance is different for different wavelengths. Therefore, the index of refraction of a material depends on wavelength. The dependence of wave speed and index of refraction on wavelength is called dispersion. The phenomenon of splitting up of white light into its constituent colors is called dispersion of light.

If a beam of white light is made to fall on one face of a prism, the light emerging from the other face of the prism consists of seven colors namely *violet, indigo, blue, green, yellow, orange and red*. The deviation suffered by the violet color is maximum, while that by the red is minimum. The band of seven colors produced at the screen is called *spectrum* **(Fig. 1.66)**.

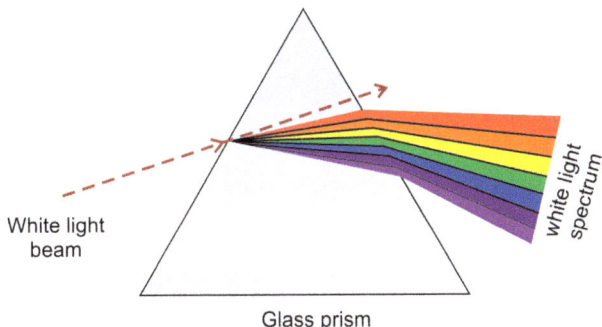

Fig. 1.66: Dispersion of sunlight or white light on passing through a glass prism. The relative deviation of different colors shown is highly exaggerated.

Scattering of Light

The sky is blue. Sunsets are red. Skylight is partially polarized; that is why the sky looks darker from some angles than from others when it is viewed through polarized sunglasses. It turns out that one phenomenon is responsible for all of these effects. When you look at the daytime sky, the light you see is sunlight that has been absorbed and then reradiated in a variety of directions. This process is called scattering. When light falls on particles of large size such as dust and water droplets, it does not get scattered. However, when light travels through the atmosphere, it gets scattered from the air molecules. The blue light (light of smaller wavelength) is scattered more than red light (light of longer wavelength), when the light travels through the atmosphere.

Sir CV Raman was awarded Nobel prize (1930) for his work on elastic scattering of light by molecules. It is popularly known as *Raman's effect*.

Wavefront

According to wave theory of light, a source of light sends out disturbances in all directions. In a homogenous medium, the disturbances reach all those particles of the medium in phase with each other and therefore at any instance, all such particles must be vibrating in phase with each other. The locus of all the particles of the medium, which at any instant are vibrating in the same phase is called the wavefront.

Depending upon the shape of the source of light, wavefront can be of following types:
- *Spherical wavefront*: A spherical wavefront is produced by a point source of light **(Fig. 1.67A)**.
- *Cylindrical wavefront*: When the source of light is linear in shape (such as a slit), a cylindrical wavefront is produced.
- *Plane wavefront*: A small part of a spherical or a cylindrical wavefront originating from a distant source will appear plane and hence called a plane wavefront **(Fig. 1.67B)**.

Huygens' Principle

Huygens' principle is a geometrical construction which is used to determine the new position of a wavefront at a later time from its given position at any instant. In other words, Huygens' principle gives a method to know as to how light spreads out in the medium.

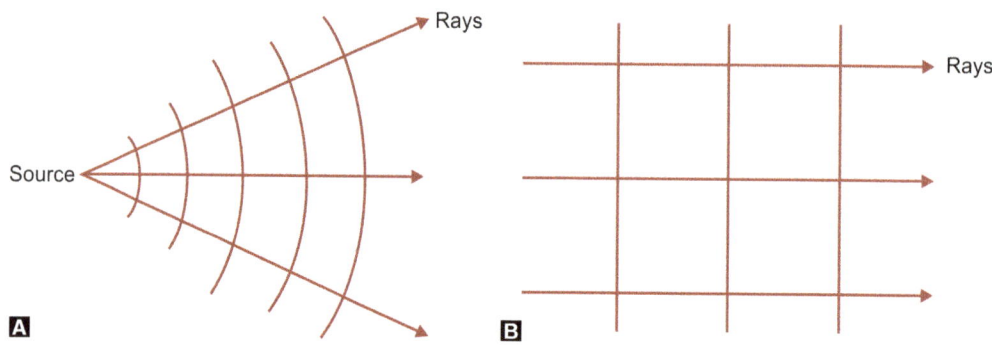

Figs. 1.67A and B: Wavefront. (A) When the wavefront is spherical, the rays radiate out from the center of the sphere; (B) When the wavefront is plane, the rays are parallel.

Huygens' principle is based upon the following assumptions:
- Each point on the given or primary wavefront acts as a source of secondary wavelets, sending out disturbances in all directions in a similar manner as the original source of light does.
- The new position of the wavefront at any instant (called secondary wavefront) is the envelope of the secondary wavelets at that instant.

Interference of Light

When a source of light emits energy, the distribution of energy is uniform in the medium, but when two sources of light lie close to each other and emit light of same wavelength and preferably of same amplitude, then due to superposition of waves from the two sources, the distribution of light energy no longer remains uniform. *The phenomenon of nonuniform distribution of energy in the medium due to superposition of two light waves is called interference of light.*

At some points in the medium, the intensity of light is maximum (constructive interference), while at some other points, the intensity is minimum (destructive interference).

Thomas Young (1801) demonstrated the interference of light experimentally. His experiment led to the conclusion that light has a wave nature.

Diffraction

The phenomenon of bending of light round the sharp corners and spreading into the regions of the geometrical shadow is called *diffraction*. The light waves are diffracted only when the size of the obstacle is comparable to the wavelength of the light. All types of wave motion exhibit diffraction effect. Sound waves or radio waves show diffraction effect in day-to-day life.

Polarization

In general, waves are of two types:
1. *Longitudinal waves*: The waves in which particles oscillate along the direction of propagation of the waves are called *longitudinal waves*.
2. *Transverse waves*: The waves in which direction of oscillation of particles is perpendicular to the direction of propagation of the waves are called *transverse waves*.

Both types of waves exhibit the phenomenon of reflection, refraction, diffraction and interference but polarization of the waves is only exhibited by the transverse waves. Polarization is characteristic of all transverse waves. This is the only phenomenon where two types of waves essentially differ from one another.

When a wave has only y-displacements, we say that it is linearly polarized in y-direction; a wave in z-displacements is linearly polarized in the z-direction. *The phenomenon due to which the vibrations of light are restricted in a particular plane is called the polarization of light.* For mechanical waves, we can build a polarizing filter, or a polarizer that permits only waves with a certain polarization direction to pass. Commonly used polarizers are tourmaline crystal or Nicol prism.

PHYSICAL PRINCIPLES OF SOUND

Ripples in a pond, musical sounds or seismic tremors triggered by an earthquake—all these exhibit a *wave phenomenon*. Waves can occur whenever a system is disturbed from equilibrium and when the disturbance can travel or propagate from one region to other. As a wave propagates, it carries energy. The energy of seismic waves can be so high that it can break the earth's crust.

Waves in a string play an important role in music. When a musician strums a wave or bows a violin, he makes waves that travel in opposite directions along the instrument's strings. What happens when those oppositely directed waves overlap is called *interference*.

Not all waves are mechanical in nature. Electromagnetic waves like light, radio waves, infrared and ultraviolet radiations, etc. can propagate in vacuum or empty spaces, where there is no medium.

Mechanical Waves

A *mechanical wave* is a disturbance that travels through some material or substance called the *medium* for the wave. As the wave travels through the medium, the particles that make up the medium undergo displacements of various kinds, depending on the nature of the wave. If the displacements of the medium are perpendicular or transverse to the direction of travel of the wave along the medium, it is called a *transverse wave*. Examples can be seen in a string or rope.

If the displacements of the medium are parallel or *longitudinal* to the direction of travel of the wave along the medium, it is called a *longitudinal wave*. Examples can be seen in a fluids (liquid) or gases.

If the displacements of the medium are both parallel and perpendicular to the direction of travel of the wave along the medium, it is called a *mixed wave*. Examples can be seen in a water canal.

These examples have three on common. First in each case the disturbance travels or propagates with a definite speed through the medium. This speed is called the speed of propagation, or simply the *wave speed*. It is determined in each case by the mechanical properties of the medium. Second, the medium itself does not travel through space; its individual particles undergo back-and-forth or up-and-down motions around their equilibrium positions. The overall pattern of the wave disturbance is what travels. Third, to set any of these systems into motion, we have to put in energy by doing mechanical work on the system. The wave motion transports this energy from one region of the medium to another. Waves transport energy, but not matter, form one region to another.

Periodic Waves

The transverse wave on a stretched string is an example of a wave pulse. The hand shakes the string up and down just once, exerting a transverse force on it. The result is a single "wiggle" or pulse that travels along the length of the string. The tension in the string restores its straight-line shape once the pulse has passed. When we give the free end of the string a repetitive or periodic motion, then each particle in the string also undergoes periodic motion as the wave propagates and we have a periodic wave.

As the wave moves, any point on the string oscillates up-and-down about its equilibrium position with simple harmonic motion. When a sinusoidal wave passes through a medium, every particle in the medium undergoes a simple harmonic motion with the same frequency.

For a periodic wave, the shape of the string at any instant is a repeating pattern. The length of one complete wave pattern is the distance from one crest to the next or from one trough to the next or from any point to the corresponding point on the next repetition of the wave shape. This is called wavelength of the wave which is denoted by λ (Greek letter *lambda*). The wave pattern travels with a constant speed v and advances a distance of one wavelength λ in a time interval of one period T. So, the wave speed v is given by:

$$v = \lambda/T$$

or because

$$f = 1/T$$
$$v = \lambda f$$

The speed of propagation equals the product of wavelength and frequency. The frequency is a property of the entire periodic wave because all points on the string oscillate with the same frequency f.

Sound Waves

Sound is a mechanical wave that is an oscillation of pressure transmitted through a solid, liquid, or gas, composed of frequencies within the range of hearing and of a level sufficiently strong to be heard, or the sensation stimulated in organs of hearing by such vibrations.

Propagation of Sound

Sound is a sequence of waves of pressure that propagates through compressible media, such as air or water. During propagation, waves can be reflected, refracted, or attenuated by the medium.

The behavior of sound propagation is generally affected by three things:
1. *A relationship between density and pressure*: This relationship, affected by temperature, determines the speed of sound within the medium.
2. The propagation is also affected by the motion of the medium itself. For example, sound moving through wind. Independent of the motion of sound through the medium, if the medium is moving, the sound is further transported.
3. The viscosity of the medium also affects the motion of sound waves. It determines the rate at which sound is attenuated. For many media, such as air or water, attenuation due to viscosity is negligible.

When sound is moving through a medium that does not have constant physical properties, it may be refracted (either dispersed or focused).

Perception of Sound

The perception of sound in any organism is limited to a certain range of frequencies. For humans, hearing is normally limited to frequencies between about 20 Hz and 20,000 Hz (20 kHz), although these limits are not definite. The upper limit generally decreases with age. Other species have a different range of hearing. For example, dogs can perceive vibrations

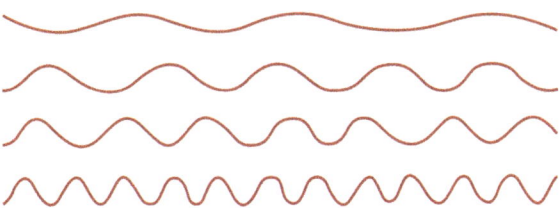

Fig. 1.68: Longitudinal and transverse waves.

higher that 20 kHz, but are deaf to anything below 40 Hz. As a signal perceived by one of the major senses, sound is used by many species for detecting danger, navigation, predation and communication. Earth's atmosphere, water and virtually any physical phenomenon, such as fire, rain wind or earthquake, produces (and is characterized by) its unique sounds. Many species, such as frogs, birds, marine and terrestrial mammals, have also developed special organs to produce sound. In some species, these produce song and speech. Furthermore, humans have developed culture and technology (such as music, telephone and radio) that allows them to generate, record, transmit and broadcast sound. The scientific study of human sound perception is known as psychoacoustics.

Physics of Sound

The mechanical vibrations that can be interpreted as sound are able to travel through all forms of matter: solid, liquid or gases. The matter that supports the sound is called the medium. Sound cannot travel through a vacuum.

Longitudinal and Transverse Waves

Sinusoidal waves of various frequencies; the bottom waves have higher frequencies than those above **(Fig. 1.68)**. The horizontal axis represents time.

Sound is transmitted through gases, plasma and liquids as longitudinal waves, also called compression waves. Through solids, however, it can be transmitted as both longitudinal waves and transverse waves. Longitudinal sound waves are waves of alternating pressure deviations from the equilibrium pressure, causing local regions of compression and rarefaction, while transverse waves (in solids) are waves of alternating shear stress at right angle to the direction of propagation.

Matter in the medium is periodically displaced by a sound wave, and thus oscillates. The energy carried by the sound wave converts back-and-forth between the potential energy of the extra-compression (in case of longitudinal waves) or lateral displacement strain (in case of transverse waves) of the matter and the kinetic energy of the oscillations of the medium.

Sound Wave Properties and Characteristics

Sound waves are often simplified to a description in terms of sinusoidal plane waves, which are characterized by these generic properties:
* Frequency, or its inverse, the period
* Wavelength
* Wave number
* Amplitude
* Sound pressure

- Sound intensity
- Speed of sound
- Direction.

Sometimes speed and direction are combined as a velocity vector; wave number and direction are combined as a wave vector.

Transverse waves, also known as shear waves, have the additional property, polarization, and are not a characteristic of sound waves.

Speed of Sound

The speed of sound depends on the medium the waves pass through, and is a fundamental property of the material. The physical properties and the speed of sound change with ambient conditions. For example, the speed of sound in gases depends on temperature. In 20°C (68°F) air at the sea level, the speed of sound is approximately 343 m/s (1,230 km/h; 767 mph). In fresh water, also at 20°C, the speed of sound is approximately 1,482 m/s (5,335 km/h; 3,315 mph). In steel, the speed of sound is about 5,960 m/s (21,460 km/h; 13,330 mph).

CHAPTER 2

Inflammation and Repair

INTRODUCTION

Before application of any treatment, it is essential for the student/clinician to ensure that his/her knowledge about anatomy, physiology and pathophysiology is sufficient to localize the site of lesion, such as depth at which damage of tissue is located or possible pathophysiology arising signs and symptoms. The selection of modality is based upon the physical and physiological effects of those modalities on the tissues and the evidence available for the efficacy of such modalities on similar types of lesions.

INFLAMMATION

Inflammation is a localized protective response, elicited by injury or destruction of tissues, which serves to destroy, dilute or wall off (sequester) both the injurious agent and the injured tissue.

The word inflammation is derived from *inflamer* a Latin word which means *to set on fire*. It begins when the normal physiology of the tissue is altered by trauma or disease. Aulus Cornelius Celsus (c. 25 BC to c. 50 AD) first described the inflammatory process which is characterized by four cardinal signs such as:
1. Calor (Heat)
2. Rubor (Redness)
3. Tumor (Swelling)
4. Dolor (Pain).

Later on, in 1871 Virchow added the fifth cardinal sign of inflammation as Function laesa (Loss of function).

Common Causes of Inflammation

Common causes of inflammation includes:
- Soft tissue injury (sprain, strain and contusion)
- Fractures (physical or pathological)
- Foreign bodies
- Autoimmune disease (rheumatoid arthritis)
- Microbial agents (bacteria, viruses, fungi, etc)
- Chemical agents (acids or alkalis)
- Thermal (Frost bite or Burns)
- Irradiation: Infrared radiation (IRR) or ultraviolet radiation (UVR)

Inflammation is Divided into Two Basic Patterns

1. ***Acute inflammation:*** It is sudden onset and early response to injury. It is designed to deliver leukocytes to the site of injury with classical signs having predominance of vascular end exudative processes.
2. ***Chronic inflammation:*** It is considered to be the inflammation of slow progress with prolonged duration (several weeks to months or even years) in which active inflammation, tissue injury and healing proceed simultaneously. It is marked chiefly by the formation of new connective tissue.

Heat results from increased blood flow through the area and is experienced only in the peripheral parts of the area such as skin. Redness is caused by the dilatation of small blood vessels across the area of injury. Fever is brought about by the chemical mediators of inflammation and contributes to the rise of temperature at the injury. Swelling called edema or edema is caused primarily by the accumulation of fluids outside of the blood vessels. The pain associated with the inflammation results in part from the distortion of tissues caused by edema and it is induced primarily by certain chemical mediators of inflammation such as bradykinins, serotonin and prostaglandins. Loss of function results from pain or swelling that inhibits mobility that prevents movement in the area.

ACUTE INFLAMMATION

Vascular Changes

Whenever any tissue is injured or damaged, there is contraction of small blood vessels momentarily which is called *vasoconstriction*. Following this transient event, which is believed to be if little importance to the inflammatory response, then the blood vessels dilate which is called *vasodilation,* increasing blood flow into the area. Vasodilation may last from about 15 minutes to even several hours.

Next, is the walls of blood vessels which normally allows only water and salts to pass through easily, becomes more permeable. Protein rich fluid called *exudates,* is now able to exit into the tissues. Important substances in the exudates includes clotting factor, which helps prevent the spreading of infectious agents throughout the body. Other proteins includes antibodies that help destroy invading micro-organisms.

As fluid and other substances leak out of the blood vessels, blood flow becomes more sluggish and white blood cells begin to fall out of the axial stream in the center of the vessel to flow nearer the vessel wall. The white blood cells then adhere to the blood vessel wall, the first step in their emigration into the extravascular space of the tissue.

As per Starling's Law, movement of fluids in and out of arterioles, capillaries and venules is regulated by the balance between:
- Intravascular hydrostatic pressure—that tends to force fluid out of vessels.
- Osmotic pressure of the plasma proteins—that tends to retain fluids within the vessels.

Cellular Changes

The most important feature of inflammation is the accumulation of white blood cells at the site of injury. Most of these cells are phagocytes, certain *cell eating* leucocytes that ingest bacteria and other foreign particles and also clean up cellular debris caused by the injury. The main phagocytes involved in acute inflammation are the neutrophils, a type of white blood cell that contains granules of cell destroying enzymes and proteins. When tissue damage is minor, an adequate supply of these cells can be obtained from those already circulating in the blood. But when the damage is extensive, stores of neutrophils (even some in immature form) are released from the bone marrow, where these are generated.

To perform their desired tasks, not only neutrophils must exit through the blood vessel wall but they must actively move from the blood vessel toward the area of tissue damage. This movement is made possible by chemical substances that diffuse form the area of tissue damage and create a concentration gradient followed by the neutrophils. The substances that create the gradient are called chemotactic factors and the one way migration of cells along with the gradient is called *Chemotaxis*.

Chronic Inflammation

Acute inflammation may progress into chronic inflammation, if the agent causing inflammation cannot be eliminated or if there is some kind of interference with the healing process. Repeated episodes of acute inflammation may give rise to chronic inflammation. The physical extent, duration, and effects of chronic inflammation vary with the cause of the injury and the body's ability to ameliorate the damage. In some cases, chronic inflammation is not a sequel to acute inflammation but an independent response.

The understanding of inflammation and then repair is essential for a clinician who treats such conditions. A physiotherapist treats a variety of inflammatory conditions like trauma, arthritis or sports injuries. The understanding of pathophysiology of inflammation helps facilitate early healing. Role of physiotherapist can be enhanced by proper understanding of the disease process and appropriate selection of modalities and physical agents along with exercises and complete therapeutic intervention of the healing process.

The process of inflammation and repair basically consists of following three phases: (i) Inflammation, (ii) proliferation, and (iii) maturation.

i. ***Phase of inflammation:*** This phase prepares the wound for healing and lasts for 1–6 days. This is the immediate protective response which attempts to destroy, dilute or isolate the cells or agents that may be at fault. It is a normal and prerequisite to healing and healing fails to occur if there is no inflammation. Though beneficial for the healing process, it is harmful for the patient in terms of pain and loss of function warranting its early resolution (acute plantar fasciitis or tennis elbow tendinitis). The role of a physiotherapist here is to get to get relief from pain and spasm and restoration of functions.

ii. ***Phase of proliferation:*** This is the second phase of tissue healing and it lasts from the third day upto 20 days. It's purpose is to cover the wound and impart strength to the injury site. The four processes occurring simultaneously in this phase are epithelialization, collagen production, wound contraction and neovascularization. In this phase careful application of certain electrophysical modalities accelerates the healing process causing early functional restoration (e.g., application of laser to plantar fascia or application of ultrasound to common extensor origin to cause healing).

iii. ***Phase of maturation:*** This phase is a transition from the phase of proliferation and produces changes in the size, form and strength of scar tissue. It is the longest phase in the healing process and can persist for over a year after the initial injury or inflammation. The ultimate goal of this phase is restoration of prior function of the injured tissue. As in this phase of tissue healing, a scar is formed and as the scar is inelastic. The collagen fibers that form the scar are largely responsible for the final function of the injured area. The aim of physiotherapy treatment in this phase is mobilization of the scar tissue, so that functional mobility can be restored.

PAIN

Pain is an experience based upon complex interaction of physical and psychological processes and is defined as "an unpleasant sensory and emotional experience associated with actual or potential tissue damage". This is the most common symptom prompting patients for medical help. It can be categorized as acute, subacute, chronic or referred pain.

Acute Pain

Acute pain is defined as pain which arises immediately after injury and resolved once the damaged tissue heals. It lasts from the onset on injury to few days or 2–3 weeks.

Subacute Pain

When acute pain persists after 2–3 weeks till about 6 months, it is called subacute pain. The goal of management here is to apply for electrophysical agents or modalities that can resolve the underlying pathology that is the source of pain.

Chronic Pain

Chronic pain is defined as the pain that does not resolve in the usual time it takes for the disorder to heal and persists for a duration greater than six months.

Referred Pain

Referred pain is the pain that feels at the location distant from its source. This is the pain which is felt in one area, when the actual tissue damage is in another area. Common examples are: A pathology in the shoulder causes referred pain in the elbow region, a pathology of hip causes referred pain in the knee or lumbar radiculopathy L5-S1 causes lateral leg pain. Also, sometimes the pain that referred from internal organs like for example involvement of heart causes lateral shoulder pain. In all these situations, the thorough knowledge of the clinician to understand the source of pain in identifying and resolving the underlying pathology by the application of suitable physical agents, modalities or exercises are important.

The course of disease, its progression, repair of tissues and treatment can be classified as follows:

Acute condition: Any condition is said to be acute if the signs and symptoms are very severe. Such conditions are usually recent in origin. This stage usually lasts for about two weeks.

Subacute condition: A condition is said to be subacute, if the signs and symptoms are less severe than what was present in acute conditions. This condition usually lasts for few weeks or a month.

Chronic condition: A condition is said to be chronic, if the signs and symptoms are less severe than what was present in subacute conditions but persists for longer duration. This condition usually lasts for few months to even years.

THE ROLE OF A PHYSIOTHERAPIST AND PHYSICAL AGENTS

The role of a physiotherapist in understanding inflammation and repair and then selecting appropriate treatment modality to reduce pain and inflammation and early restoration of physical functions are important. The modalities that can be used to reduce inflammation, e.g., cold (cryotherapy); accelerate healing, e.g., laser, ultrasound, heat, etc; mobilize scar tissue by softening collagen fibers, e.g., paraffin wax bath, ultrasound, diathermy etc. and then reducing pain, e.g., TENS, interferential therapy, heat and cold, etc. The evidence on the efficacy of treatment modality like in reducing inflammation, for example, cold and in accelerating healing process like using ultrasound and increasing functions like using nerve muscle electrical stimulation is important. Adequate precaution needs to be taken while application of these modalities over sensitive tissues. Proper preparation of patient before using any modality is important and will be covered in further chapters.

CHAPTER 3

Low Frequency Currents

FARADIC TYPE CURRENT

Faradic type current is short duration interrupted direct current (DC) with pulse duration of 0.1–1 ms and frequencies between 50 and 100 Hz, used for the stimulation of innervated muscles. The term faradism was previously used to signify the type of current produced by the first faradic coil and was unevenly alternating current (AC) with each cycle consisting of two unequal phases **(Fig. 3.1)**:
1. Low-intensity long duration current
2. High-intensity short duration current

Faradic coils have now been replaced by electronic stimulators **(Figs. 3.2A and B)** which almost have the same physiological effect but differs in the waveform **(Fig. 3.3)**. The features essential for the production of these physiological effects are the impulses with duration of 0.1–1 ms with a frequency of 50–100 Hz.

Modified Faradic Current

For better results in the treatment, faradic current is always surged to produce a near normal tetanic-like contraction and relaxation of the muscle. The apparatus should have sufficient control to surge the current so that the intensity of successive impulses increases gradually with surges varying in waveform to provide satisfactory muscle contraction and relaxation.

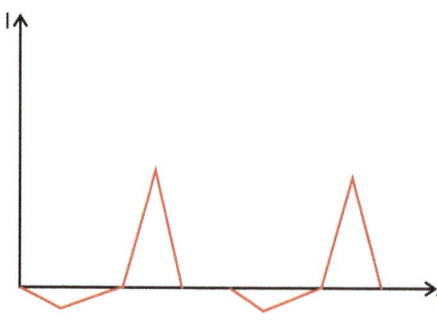

Fig. 3.1: Pure faradic current.

Chapter 3: Low Frequency Currents

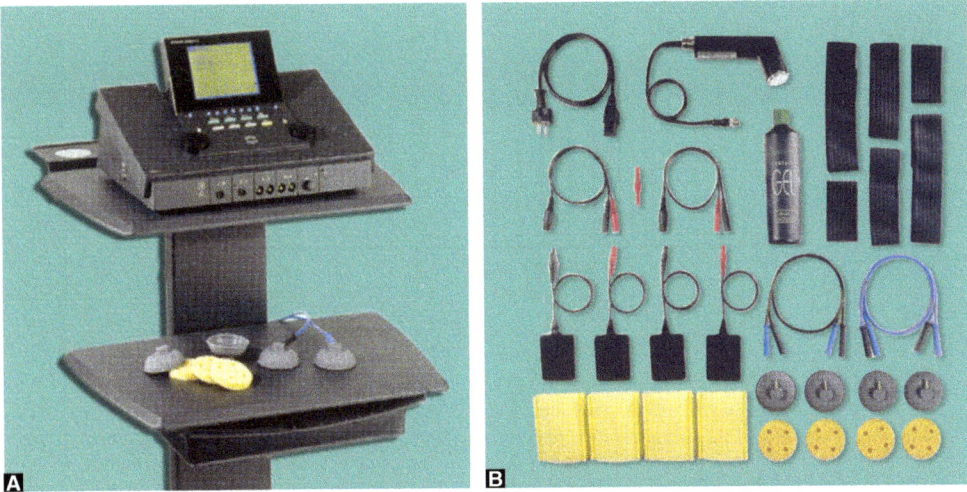

Figs. 3.2A and B: (A) Low frequency current apparatus; (B) Treatment accessories.

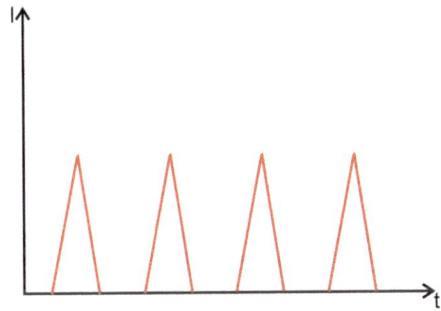

Fig. 3.3: Faradic current from electronic stimulator.

In the original faradic coils, the current was surged by hand but in modern stimulators an electronic device is used. The circuit can be modified to give surges of various durations, frequencies and waveforms. Various forms of surge are available, such as trapezoidal, triangular and saw-tooth impulses, and that most suitable for each patient must be selected **(Fig. 3.4)**.

ELECTROTHERAPEUTIC CURRENTS

Alternating, Direct and Pulsed Currents

Electrotherapeutic currents are basically of three types. These are: (1) *AC*, (2) *DC, or* (3) *pulsed*. Specific therapeutic effects are produced by these electrotherapeutic currents, which are capable of producing specific physiologic changes when introduced into the biological tissues.

Direct current also referred as galvanic current or *constant galvanism* which has a unidirectional flow of electrons toward the positive pole **(Fig. 3.5A)**. In modern devices, the polarity and thus the direction of the flow of current, can also be reversed. The therapeutic use

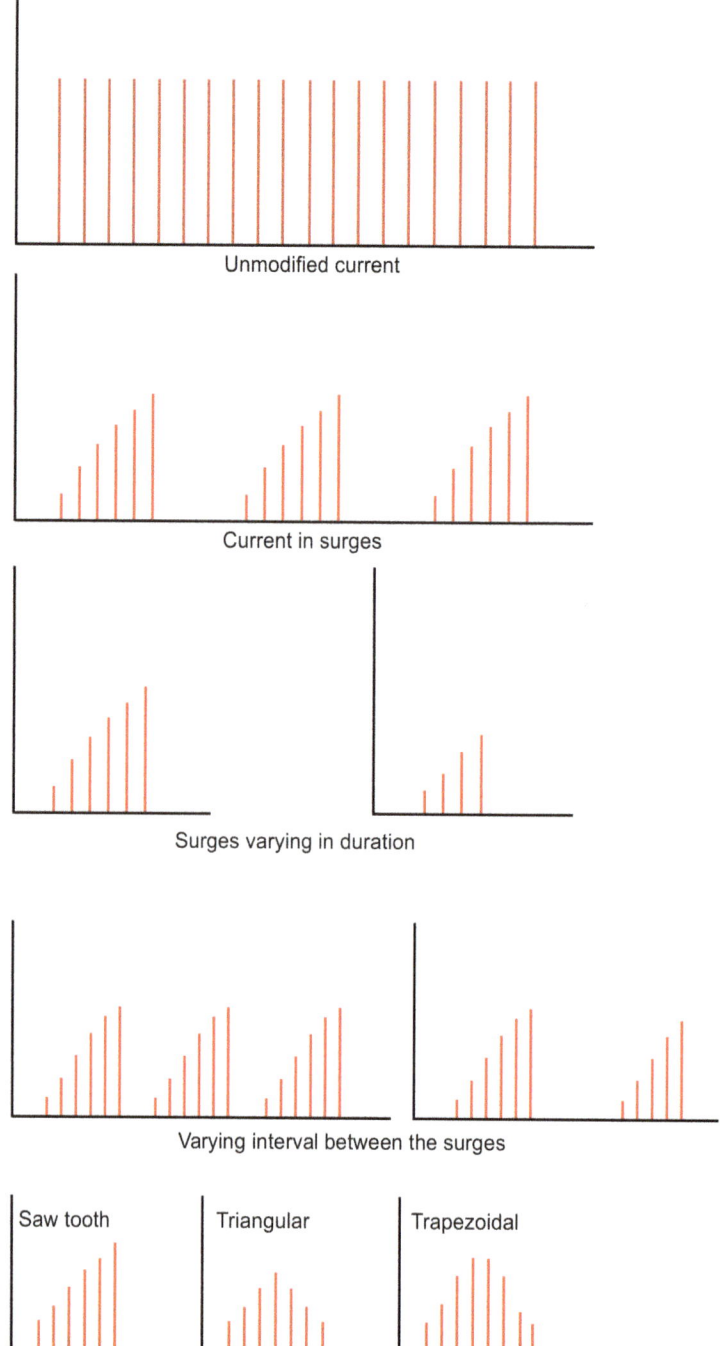

Fig. 3.4: Unmodified and modified (surged) form of faradic current.

of this unidirectional flow of current is to introduce medication into the body tissues is called as iontophoresis (*LeDuc*, 1903). Some apparatus have the capability of automatically reversing polarity, in which case the physiologic effects will be similar to AC.

Interrupted Direct Current

If the continuous unidirectional current is interrupted, it gives rise to series of pulses or phases of unidirectional current. A current, which varies sufficiently in magnitude, can stimulate a motor nerve and so produces contraction of the muscles to which it supplies. Suitable current can also stimulate denervated muscle. Intermittent DCs are used in these cases, which ranges from 0.01 to 3 ms. The equipment commonly provides duration of 0.01, 0.03, 0.1, 0.3, 1, 3, 10, 30, 100 and 300 ms.

In an AC, the flow of electrons constantly changes direction, or stated differently, reverses its polarity. Electrons flowing in an AC always move from the negative to positive pole, reversing direction, when polarity, if reversed **(Figs. 3.5B and C)**.

Evenly Alternating Currents

Sinusoidal currents: Sinusoidal currents are evenly alternating sine wave currents of 50 Hz. This gives 100 pulses or phases in each second of 10 ms each, 50 in one direction and 50 in another **(Fig. 3.6)**.

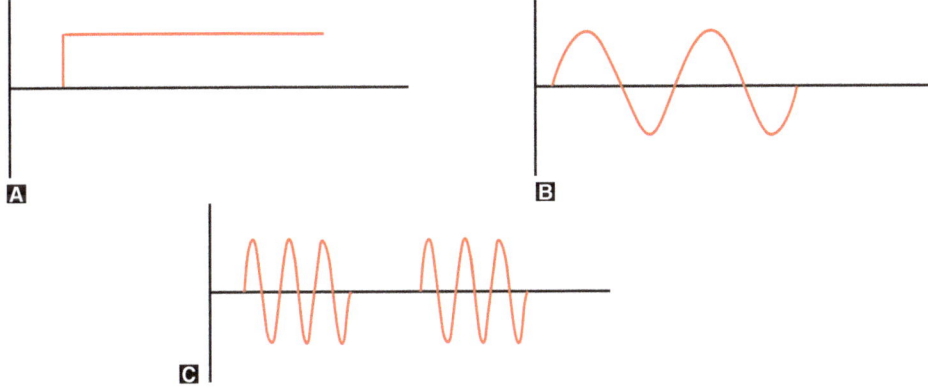

Figs. 3.5A to C: (A) Direct monophasic current; (B) Alternating biphasic current; (C) Pulsed polyphasic current.

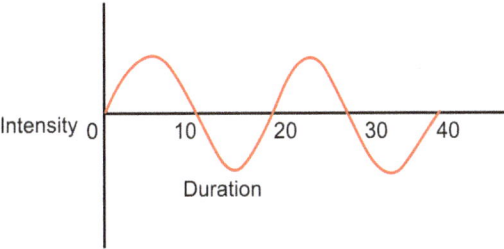

Fig. 3.6: Sinusoidal current.

It is produced from the mains by reducing the voltage to 60–80 V with a step-down transformer. It is usually surged to cause rhythmical muscle contractions. It relieves pain and reduces edema.

Because of marked sensory stimulation this current is often applied to large areas and rarely used for local muscle stimulation.

Diadynamic currents: Introduced by Pierre Bernard nearly 70 years ago, they are sinusoidal, DCs being rectified mains type currents with frequency of 50–100 Hz. There are six different types of currents, which are each used for different purposes:

1. The *MF (monophase)* is a half-sinusoidal AC, which is created by a one-way DC converter of 50 Hz, with an impulse length and interruption of 10 ms each. The primary effect of this type of current is muscle stimulation **(Fig. 3.7A)**.
2. The *DF (diphase)* type of current is created by an AC of 50 Hz by means of a two-way DC converter, so that a current of 100 Hz is achieved. The patient feels a stabbing sensation in the treated area. The stimulus is less than that of the MF and primarily affects the autonomic nervous system in the sense of lowering the increased sympathetic tone **(Fig. 3.7B)**.
3. The *short-period (SP) current* involves a sudden alternation of MF and DF currents. The patient senses the abrupt change between the tensing MF current and relaxing DF current **(Fig. 3.7C)**.
4. In the *long-period (LP) current*, the MF current is mixed with a second modulated MF. The gradual raising and lowering of the amplitude is experienced by the patient as a more pleasant sensation than that produced by SP **(Fig. 3.7D)**.
5. In the *syncopated rhythm (RS)* the current is interrupted by a pause of 0.9 second after a current flow of 1.1 second. This type of current is used for the electrical stimulus of the muscles **(Fig. 3.7E)**.
6. The *modulated monophase (MM)* current not listed by Bernard is a logical extension of his currents. In the MM the RS is gradually reduced in stepwise fashion. Like the RS, the MM is suited for the treatment of muscular atrophies, but the faradic excitability of the particular muscles must be maintained **(Fig. 3.7F)**.

The therapeutic effects of the diadynamic currents have been researched and established in numerous studies (Bernard).

Therapeutic Effects (Rennie, 1988)

- Pain relief
- Decrease inflammation and swelling
- Muscle reeducation
- Increase local circulation
- Facilitation of tissue healing

Interrupted Galvanic Current

It is called as long duration current having duration of more than 1 ms up to 300 or 600 ms. Interruption is the most usual modification of DC, the flow of current commencing and ceasing at regular intervals. The rise and fall of intensity may be sudden and may be of rectangular, sawtooth, triangular and trapezoidal type **(Fig. 3.8)**.

Chapter 3: Low Frequency Currents

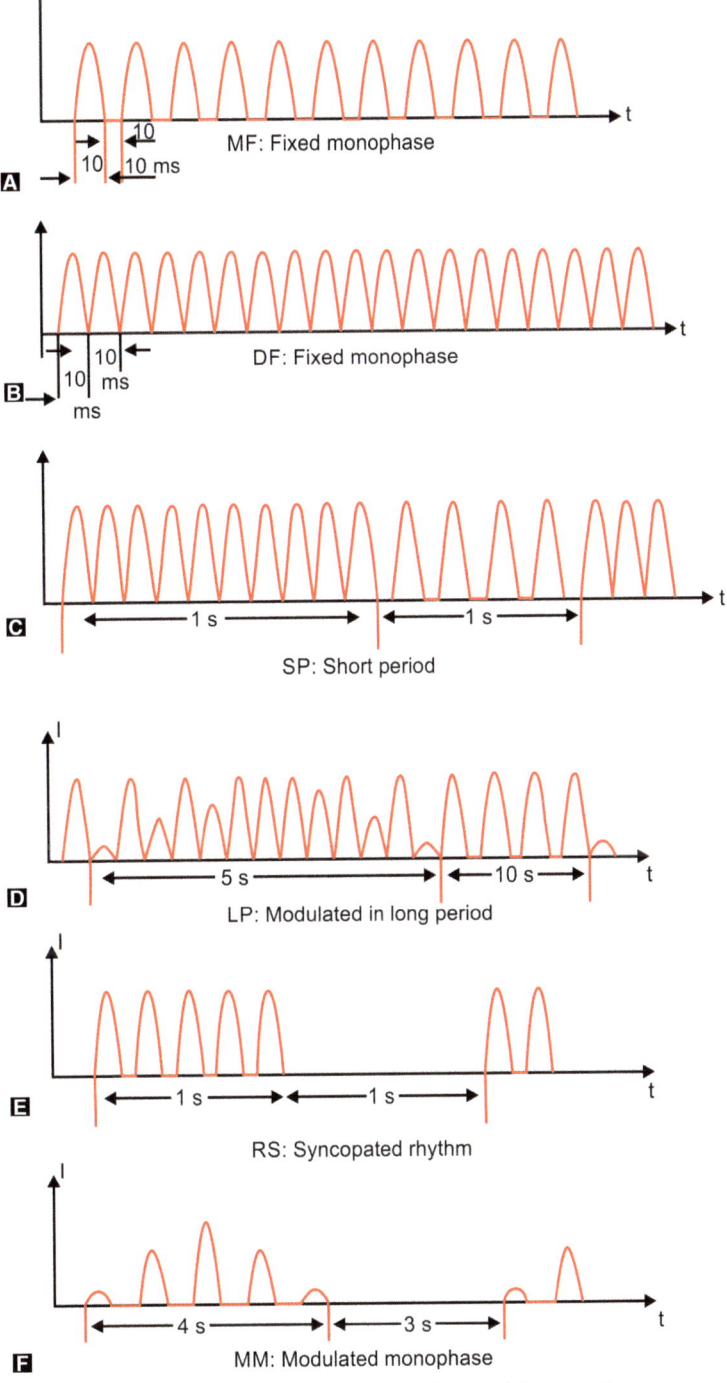

Figs. 3.7A to F: Modulations of various phases of diadynamic currents.

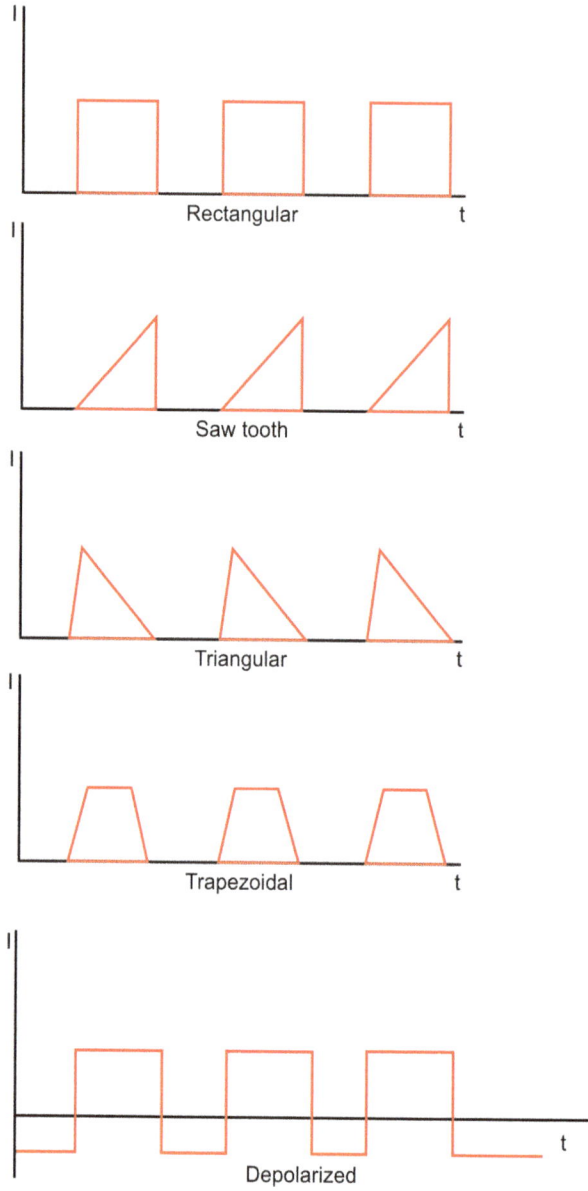

Fig. 3.8: Modified direct current impulses.

The impulse in which the current rises gradually are often termed "selective" because a contraction of denervated muscle can often be produced with an intensity of current that is insufficient to stimulate the motor nerve. This occurs due to accommodation. It is often found that the more long-standing the denervation, the slower the rise in intensity of current that is required.

An impulse of 100 ms duration is often used which requires frequency of 30 Hz. But as you increase the duration, frequency must be reduced.

To eliminate the danger of chemical burn reverse wave of current, i.e., depolarized impulses should be used, which also reduces the skin irritation.

Production of interrupted DC is usually accomplished in modern apparatus by circuits, which employ transistors and timing devices. Current is always applied to the patient via potentiometer as this allows the intensity of current to be turned up from zero.

NERVE TRANSMISSION

In normal nerve, there is difference of concentration of ions inside and outside the nerve. Due to this there is difference of potential called as potential difference (PD) between inside and outside of the nerve.

Nerve remains in two states:
1. Resting state
2. Stimulated state

In resting state, the nerve is *positive outside* and *negative inside* (**Fig. 3.9**). At this time, the nerve is not permeable to Na$^+$ ions, so it is called as polarized state of nerve.

When a nerve is stimulated, it causes fall in PD. When the fall reaches to a certain level, it provides the permeability of sodium ions. This permeability causes the difference in concentration of ions inside and outside the nerve and thus further fall of PD until reversal of polarity occurs. Now the membrane is positive inside and negative outside (**Fig. 3.10**).

Immediately after this activity the Na$^+$ ions are pumped again and the stimulated part again comes to resting state.

Now the difference between the active and resting part of the nerve causes the local electron flow between the active and resting part of the nerve. The direction of electron flow through the membrane is opposite to the PD across the fiber.

The fiber acts as a resistance to current so that current flow lowers the PD, this again make the membrane permeable to Na$^+$ ions and cause the reversal of PD as before. These changes of PD are then propagated along the length of nerve fiber. This change of polarized stage causes the travel of impulse.

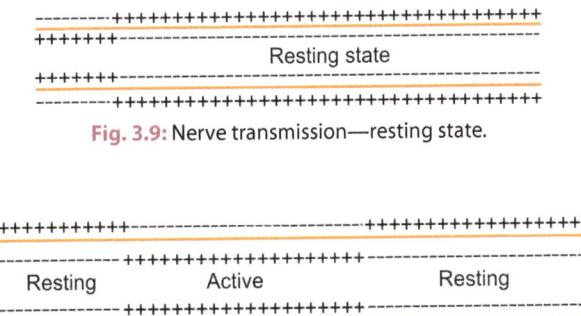

Fig. 3.9: Nerve transmission—resting state.

Fig. 3.10: Nerve transmission—stimulated state.

Electrical Stimulation of Nerves

To initiate the nerve impulse, varying current of adequate intensity must be applied. PD is being formed when current flows in plasma membrane of nerve fibers and resistance lies in series with other tissues. The membrane nearer to cathode will be negative and is denoted by "n", whereas, surface nearer to anode will be positive and is denoted as "p" (**Fig. 3.11**).

Increase in PD occurs on the nerves nearer to anode, whereas the PD decreases in the membrane nearer to the cathode because of opposite polarity.

When the membrane becomes permeable to Na^+ ions by fall in PD to a certain level, then the ions enter the axon and initiate the nerve impulse.

When cathode is applied to superficial nerve then nearest side will get activated but the anode can only initiate the nerve impulse. Therefore, further aspect of anode is activated. Due to this, the density of current is less in further aspect of nerve fiber than near one. So for initiating impulse cathode is more effective than anode. In some apparatus, polarity of terminals is marked which is beneficial for high peak of current for effective stimulus. To get contraction of innervated muscle in less current, cathode should be connected to active electrode.

Accommodation

When a constant current flows, the nerve adapts itself. This phenomenon is known as *accommodation*.

Effect of Frequency of Stimulation

The muscle responds with a large contraction and then rotates to its resting state. It is called twitch contraction. When single stimulus is applied per second then there is contraction followed by immediate relaxation. Increase in the frequency of stimuli up to 20 Hz shortens the period of relaxation.

If stimuli are given more than 20 Hz then there is no time for complete relaxation between the contraction and another impulse. At more than 60 Hz, there is no relaxation at all and current flows smoothly leading to tetanic contraction.

Strength of Contraction

It depends on:
* Quantity of motor nerve activated
* Rate of change of current

If intensity of current rises suddenly, less intensity is required for muscle contraction as there is no time for accommodation but if current rises slowly greater intensity is required as in trapezoidal, triangular current, etc.

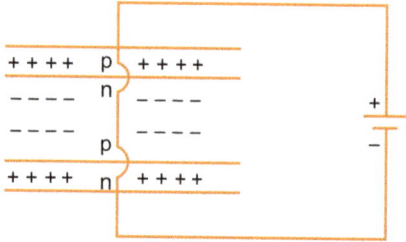

Fig. 3.11: Potential difference across a nerve fiber.

Pathological Changes in Peripheral Nerve

Peripheral nerves may be damaged by injury or disease in many different ways and the nerve fiber is affected in following ways:
- It can be stopped over a small section of the nerve fiber a local block, so that conduction above and below is normal (in neuropraxia).
- It can be slowed which is usually due to the myelin sheath being affected.
- It can be stopped over a small section of the nerve fiber, a local block. It can be stopped over the whole distal length of nerve from site of injury to the skin and muscle, as in neurotmesis and axonotmesis or damage to nerve cell.

Seddon's Classification

Neuropraxia

Temporary mild compression of the nerve will lead to a conduction block called as *neuropraxia*. It causes displacement of the myelin sheath and local edema of the nerve fiber. The damage is not so severe to cause degeneration of the fiber. As there is no permanent damage so recovery occurs rapidly in a few days or weeks. Since only a section of a nerve fiber is affected, conduction beyond the blockage is normal, thus electrical stimulation of motor nerve fiber beyond the block will cause muscle contraction. Electrical stimulation applied proximal to the block does not result in muscle contraction.

Axonotmesis

More severe compression injury may cause sufficient damage to the nerve axon. This is called *axonotmesis*. Degeneration of the axon takes place including the myelin sheath. Example of this type of lesion is—radial nerve palsy in fractured shaft of humerus. Once the nerve fiber has degenerated, alteration in electrical reaction occurs.

Neurotmesis

Instead of compression if the injury is such as to disrupt all tissues of the nerve fiber such as a cut through the nerve, then the distal segment will degenerate completely. Since the tissue is totally disrupted the axon filament will not readily find correct channels down to regrow, so that recovery is at best imperfect. This is called as *neurotmesis*. Such lesion often requires surgery to ensure that the two cut ends are sufficiently approximated to allow successful growth.

Process of Denervation

Severe injury to the nerve causes damage to the nerve axon so that it is unable to support the metabolic process of its distal part resulting in degeneration of the whole length of the new fiber including the myelin sheath distal to the lesion. This process is called *Wallerian degeneration*. It takes as long as 14 days to degenerate. The distal section of nerve remains excitable and can conduct impulse before degeneration has taken place.

Because of this it may not be possible to make full assessment of the lesion till 3 weeks, after suspected nerve injury.

Regeneration of Nerve

In axonotmesis, the fibrous framework of the bundle of nerve fibers remain intact and fills a chain of Schwann cells so that ultimately nerve fibrils sprouting from the intact proximal part of the nerves are guided in their proper channels to reform the complete nerve process.

The duration needed for full recovery will depend on the site of the lesion and the length of nerve that has to regrow. The rate of regrowth is somewhat variable, being more rapid at first, up to 5 mm per day, but is usually considered to be an average 1-2 mm per day.

When there is degeneration of the nerve fiber the normal response is reduced or lost and the changes become evident 3 or 4 days after injury. Changes in the reaction obtained on stimulation over the muscle, may be observed before the end of 1st week.

WAVEFORMS

The term waveform means the graphical representation of the direction, shape, amplitude, duration and pulse frequency of the electrical current produced by the electrotherapeutic device. The instrument which is used to display the electric current is called an oscilloscope.

Pulses, Phases and Direction of Current Flow

The individual waveform as shown by an oscilloscope is referred to as a *pulse*. A pulse may contain either one or two *phases* (**Fig. 3.12**). It rises above or goes below the baseline for some specific period of time. DC also referred to as monophasic current, produces waveforms that have only a single phase in each pulse. Current flow is unidirectional, always flowing in the same direction toward either the positive or negative pole. Conversely, AC, also referred to as biphasic current, produces waveforms that have two separate phases during each individual pulse. Current flow is bidirectional, reversing direction or polarity once during each pulse.

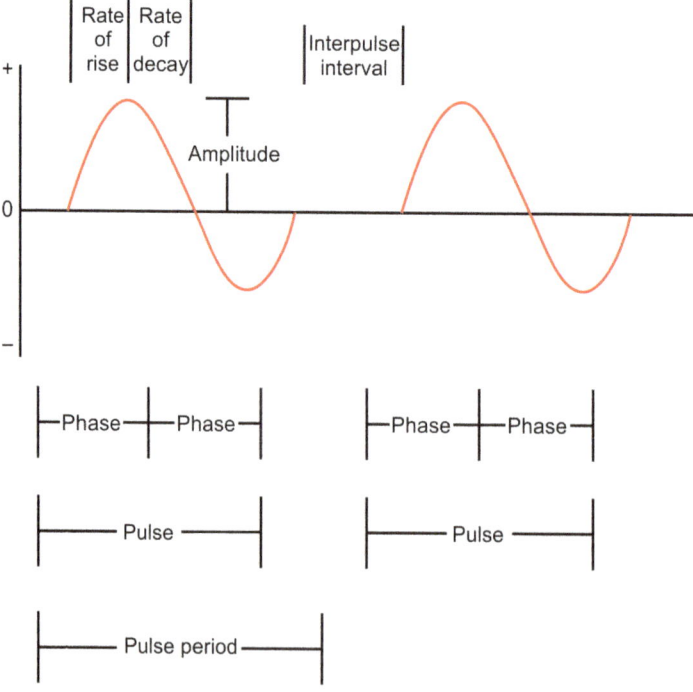

Fig. 3.12: Waveform—biphasic pulse.

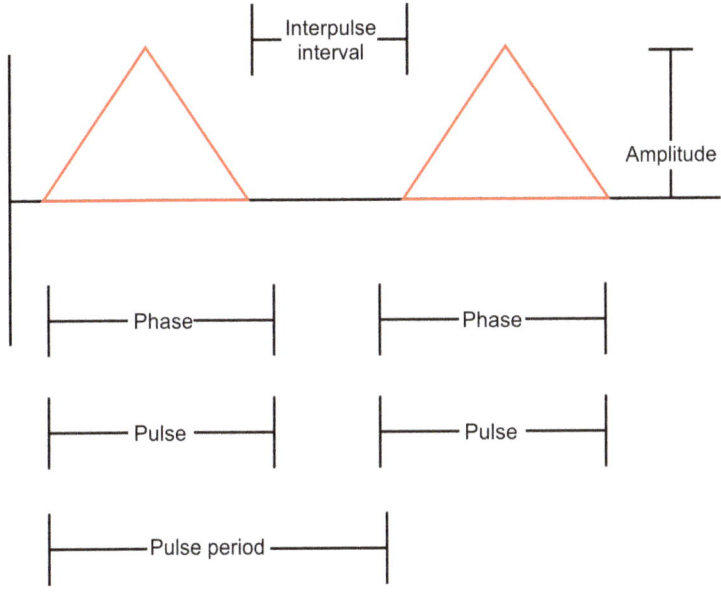

Fig. 3.13: Waveform—monophasic pulse.

Biphasic waveforms may be symmetrical or asymmetrical. If both phases of the waveform may be symmetrical, the shape and size of each phase is identical **(Fig. 3.13)**. Pulsed current waveforms are called polyphasic currents and are representative of electrical current that is conducted as a series of pulses of short duration followed by a SP of time, when current is not flowing called the *interpulse interval*. Single current may flow in one direction as in DC or may reverse direction of flow as in AC. With pulsed currents, there is always some interruption of current flow.

Waveform Shape

It could be of any type like sine, rectangular, or triangular waveform depending on the capabilities of the generator producing the current. Alternating, direct and pulsed currents may be of the following waveform shapes as shown in **Figure 3.14**.

Pulse Amplitude

The maximum amplitude of a pulse can be shown by the tip of highest point of each phase. The amplitude of each pulse reflects the intensity of the current. The term amplitude is synonymous with the terms voltage and current intensity. The higher the amplitude, the greater is the voltage or intensity.

The total current cannot be confused with the tip of highest point of a phase. The total current delivered to the tissues can only be calculated by averaging the current flowing per unit time including the interpulse intervals. The electrical generators that produce short duration pulses, the total current produces (coulomb/s) is low compared to peak current amplitudes due to long interpulse intervals. Thus, the average current or the amount of current flowing per unit of time is relatively low. Average current can be increased by either increasing pulse duration, increasing pulse frequency, or by some combination of the two.

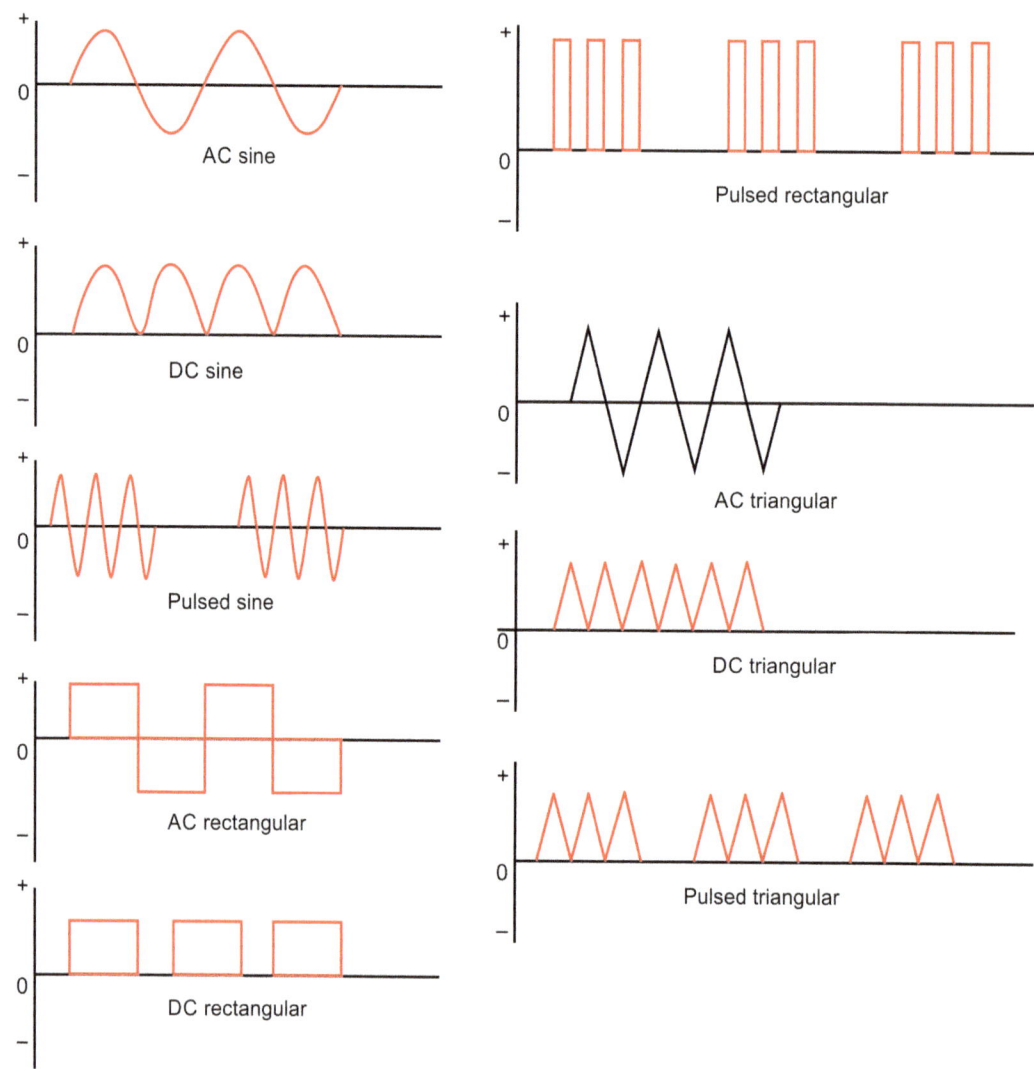

Fig. 3.14: Waveform shapes.

Pulse Charge

The term pulse charge indicates the total amount of electricity that is delivered to the patient during each pulse. In monophasic currents, the phase charge and the pulse charge are the same and are greater than zero. With biphasic currents the pulse charge is equal to the algebraic sum of the phase charges. If the pulse is symmetrical the net pulse charge is zero. In asymmetrical pulses, the net pulse charge cannot be zero.

Rise and Decay Time

The rate of rise in amplitude or the rise time indicates the time taken by a pulse to reach its maximum amplitude in each phase. Conversely, decay time refers to the time taken by a pulse to return to neutral. The rate of rise is important therapeutically so as to avoid accommodation of the nerves to the constant amplitude current, which results in constant level of depolarization and nerves become unexcitable at that same intensity or amplitude. Rate of rise and decay times are generally short, ranging from nanosecond to millisecond.

By observing the three different waveforms, it is apparent that the sine wave has a gradual increase and decrease in amplitude for both alternating and DCs. The rectangular wave has an almost instantaneous increase in amplitude, which plateaus for a period of time and then abruptly falls off. The shape of these waveforms as they reach their maximum amplitude or intensity is directly related to the excitability of the nervous tissue. The more rapid the increase in amplitude or the rate of rise, the greater the current's ability is to excite nervous tissue.

Most modern DC generators make use of a twin-peak triangular pulse of very short duration and peak amplitudes as high as 500 V. Combining high-peak intensity with a short-phase duration produces a very comfortable type of current as well as an effective means of stimulating sensory, motor and pain fibers.

Asymmetric Waveforms

The use of asymmetrical waveforms for therapeutic purposes is now of the past. The true faradic waveform is also no longer being used. The so-called true faradic current is like a biphasic pulsed current with asymmetric waveform. The original faradic current is like an AC because there was always a reversal of direction of current flow. The amplitude of the portion of the wave in the negative direction was not great enough to produce any physiologic response.

In the monophasic saw-tooth or exponential waveform the amplitude rises very gradually and then falls abruptly. Current that uses this waveform stimulates denervated muscle without affecting normally innervated muscle, since the gradual rise in amplitude allows for accommodation of the normal muscle.

Exponential Current

The basic phenomenon is to rise the current impulses gradually. When represented graphically, these impulses display a similarity to a triangle, which is why this form of current is called triangular current. As the current does not increase in a straight line, but rather in accordance with a mathematical exponential equation, the current is also called *exponential current*.

Pulse Duration

The length of time that current is flowing in one cycle indicates duration of each pulse. With monophasic current the phase duration is the same as the pulse duration. It is the time from initiation of the phase to its end. With biphasic current the pulse duration is determined by the combined phase durations. In some devices, it is prefixed and in some the uses can alter it. The phase duration as well as pulse duration may be as short as few microseconds or may be a long duration DC that flows for several minutes.

In pulsed currents and also in some cases with alternating and DCs, the current flow can be off for some period of time. The combined time of the pulse duration and the rest duration or interpulse interval is known to as the pulse period.

Pulse Frequency

Pulse frequency is the number of pulses per second. Each individual pulse either rises or falls from its base value. As the frequency of any waveform is increased, the amplitude tends to increase and decrease more rapidly. The muscular and nervous system responses depend on the length of time between pulses and on how the pulses or waveforms are modulated. Muscle will respond with individual twitch contraction to pulse rates of less than 50 pulses per second. At 50 pulses per second or greater, a tetany will result, regardless of whether the current is biphasic, monophasic, or polyphasic.

CURRENT MODULATION

The current modulation is an important phenomenon because the physiologic response to the various waveforms depends largely on *current modulation*. Modulation refers to any alteration in the magnitude or any variation in duration of these pulses. Modulation may be continuous, interrupted, burst, or ramped. According to various treatment goals the parameters of current modulation must be established.

Continuous Modulation

Continuous modulation means that the amplitude of current flow remains the same for several seconds or minutes. Continuous modulation is usually associated with long-pulse duration DC **(Fig. 3.15A)**. With DC, flow is always in a uniform direction. The positive and negative accumulation of charged ions over a period of time creates either an acidic or alkaline environment that may be of therapeutic value. This therapeutic technique has been referred to as medical galvanism. The technique of iontophoresis also uses continuous DC to drive ions into the tissues. If the amplitude is great enough to produce a muscle contraction, the contraction will occur only when the current flow is turned on or off. Thus with DC continuous modulation, there will be a muscle contraction both when the current is turned on and when it is turned off. Continuous modulation is also used with AC primarily to elicit muscle contractions.

Interrupted Modulation

In interrupted modulation, current flows for some period of time called the on-time, and is then periodically turned off during the off-time. On-time and off-time can be prefixed in some devices or can be altered by the operator. Interrupted modulation is used with monophasic as well as for biphasic currents. Currents with sine, rectangular, or triangular-shaped waveforms may be interrupted. Interrupted modulation is used clinically for muscle reeducation and strengthening and for improving range of motion **(Fig. 3.15B)**.

Burst Modulation

Burst modulation occurs when pulsed current flows for a short duration and then is turned off for a short duration and in a repetitive cycle. With polyphasic current, sets of pulses are combined. These combined pulses are most commonly referred to as bursts. These are also called pulse packets, envelopes, pulse trains, or beats **(Fig. 3.15C)**. The interruptions between individual bursts are called interburst intervals. The interburst interval may be too short to have any effect on a muscle contraction. Thus, the physiologic effects of a burst of pulses will be the same as with a single pulse. Bursts may be used with monophasic and biphasic currents as well.

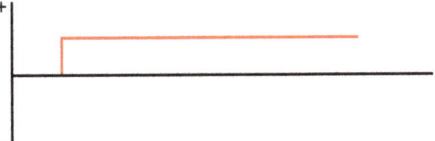

Fig. 3.15A: Continuous modulation.

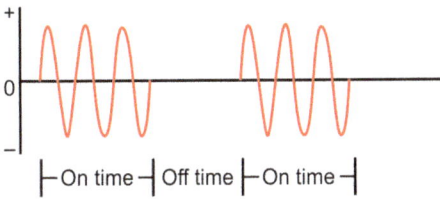

Fig. 3.15B: Interrupted modulation.

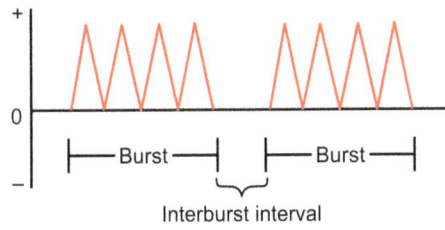

Fig. 3.15C: Burst modulation.

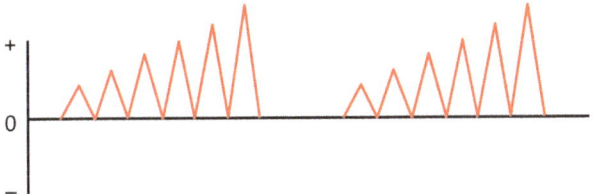

Fig. 3.15D: Ramping modulation.

Ramping Modulation

In ramping modulation which is also called sometimes as surging modulation, current amplitude increases gradually or decreases gradually in its intensity. It is also called ramping- up or ramping-down of current modulation **(Fig. 3.15D)**. Ramp-up time is usually preset at about one-third of the on-time. The ramp-down option is not available on all machines. This type of modulation gives the patient a very comfortable feeling because of the very gradual rise of intensity of the current. Ramping modulation is used clinically to elicit muscle contraction and is generally considered to be a very comfortable type of current.

INDICATIONS FOR THE USE OF LOW FREQUENCY CURRENTS

- *Facilitation or initiation of the muscle action:* When the patient is unable to produce muscle contraction or finds it difficult to do so, electrical stimulation may be required in assisting to produce voluntary contraction. In cases of pain, electrical stimulation of motor neurons reduces the inhibition, which acts on larger anterior horn cells, so as to facilitate the transmission of voluntary impulses to the muscles and helps in inducing relaxation to its antagonists.

  Initially treatment should be given in pain-free range so that no movement causing pain is produced. Patient is advised to produce voluntary contraction along with the electrical stimulation. The amount of voluntary contraction is increased gradually and electrical stimulation is reduced until the muscles produce full voluntary contraction.

- *Reeducation or relearning of muscle action:* According to Beavor's theory, the brain appreciates movements and not individual muscle action. In some situations where muscle is not under voluntary control reeducation or relearning of muscle action is required. These situations could be:
  - Prolonged disuse
  - Incorrect use

  In these circumstances faradic stimulation may be used to produce contraction and thus help to restore the sense of movement.

  Due to prolonged disuse person is not able to contract muscle voluntarily as in cases of long-standing flat foot, reeducation of intrinsic muscles of foot is done by faradic stimulation.

  In cases where person is using incorrect pattern of movement, correct pattern is taught by faradic stimulation, e.g., stimulation of abductor hallucis muscle in hallux valgus.

  Active contractions should be attempted at the same time along with the electrical stimulation.

- *Training/teaching of a new muscle action:* For training or teaching a new muscle action faradic current is used. The cases where teaching a new muscle action is required, could be:
  - Tendon transplantation surgery
  - Reconstructive operations

  In tendon transplantation and reconstructive operations a muscle is required to perform a different or new action from which it was previously doing. For this, faradic type current is required and muscle is stimulated in a new pattern. During this treatment the patient must concentrate on a new movement and try to assist it along with voluntary contractions.

- *Loosening and prevention of adhesion:* Effusions in the tissues when stays there form adhesion. Adhesions are formed where there is no proper muscle contraction. If adequate active exercise is not possible, electrical stimulation in the form of faradic current may be used to prevent adhesions. Muscle contraction loosens and stretches the adhesions, which have already formed.

- *Improvement in venous and lymphatic drainage:* Alternative contraction and relaxation of muscles produces pumping action, which leads to venous and lymphatic drainage. Effect of faradic current for improving venous and lymphatic drainage is described as *faradism under pressure,* this is a very effective treatment of edema and gravitational ulcer.

- *Maintaining or increasing in range of movement:* The movement may be limited by shortening of different tissues and from different causes. Faradic stimulation of muscle to stretch the shortened tissue is used in:

- *Contracture of fibrous tissue and scaring:* Limitation of joint movement due to shortening of soft tissue on one side of the joint has been treated by electrical stimulation of the muscle that stretches the contracture.
- *Deformities like scoliosis:* In scoliosis lateral trunk muscles on the convexity of the curve are stimulated electrically. Electrodes are placed at the patient's back and muscle contraction is obtained by stimulating the muscles in order to reduce convexity.
- *Neuropraxia of a motor nerve:* In neuropraxia, the impulses from brain are not able to reach up to the muscles supplied by affected nerve through site of lesion. In neuropraxia, there is no degeneration of nerve so if we stimulate the nerve below site of lesion, the impulses will easily pass to the muscle and cause the contraction. Electrical stimulation is not usually necessary in neuropraxia because recovery takes place with any marked changes in the muscle tissue.
- *Severed motor nerve:* When any nerve is damaged severely there occurs degeneration of axons. Degeneration takes several days to complete, and for a few days after the injury a muscle contraction may be obtained by faradic type current. But after degeneration, muscles can be stimulated by interrupted DC or modified DC.
- *For replacing orthosis:* Low frequency stimulation may be used to enhance the function of a paralyzed or weak muscles thus eliminating the need for a splint or brace or orthosis.
- *Stimulation of denervated muscle:* For stimulation of denervated muscle, interrupted DC or galvanic current is used which directly stimulate the muscle fiber. In denervated muscle there occurs wasting and then fibrosis. Muscle looses its property of contractility, excitability, elasticity and irritability. By electrical stimulation the process of muscle wasting slows down, but it needs strong electrical impulses for this purpose. Approximately 300 contractions per session are required, but this also is not always practically possible due to muscle fatigue. So for treatment to be effective at least 90 contractions need to be performed in a session. If fatigue occurs soon, number of contractions may be reduced and treatment time prolonged.

PHYSIOLOGICAL EFFECTS OF LOW FREQUENCY CURRENTS

- *Effect on body tissues:* Tissues contain fluids, which contain ions and thus are good conductor of electricity. Current passing through the body tissues consists a two-way migration of ions and the conductivity of different body tissues varies according to the amount of fluid they contain. Muscle is having good blood supply and so is a good conductor while fat is a poor conductor. The epidermis has a high resistance and thus is a bad conductor. So for having better conduction of electricity, we use some media like water or gel to lower the resistance for treatment purposes.
- Stimulation of sensory nerves:
  - *Faradic current:* When applying a faradic type current mild prickling sensation is felt due to stimulation of sensory nerves. This stimulation is not very marked because the stimuli are of fairly short duration.
  - *Interrupted galvanic current:* This also stimulates sensory nerves and results in stabbing or burning sensation. This stimulation is very marked because the stimuli are long-duration impulses.

  When sensory nerve is stimulated either by faradic or interrupted galvanic current, it also produces reflex vasodilatation of superficial blood vessels. So slight erythema is seen, this vasodilatation is limited up to superficial area only.

- *Stimulation of motor nerves by faradic current:* Faradic current stimulates the motor nerves and if it is of sufficient intensity, it stimulates muscle to which the nerve supplies. The contraction produced is thus a *tetanic contraction* because stimuli are repeated 50 times per second. This type of contraction if maintained for a longer period may result in muscle fatigue. So to avoid this, current is commonly *surged* to allow muscle relaxation. When the current is surged the contraction gradually increases and decreases in strength, in a manner similar to a voluntary contraction.
  - *By galvanic current:* If we stimulate motor nerve with interrupted galvanic current it also produces muscle contraction but because of frequent repeated stimuli it produces muscle twitch followed by immediate relaxation. Effect of this type of current is thus less beneficial on the muscles.
- *Effect on muscle contraction:* Electrical stimulation of motor nerves causes muscle contraction and results in changes similar to those associated with voluntary contraction. These contractions help in regaining the *properties of muscles* as such and also helps in:
  - *Increasing metabolism:* The contraction and relaxation of muscles results in pumping action on the blood vessels within the muscles and around it.
    This pumping action provides more blood supply to the muscles and also results in increased demand and supply of oxygen and nutrition.
  - *Removal of waste products:* If the muscle contraction and relaxation is sufficient enough to cause pumping effect on venous and lymphatic vessels it results in removal of waste products.
- *Stimulation of denervated muscle:* For contraction of denervated muscle the impulse more than 1 ms is required. This impulse is usually not tolerable by the patient for treatment purposes. Thus faradic type current is not used for stimulation of denervated muscle. Interrupted DC is used for stimulation of denervated muscle therapeutically, when it is of sufficient intensity and duration. Effective contraction is obtained only when current rises slowly rather than rising suddenly. An impulse of 100 ms is the shortest impulse for satisfactory treatment of denervated muscle. So, intensity and duration of the impulse are important factors for stimulation of denervated muscle.
- *Chemical effects following stimulation:* Chemical effects are produced at the electrodes due to passing of DC through the electrolyte. It results in formation and accumulation of chemicals at the electrode site resulting in chemical or electrolytic burn. The risk is comparatively less with an intermittent current than with a DC. When an alternative current is used, chemicals formed during one phase are neutralized during the next phase as the ions move one way during one phase and in reverse direction during the other phase. In a condition, where the two phases are equal, chemicals formed during one phase are neutralized during the next phase.

METHODS OF TREATMENT

TREATMENT OF PATIENT'S CONDITION
- Median nerve stimulation
- Ulnar nerve stimulation
- Radial nerve stimulation

Chapter 3: Low Frequency Currents

- Erb's paralysis
- Facial nerve stimulation
- Deltoid inhibition
- Quadriceps inhibition
- Lateral popliteal nerve stimulation
- Faradism under pressure
- Faradic foot bath
- *Common motor points*

PROFORMA FOR PATIENT'S ASSESSMENT

- *Receiving the patient:* Good morning, I am a physiotherapist and I am going to treat you. Please, cooperate with me during the treatment and wait until I go through your case sheet.
- *History taking or going through the case sheet:*
  - Name
  - Father's and mother's name
  - Age
  - Sex
  - Occupation
  - *Address:* Correspondence and permanent
- *Chief complaints:*
  - History of present illness
  - History of past illness
  - Family history
  - Social and occupational history
  - Treatment history
  - Prognosis of the treatment
  - *Investigations:*
    - Hematological tests
    - Radiological tests: X-rays, magnetic resonance imaging (MRI) scan, etc.
    - Others
- *Checking for general contraindications:*
  - Hyperpyrexia/Fever
  - Hypertension
  - Anemia
  - Severe renal and cardiac failure
  - Deep X-ray and cobalt therapy
  - Epileptic patients
  - Noncooperative patients
  - Mentally retarded patients
  - Very poor general condition of the patient, etc.
- *Checking for local contraindications:*
  - Open wounds
  - Very recent fractures
  - Skin grafts
  - Severe edema

- Hairy surface
- Acute inflammation
- Metal in the part
- Malignant growth
- Hypersensitive skin
- Loss of sensation, etc.

❖ *Preparation of trays:*
- Skin resistance lowering tray
- Treatment tray

Skin Resistance Lowering Tray

❖ Saline water
❖ Soap
❖ Cotton
❖ Vaseline
❖ Towels, etc.

Treatment Tray

❖ Mackintosh
❖ Lint pads
❖ Pad or plate electrodes and pen electrode
❖ Leads
❖ Straps
❖ Cotton
❖ Powder
❖ Gel, etc.

Preparation of Treatment Tray

❖ *Mackintosh:* The Mackintosh is to be kept under the patient's treatment part to prevent earth shock and to prevent dripping of water.
❖ *Lint pad:* The lint pad is made up of lint cloth and it is used to prevent accumulation of chemicals in the tissues formed during the treatment which if not prevented leads to burn. It must be in 8 or 16 layers. More the layers of lint pad, less the chance of accumulation of chemicals, less the chance of burn.

 To stimulate more number of motor points, two different electrodes covered with lint pads are used. If stimulation of individual muscle is required, pen electrode is used (active) **(Fig. 3.16)**.

 Always to use indifferent pad proximally (nerve trunk or plexus) and active pad distally (individual muscle).
- *Active pad:* It is the place where the electrons enter the circuit. It is smaller than the indifferent pad always. It should be placed on the motor point distally (pen electrode).
- *Indifferent pad:* It is the place where electrons leave the circuit. It is placed proximally. This helps to complete the circuit.

❖ *Electrodes:* It could be of pad or plate type or pen type. Pad or plate electrodes are kept in between the lint pads for even distribution of current. The edges of plate electrode should

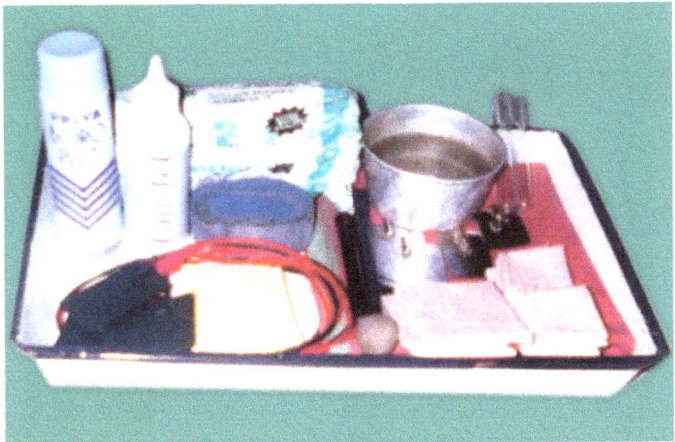

Fig. 3.16: Treatment tray.

be blunt. It should be smaller than the lint pad so that it cannot come in contact with the skin. Pen electrode is used for smaller muscles or for specific motor points.
- *Leads:* Used to connect the electrodes with the stimulator.
- *Straps:* Usually rubber straps are used. It should be placed over the pad. It should be fixed with the help of jaconet piece.
- *Cotton:* Used to prevent dripping of water and for cleaning the surface.
- *Powder:* Used to apply over the skin if there is any redness after the treatment. Redness occurs due to erythema. It gives soothing effect.
- *Gel:* Used for pad electrodes where lint pads are not used. Gel is used for proper contact of electrodes with the patient's surface.

Preparation of Skin Resistance Lowering Tray

- *Saline water:* Prepared by adding the pinch of salt to the bowl of water. The aim of preparing saline water is to prepare more ions so that minimum amount of current that is enough to get the brisk contraction. If we use more than 1% saline there will be lowering of ions and less amount of current passes since there will be restriction of ions.
- *Soap:* It is used for cleaning the part to be treated to remove dirt, dust or sebum, etc. thus lowering the skin resistance **(Fig. 3.17)**.
- *Cotton:* It is used for cleaning the surface.
- *Vaseline:* It is applied over scar tissue. It prevents the concentration of more current on the scar tissue.
- *Towels: They* are used for covering the body part. Neat and clean towels should be used every time.
- *Lowering skin resistance:* By removing dust particles, sebum or sweat, skin resistance can be lowered. In the presence of all these dust particles, sebum or sweat greater intensity of current is required to get the contraction. It provides some resistance to the passage of current.
- *Preparation of apparatus:*
  - Check whether all the knobs are at zero.
  - Checking the pins of the plug and check whether the switch is turned off.

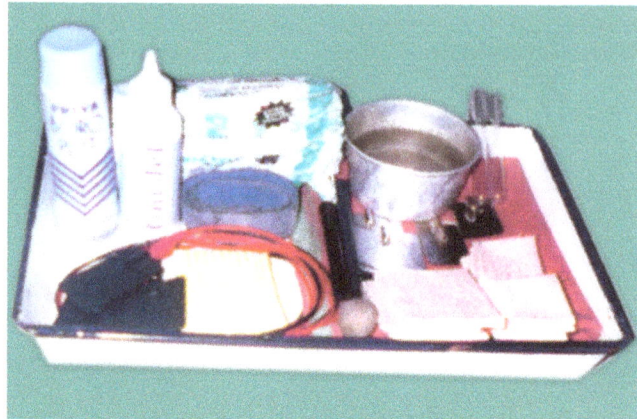

Fig. 3.17: Skin resistance lowering tray.

- Check the insulation of the wire.
- Check whether the switch in the stimulator is working.
- Check whether fuse is present in the apparatus; see that it is not blown out.
- Check whether hand switch for patients use is intact and is working.

❖ *Correct positioning of the patient:*
  - Position the patient in such a way that it is comfortable to the patient.
  - Part to be treated must be exposed and should be at adequate distance from the modality.

❖ *Correct positioning of physiotherapist:*
  - Position of physiotherapist should also be comfortable so that he/she may not get tired after the treatment.
  - Position should be such that it provides maximum accessibility to the treatment part and to the modality.

❖ *Checking of apparatus:* Self test to be done.
  - Apparatus must be checked once in front of the patient.
  - Place the electrodes on yourself on palmar or dorsal aspect of hand or forearm.
  - Switch "on" the apparatus and gradually increase the current.
  - Explain the patient the feel of the current.
  - This will increase the confidence of the patient and will reduce its apprehension.

❖ Correct placing of pads and electrodes.

❖ *Instructions to the patient:* I am going to start the treatment.
  - Be relaxed
  - Do not touch anything around you
  - Do not pull the leads
  - Do not touch the walls or ground
  - If you feel uneasy switch off from the patients switch

❖ *Regulating the current:*
  - Gradually increase the current.
  - Keep talking with the patient about the feel of the current.
  - Tell him to inform you immediately about any inconvenience, discomfort or burning.

- *Palpating tendon:* Feel the contraction by palpating the tendon.
- *Selection of current:*
  - Faradic current
  - Galvanic current
  - Other
- Selection of pulse, frequency, duration and treatment time
- Treatment
- *Explanation to the patient:*
  - Explain the patient the advantages of the treatment.
  - Explain the patient the course or duration of the treatment.
  - Explain the patient the do's and don'ts in home and otherwise.

MEDIAN NERVE STIMULATION

- *Receiving the patient:* Good morning, I am a physiotherapist and going to treat you. Please, cooperate with me during the treatment and wait until I go through your case sheet.
- *History taking or going through the case sheet:*
  - Name
  - Father's and mother's name
  - Age
  - Sex
  - Occupation
  - *Address:* Correspondence and permanent.
- *Chief complaints:*
  - History
  - History of any previous treatment taken.
- *Examination:* To the examiner
  - *Side:* Right or left
  - Site
- *Checking for any general and local contraindications:*
  - Fever
  - Hypertension
  - General condition of the body
  - Open wound
  - Hypersensitive skin
  - Metal in the tissue or in surrounding area
  - Loss of sensation, etc.
- *Course of nerve:* The median nerve arises in the axilla from the medial and lateral cords of brachial plexus with root values C5, C6, C7, C8 and T1. It supplies the following muscles:
  - Pronator teres
  - Flexor carpi radialis
  - Palmaris longus
  - Flexor digitorum superficialis
  - Flexor digitorum profundus
  - Flexor pollicis longus (FPL)
  - Pronator quadratus

- Abductor pollicis
- Flexor pollicis
- Opponens pollicis
- First and second lumbricals

It runs down in front of the elbow and supplies muscular branches in the forearm and enters the palm deep to the flexor retinaculum of the wrist. Its main sensory supply is to thumb, index, middle and radial half of ring finger.

Indications

- ❖ *Injury at the level of elbow:*
  - *Cause:*
    - Supracondylar fracture
    - Dislocation of elbow joint
  - *Clinical features:* All the muscles are paralyzed supplied by the nerve.
- ❖ *Injury at the wrist level:*
  - *Cause:*
    - Glass cut injury.
    - *Carpal tunnel:*
      - Dislocated lunate bone
      - Chronic compression by swelling in the tunnel
      - Compound palmar ganglion
      - *Clinical features:* Hand muscles supplied by the nerve are paralyzed.
- ❖ *Deformity:*
  - *Pointing index finger:* Because of paralysis of long flexor tendons of index finger.
  - Simian hand or ape thumb deformity—Opponens and short flexor paralysis.
  - Inability of flex the interphalangeal (IP) of thumb due to paralysis of FPL.
  - *Opponens palsy:* To oppose thumb to touch tip of other fingers.
  - Paralysis of abductor pollicis brevis.
  - *Sensory signs:* Loss of sensation in the thumb, index, middle and radial half of ring finger.
- ❖ *Treatment:*
  - Preparation of trays
  - Preparation of apparatus
  - *Position of the patient:* The patient is made to sit in a wooden chair, provided with backrest, he places his hand on the table with arms abducted and forearm supinated and elbow semiextended.
  - *Position of therapist:* Walk standing
  - Checking of local contraindications
  - Reducing skin resistance
  - Checking apparatus (self test)
  - *Correct placing of pads:*
    - For forearm muscles:
      - *Inactive:* Over medial epicondyle of humerus
      - *Active:* Over the motor point.
    - For hand muscles:
      - *Inactive:* Over wrist
      - *Active:* Over the motor point **(Fig. 3.18)**.

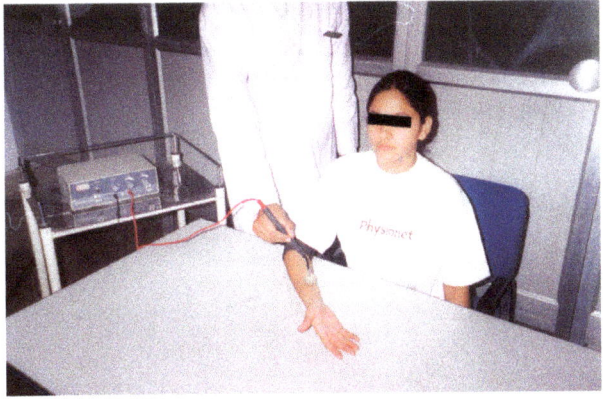

Fig. 3.18: Median nerve stimulation.

- ❖ *Instructions to the patient*:
  - Feel of current
  - Instruction to the patient to inform if any burning
  - *Warning:* Not to touch anything.
- ❖ Regulating current
- ❖ *Palpating tendon:* Feel the contraction by palpating the tendon.
  - Gradually increasing the current.
  - Keep talking with the patient about the feel of the current.
- ❖ *Home programs:*
  - Grasping and squeezing a rubber ball
  - Closing the hand then opening gently
  - Touching the tip of each finger in turn with tip of thumb making O's
  - Touching the 2nd phalanx of each finger with tip of thumb
  - Piano playing movements of fingers with hand halfway between pronation and supination
  - Abduction of wrist hand on block fingers flexed over edge push away weight by abducting hand.
  - Wrist machine for supination and pronation when strong enough.

Picking up and putting down small objects, balls, dice, marbles, coins held by fingers, also exercises with sand tray.

ULNAR NERVE STIMULATION

- ❖ *Receiving the patient:* Good morning, I am a physiotherapist and going to treat you. Please, cooperate with me during the treatment and wait until I go through your case sheet.
- ❖ *History taking or going through the case sheet:*
  - Name
  - Father's and mother's name
  - Age
  - Sex
  - Occupation
  - *Address:* Correspondence and permanent

- ❖ *Chief complaints*:
    - History
    - History of any previous treatment taken.
- ❖ *Examination:* To the examiner
    - *Side:* Right or left
    - Site
- ❖ *Checking for any general and local contraindications*:
    - Fever
    - Hypertension
    - General condition of the body
    - Open wound
    - Hypersensitive skin
    - Metal in the tissue or in surrounding area
    - Loss of sensation, etc.
- ❖ *Indications of treatment*:
    - *Injury at the level of elbow region:*
        - Traction injury resulting from violent valgus stress to the elbow
        - Avulsion fracture of medial epicondyle
        - Dislocation of elbow
        - Supracondylar fracture of humerus
        - Tardy or late ulnar neuritis—caused by increasing valgus deformity due to nonunion of the fracture of lateral condyle of humerus.
    - *Injury at the level of wrist:* The ulnar nerve arises in the axilla from the medial cord of brachial plexus with root values C7, C8, T1. It runs along the medial epicondyle of humerus at the elbow to enter the forearm. It enters the palm by passing in front of the flexor retinaculum through a fibrous canal. It supplies the following muscles of the forearm and the intrinsic muscles of hand:
        - Flexor carpi ulnaris
        - Flexor digitorum profundus
        - Adductor pollicis
        - Flexor pollicis brevis
        - First dorsal interosseous
        - First palmar interosseous
        - Abductor digiti minimi
        - Flexor digiti minimi
        - Opponens digiti minimi
        - Third and fourth lumbricals
- ❖ *Clinical features*:
    - All the muscles are paralyzed. When there is injury at the elbow—typical ulnar claw hand of ring and little fingers, wasting of hypothenar muscles and depression in the interosseous spaces in dorsal aspect of the hand. Adduction of thumb is not possible.
    - *Sensory loss:* Confined to the little finger and medial half of the ring finger and the ulnar border of the hand.
    - *Injury at wrist:* Flexor carpi ulnaris, flexor digitorum profundus usually escapes **(Fig. 3.19)**.
- ❖ Preparation of trays
- ❖ Preparation of apparatus

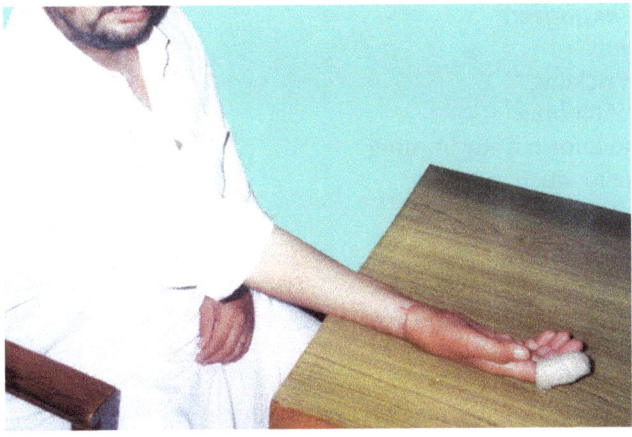

Fig. 3.19: Patient with ulnar nerve injury.

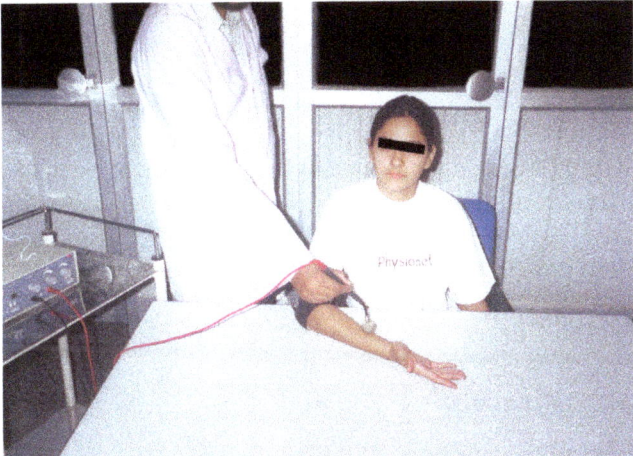

Fig. 3.20: Ulnar nerve stimulation.

- *Positioning of patient:* The patient is made to sit in a wooden chair, provided with backrest, he places his hand on the table with arms abducted and forearm supinated and elbows semiextended **(Fig. 3.20)**.
- *Position of physiotherapist:* Walk standing by the side of the patient.
- Reducing skin resistance
- *Treatment:*
    - Checking of apparatus
    - Correct placing of pads and electrodes.
    - *For stimulating forearm muscles:*
        - *Inactive electrode:* Over wrist/over carpal bones
        - *Active electrode:* Over the motor point.
    - *For adductor pollicis and interossei:* Stimulate on the dorsum of hand.
        - *Neuropraxia:* Above the site of lesion
        - *Axonotmesis/Neurotmesis:* Below the site of lesion.

- *Instructions to the patient:*
  - *Feel of current:*
    - *Faradic:* Prickling
    - *Galvanic:* Stabbing.
  - Instruction to inform if any burning
  - *Warning:* Not to touch anything
  - Regulating current
  - Palpating tendon
  - Winding up. Check the treated area after treatment
  - *Other special points:* Comfort of the patient.
- *Selection of current:*
  - *Neuropraxia:* Surged faradic
  - *Axonotmesis/Neurotmesis:* Interrupted galvanic current.
- Reason for procedure.
- *Home programs:*
  - Finger parting and closing (hand in supination table).
  - Grasping a sheet of paper with both hand between thumb and its finger keeping metacarpophalangeal (MCP) flexed and IP extended.
  - *Adult:* Finger tips and thumb of both hands placed together, fingers slightly abducted and thumb between abduction and adduction, bring the four finger tips close together flexing the MCP and bring thumb tip into contact with index finger exercises.
  - Finger stretching, hands pronated on table, fingers flexed, stretch each finger forward in turn.
  - Hands side by side on table supinated approximation in succession tips of two little finger, two ring, two middle and two index.
  - Place index and little finger in front of middle and ring fingers.

RADIAL NERVE STIMULATION

- *Receiving the patient:* Good morning, I am a physiotherapist and going to treat you. Please, cooperate with me during the treatment and wait until I go through your case sheet.
- *History taking or going through the case sheet:*
  - Name
  - Father's and mother's name
  - Age
  - Sex
  - Occupation
  - *Address:* Correspondence and permanent
- *Chief complaints:*
  - History
  - History of any previous treatment taken.
- *Examination:* To the examiner
  - *Side:* Right or left
  - Site
- *Duration:*
  - Within 21 days FG test
  - After 21 days standard deviation (SD) curve

- ❖ *Checking for any general and local contraindications:*
  - Fever
  - Hypertension
  - General condition of the body
  - Open wound
  - Hypersensitive skin
  - Metal in the tissue or in surrounding area
  - Loss of sensation
- ❖ *Knowledge of anatomy:*
  - *Course of nerve:* Radial nerve is formed from the posterior cord of brachial plexus in the axilla with root values C5, C6, C7, C8 and T1. It winds around the mid shaft of humerus in the spiral groove and give the posterior interosseous nerve just above the elbow and continues as the superficial branch of radial nerve.
    It supplies:
    - Triceps
    - Anconeus
    - Brachioradialis
    - Extensor carpi radialis brevis
    - Extensor carpi radialis longus
    - Extensor carpi ulnaris
    - Extensor digitorum
    - Supinator
    - Extensor digiti minimi
    - Abductor pollicis longus
    - Extensor pollicis brevis
    - Extensor pollicis longus
    - Extensor indicis.
    - *Level of lesion:*
    - *Axilla:* Old type of crutch with T type support at the top—injury at this level all the muscles are paralyzed.
    - Humerus—Saturday night palsy or drunkard palsy Tourniquet palsy—compression of blood vessels and nerves Chemical neuritis (postinjection palsy).
  - *Elbow:*
    - Supracondylar fracture
    - Dislocation of head of radius
    - Surgical excision of the head of radius (accidentally).
- ❖ *Clinical features:*
  - *Motor:*
    - Wrist drop depending upon the level
    - Finger drop of injury
    - Thumb drop
    - *Paralysis at axilla:* Active extension at the elbow is also affected with all the earlier.

Sensory: Small area in the dorsum of the hand over the metacarpal bones of the thumb and index finger.
- ❖ *Preparation of trays:*
  - Skin resistance lowering tray
  - Treatment tray

- Preparation of apparatus.
- *Position of the patient:*
  - The patient is made to sit in a wooden chair, provided with backrest; he places the hand on the table with arms abducted and elbows flexed to a 90°. The wrist is supported with a pad to:
    - Keep the wrist in normal functional position
    - Prevent over stretching of paralyzed muscle
    - Eliminate gravity.
- *Position of the physiotherapist:* Walk/stride standing position by the side of the patient
- *Checking for local contraindications:* Reducing skin resistance.
- *Treatment:*
  - Checking of apparatus
  - *Placement of electrodes:*
    - *Inactive:* Radial groove
    - *Active:* Over the motor points.
  - *Neuropraxia:*
    - *Indifferent electrode:* Just above the site of lesion
    - *Active electrode:* Over the motor point.
  - *Axonotmesis/Neurotmesis:*
    - *Indifferent electrode:* Just below the site of lesion
    - *Active electrode:* Over the motor point.
- *Selection of current:*
  - *Neuropraxia:* Surged faradic current
  - *Axonotmesis/Neurotmesis:* Interrupted galvanic current 10-30 contraction.
- *Instructions to the patient:*
  - *Feel of current:*
    - *Faradic current:* Prickling sensation
    - *Galvanic current:* Stabbing sensation.
  - Inform if any burning sensation
  - *Warning:* Not to touch anything.
- Regulating current
- Palpating tendon
- Winding up
- *Other special points:* Comfort and consideration.
- *Splint:* Dynamic cock up splint.
- *Home programs:*
  - *Active assisted exercise:* With the other hand wrist extension is done.
  - Grasp and squeeze tennis ball.
  - *Five finger exercise:* Hand pronated to the table, finger flexed and raise each finger separately and later altogether.
  - Finger parting and closing.

ERB'S PARALYSIS

- *Receiving the patient:* Good morning, I am a physiotherapist and going to treat you. Please, cooperate with me during the treatment and wait until I go through your case sheet.
- *History taking or going through the case sheet:*
    - Name
    - Father's and mother's name
    - Age
    - Sex
    - Occupation
    - *Address:* Correspondence and permanent
- *Chief complaints:*
    - History
    - History of any previous treatment taken.
- *Examination:* To the examiner
    - *Side:* Right or left
    - Site
- *Checking for any general and local contraindications:*
    - Fever
    - Hypertension
    - General condition of the body
    - Open wound
    - Hypersensitive skin
    - Metal in the tissue or in surrounding
    - Loss of sensation, etc.
- *Knowledge of anatomy:* When there is injury at the level of Erb's point C5, C6 it causes paralysis of the deltoid, supraspinatus, infraspinatus, biceps and brachialis muscle. The arms hang by the side with shoulder in internal rotation, elbow in extension and the forearm pronated with the palm facing backwards, the so called "policeman tip" position. The hand and finger functions are preserved.
    - *Causes:*
        - Breech delivery
        - Undue separation of the head of the humerus.
- Preparation of trays.
- Preparation of apparatus.
- *Correct positioning of the patient:*
    - *Child:* Sitting position with arm slightly abducted and forearm supinated
    - *Infant:* On the mother's lap resting on a pillow.
- Correct position of physiotherapist.
- Checking of apparatus (self test)
- *Treatment:*
    - *Placement of electrodes:*
        - Child:
          Inactive: Over the nape of the neck
          Active: Over the motor point.

The inactive pad electrode can be tied on the dorsum of the physiotherapist's hand.
- *Selection of current:* Surged faradic or interrupted galvanic current is used.
- Explaining feel and purpose
- *Instructions to the patient:*
  - Inform if any burning
  - Not to touch anything.
- Regulating current
- Palpating tendon
- *Winding up:* Check the treatment area.
- *Home program:*
  - Exercises taught to the mother (abduction of the shoulder external rotation of the shoulder)
  - *Splint:* Aeroplane splint can be used.

FACIAL NERVE STIMULATION

- *Receiving the patient:* Good morning, I am a physiotherapist and going to treat you. Please, cooperate with me during the treatment and wait until I go through your case sheet.
- *History taking or going through the case sheet:*
  - Name
  - Father's and mother's name
  - Age
  - Sex
  - Occupation
  - *Address:* Correspondence and permanent.
- *Chief complaints:*
  - History
  - History of any previous treatment taken.
- *Examination:* To the examiner
  - *Side:* Right or left
  - Site
- *Checking for any general and local contraindications:*
  - Fever
  - Hypertension
  - General condition of the body
  - Open wound
  - Hypersensitive skin
  - Metal in the tissue or in surrounding area
  - Loss of sensation, etc.
- *Knowledge of anatomy:*
  - *Bell's palsy:* This is the lower motor neuron lesion of the facial nerve and resultant paralysis of the muscles that it supplies.
  - *Course of the nerve:* It starts from seventh cranial nerve nucleus. It is situated in the ventral part of tegmentum of pons, rounds VI nucleus along its course expands to form geniculate

ganglion, it gives a branch to stapedius muscle, a branch supplying anterior two-thirds of tongue. Emerging from stylomastoid foramen it enters the parotid gland and divides into:
- Temporal
- Zygomatic
- Mandibular
- Buccal
- Cervical branches.
- *Muscles supplied:*
  - Occipitofrontalis
  - Orbicularis oculi
  - Corrugator and procerus
  - Zygomaticus major and minor
  - Levator anguli oris
  - Levator labii superioris
  - Buccinator
  - Orbicularis oris
  - Risorius
  - Mentalis
  - Depressor anguli oris
  - Depressor labii inferioris.
- ❖ *Causes:*
  - Idiopathic
  - Exposure to chill weather
  - Fracture of mandible
  - Fracture of mastoid process
  - Dislocation of temporomandibular joint
  - Middle ear infection
  - Anesthesia during middle ear surgery
  - Trauma to jaw, parotid region
  - Cerebellopontine angle tumors
  - Hemorrhage at the site of the nucleus of the nerve.
- ❖ *Clinical features:*
  - Bell's phenomenon
  - Loss of facial expression.
- ❖ Receiving the patient.
- ❖ Knowing details of condition.
- ❖ Preparation of trays.
- ❖ Preparation of apparatus.
- ❖ *Preparation and position of the patient:* Supine lying position with the hair duly tied up **(Fig. 3.21)** and eyes closed, ask the patient to wash his face before treatment.
- ❖ *Position of therapist:* Stride/walk standing position at the side of the patient.
- ❖ *Checking for local contraindications:*
  - Acne
  - Tooth clips
  - Eye infections

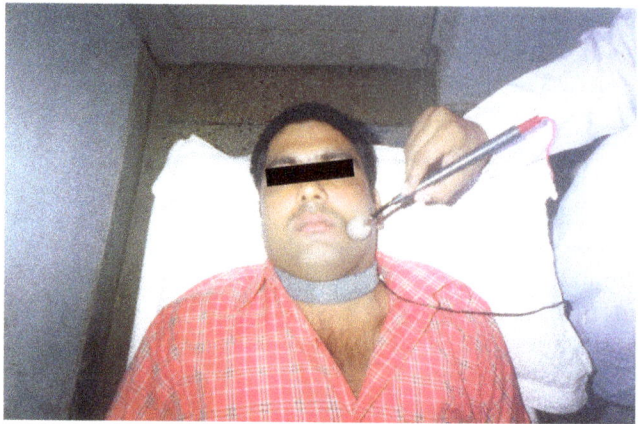

Fig. 3.21: Facial nerve stimulation.

- Hairy surface
- Mouth ulcers
- Mumps, measles, etc.
❖ Checking of apparatus.
❖ *Correct placing of electrodes:*
  - *Inactive:* Over the nape of neck
  - *Active:* Over the motor point.
❖ *Instructions to the patient:*
  - Feel of current
  - Inform if any burning
  - *Warning:* Not to touch anything.
❖ *Treatment:*
  - *Selection of current:*
    ♦ *For the muscles:* Interrupted galvanic
    ♦ *For the nerve trunk:* Surged faradic.
❖ Regulating current
❖ Winding up
❖ *Home programs:*
  - Look surprised and then "frown".
  - Smile, grin, say "O"
  - Say a, e, i, o, u
  - Squeeze eyes closed then make wide open
  - Hold straw in mouth, suck and blow
  - Whistle
  - *Advice:*
    ♦ Avoid intake of cold substances
    ♦ Cover up the head and face with a scarf
    ♦ Avoid taking in hot substances when there is sensory loss in anterior two-thirds of tongue.

Chapter 3: Low Frequency Currents

DELTOID INHIBITION

- *Receiving the patient:* Good morning, I am a physiotherapist and going to treat you. Please, cooperate with me during the treatment and wait until I go through your case sheet.
- *History taking or going through the case sheet:*
  - Name
  - Father's and mother's name
  - Age
  - Sex
  - Occupation
  - *Address:* Correspondence and permanent.
- *Chief complaints:*
  - History
  - History of any previous treatment taken.
- *Examination:* To the examiner
  - *Side:* Right or left
  - Site
- *Checking for any general and local contraindications:*
  - Fever
  - Hypertension
  - General condition of the body
  - Open wound
  - Hypersensitive skin
  - Metal in the tissue or in surrounding
  - Loss of sensation, etc.
- *Condition:* Due to fear of pain, the patient keeps the deltoid muscle in contracted position. Abduction and flexion of shoulder are limited.
- *Causes:*
  - Fracture shaft of humerus
  - Traumatic synovitis
  - Any soft tissue injury around the shoulder joint
  - Dislocation of shoulder, etc.

  Deltoid is supplied by axillary or circumflex nerve (root value C5).
- Preparation of trays.
- Preparation of the apparatus.
- *Position of the patient:* The patient sitting in a chair with back support, the arm support.
- *Position of therapist:* Stand by the side of the patient.
- *Checking of local contraindications:* Reducing skin resistance.
- Checking of apparatus (self test).
- *Placement of electrodes:*
  - *Inactive:* Nape of neck (pad electrode)
  - *Active:* Anterior, middle or posterior fibers of deltoid (pen electrode).
- *Selection of current:* Surged faradic current.

- *Instructions to the patient:*
  - To inform any burning
  - *Warning:* Not to touch anything.
- Regulating current
- Winding up
- Check the treatment area after treatment.

Faradic current is selected as it has the property of reeducation of muscles.

QUADRICEPS INHIBITION

- *Receiving the patient:* Good morning, I am a physiotherapist and going to treat you. Please, cooperate with me during the treatment and wait until I go through your case sheet.
- *History taking or going through the case sheet:*
  - Name
  - Father's and mother's name
  - Age
  - Sex
  - Occupation
  - *Address:* Correspondence and permanent.
- *Chief complaints:*
  - History
  - History of any previous treatment taken.
- *Examination:* To the examiner
  - *Side:* Right or left
  - Site
- *Checking for any general and local contraindications:*
  - Fever
  - Hypertension
  - General condition of the body
  - Open wound
  - Hypersensitive skin
  - Metal in the tissue or in surrounding area
  - Loss of sensation, etc.
- *Condition:* Due to fear of pain the patient cannot contract the quadriceps. He holds the muscle in a tensed position; extension of knee is limited.
- *Causes:*
  - Fracture shaft of femur
  - Meniscectomy
  - Traumatic synovitis of knee
  - Surgical intervention
  - Soft tissue injury around the knee
  - Postoperative, (i.e.,) after arthroscopy.
- Preparation of trays (two pad electrodes).
- Preparation of apparatus.
- *Position of the patient:* Half lying position.

The knee is flexed 20-30°. The patient should be able to watch the contraction, the knee is supported by placing a pillow.
- *Position of therapist:* Stride standing by the side of the patient.
- Checking the local contraindications.
- Checking of apparatus.
- Correct placing of pads and electrodes:
  - *(Pad) in different:* Upper one-third of thigh (femoral triangle)
  - *(Pad) active:* Kept over the lower part of thigh (so that it cover all the motor points of quadriceps).
  - *By using two pen electrodes:*
    - Vastus medialis and vastus lateralis
    - Vastus lateralis and rectus femoris
    - Vastus medialis and rectus femoris
- *Selection of current:* Surged faradism, duration—10 minutes.
- *Instructions to the patient:*
  - Explaining the feel and purpose
  - Instruction to inform any burning
  - *Warning:* Not to touch anything.
- Regulating current
- Winding up
- Check the treatment area. If erythema—apply powder.

Surged faradic current is used; as the muscle is innervated and as the faradic current is helpful in the reeducation of muscle.

LATERAL POPLITEAL NERVE INJURY

- *Receiving the patient:* Good morning, I am a physiotherapist and going to treat you. Please, cooperate with me during the treatment and wait until I go through your case sheet.
- *History taking or going through the case sheet:*
  - Name
  - Father's and mother's name
  - Age
  - Sex
  - Occupation
  - *Address:* Correspondence and permanent
- *Chief complaints:*
  - History
  - History of any previous treatment taken.
- *Examination*: To the examiner
  - *Side:* Right or left
  - Site
- *Checking for any general and local contraindications:*
  - Fever
  - Hypertension
  - General condition of the body

- Open wound
- Hypersensitive skin
- Metal in the tissue or in surrounding
- Loss of sensation, etc.

❖ *Course of nerve:* The lateral popliteal nerve arises at the upper part of the popliteal fossa as the lateral division of sciatic nerve. It winds around the neck of the fibula to enter the leg. It divides into two branches:
  i. The superficial branch supplies:
     ◆ Peroneus longus
     ◆ Peroneus brevis.
  ii. The deep branch supplies:
     ◆ Tibialis anterior
     ◆ Extensor hallucis longus
     ◆ Extensor digitorum longus
     ◆ Extensor digitorum brevis.

❖ *Causes of injury:*
  - Cuts and lacerations over the neck of fibula.
  - Fracture neck of fibula associated with fracture lateral tibial condyle as in abduction injuries to the knee.
  - Traction injury due to adduction violence of knee associated with medial tibial condyle fracture.

❖ *Clinical features*:
  - Foot drop
  - Loss of sensation in the outer aspect of the leg and dorsum of the foot.

❖ Preparation of trays.
❖ Preparation of apparatus.
❖ *Position of patient:* Half lying position with pillow under the leg and sand bag placed under the foot.
❖ *Position of therapist:* Walk standing/stride standing.
❖ Checking of apparatus.
❖ *Placement of pads:*
  - *Inactive:* Neck of fibula
  - *Active:* Over the motor point.
❖ *Instructions to the patient:*
  - Explaining the feel and purpose.
  - Instruction to inform if any burning.
  - *Warning:* Not to touch anything.
❖ Regulating current
❖ Palpating tendon
❖ Winding up
❖ *Home programs:*
  - Foot drop splint to be used.
  - Placing the foot over edge of plinth, dorsiflexion and plantar flexion is advised.
  - Also in sitting legs crossed dorsiflexion and plantar is advised.

FARADISM UNDER PRESSURE

- *Receiving the patient:* Good morning, I am a physiotherapist and going to treat you. Please, cooperate with me during the treatment and wait until I go through your case sheet.
- *History taking or going through the case sheet:*
  - Name
  - Father's and mother's name
  - Age
  - Sex
  - Occupation
  - *Address:* Correspondence and permanent
- *Chief complaints*:
  - History
  - History of any previous treatment taken.
- *Examination:* To the examiner
  - *Side:* Right or left
  - Site
- *Checking for any general and local contraindications*:
  - Fever
  - Hypertension
  - General condition of the body
  - Open wound
  - Hypersensitive skin
  - Metal in the tissue or in surrounding area
  - Loss of sensation, etc.
- *Purpose:* Electrical stimulation of the muscles that generally acts as the muscle pump may be combined with compression and elevation of the limb to increase venous and lymphatic return and so relieve edema, especially when treated with faradic type current.
- *Indications*:
  - Soft tissue injury of the extremities
  - Gravitational edema
  - Lymphedema
  - Postphlebitic syndrome
  - Varicose ulcers, etc.
- Preparation of trays (include crepe bandage).
- Preparation of apparatus.
- *Position of the patient*:
  - *Upper limb:* The patient is made to sit in a chair with support, the arm is slightly abducted and forearm supinated with palm facing upwards. The whole limb should be placed in elevation. So that gravity assists the venous and lymphatic return.
- *Position of the therapist*:
  - By the side of the patient walk/stride standing.
  - Checking of local contraindications.
  - Reducing skin resistance.
- Checking of apparatus (self-test).

- *Placement of pads and electrodes:*
  - *Upper limb:* Flexor aspects of arm and forearm.
  - *Lower limb:*
    - *Active electrode over:* Calf muscles
    - *Inactive electrode over:* Neck of fibula.
  - Fix the pads in position firmly, with straps, if necessary test the contraction produced. Adjust the pads as necessary. Then apply an elastic bandage, starting distally. It should be firm but not too tight, avoid gaps between the turns of the bandage.
- *Instructions to the patient:*
  - Explaining feel and purpose.
  - Instruction to inform if any burning.
  - *Warning:* Not to touch anything.
- *Selection of current:* Surged faradic current as it helps in increasing the venous and lymphatic return.
- Regulating current
- Winding up
- Checking the treatment part

FARADIC FOOT BATH

- *Receiving the patient:* Good morning, I am a physiotherapist and going to treat you. Please, cooperate with me during the treatment and wait until I go through your case sheet.
- *History taking or going through the case sheet:*
  - Name
  - Father's and mother's name
  - Age
  - Sex
  - Occupation
  - *Address:* Correspondence and permanent.
- *Chief complaints:*
  - *History of illness:* Present or past
  - History of any previous treatment taken.
- *Examination:* To the examiner
  - *Side:* Right or left
  - Site.
- *Checking for any general and local contraindications:*
  - Fever
  - Hypertension
  - General condition of the body
  - Open wound
  - Hypersensitive skin
  - Metal in the tissue or in surrounding area
  - Loss of sensation, etc.

Also,
- Infection of nails
- Recent metatarsal fracture
- Eczema or fungal infection
- Crack foot
- Open-unhealed wounds.

❖ *Indications*:
- Flatfoot (pes planus)
- Chronic retrocalcaneal bursitis
- March fracture
- Pott's fracture
- Metatarsalgia
- Plantar fasciitis
- Plantar digital neuritis
- Calcaneal spur
- Sudeck's atrophy
- Hallux valgus
- Hallux rigidus
- Osteochondritis
- Rheumatoid arthritis of foot
- Poor musculature of arch of foot.

❖ *Preparation of trays:* Only treatment tray, skin resistance lowering tray is not needed. Patient should be asked to wash his foot before the treatment.

❖ *Treatment tray*:
- Lint pads
- Mackintosh
- Tray with saline/tap water
- Straps
- Pad electrode and pen electrode
- Leads
- Vaseline
- Salt
- Therapeutic electrical stimulator
- Wooden footstool

❖ Preparation of apparatus.

❖ *Positioning of the patient:* Patient sitting over the wooden stool. Foot is placed in treatment tray kept over the spread Mackintosh. Hip and knee are flexed to about 90°. Patient is asked to hold hip knee firmly to maintain contact by using body weight. Place the foot in a bath containing enough warm water to cover the toes **(Fig. 3.22)**.

❖ *Position of physiotherapist:* The physiotherapist should position himself in such a way that she/he does not get entangled and he must be free to reach the patient and machine. Sitting on stool and treating the patient is ideal. Sit on the stool in front of patient at the controls of the machine and at the same time observe the muscle contraction.

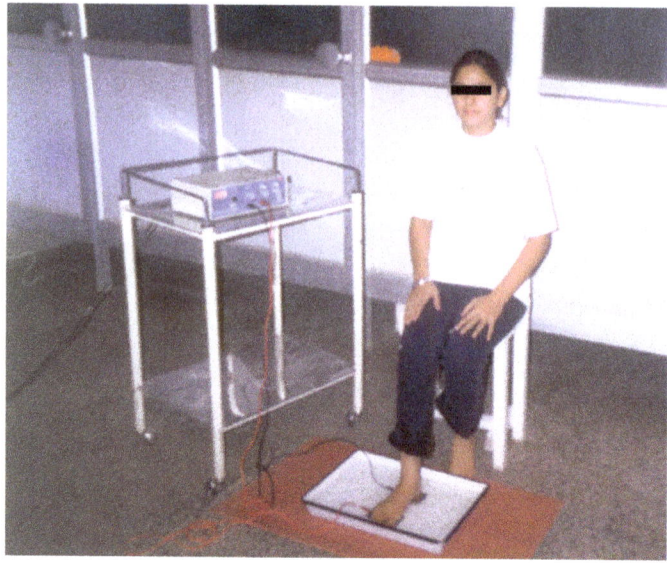

Fig. 3.22: Faradic foot bath.

- ❖ *Checking of apparatus:* Self-test to be done under water.
- ❖ *Correct placing of pads and electrode*:
  - *Lumbricals:* Two electrodes placed transversely across the bottom of the bath, one under the heel and other obliquely under the metatarsal heads.
  - *Plantar interossei:* Place one electrode on each side of the foot at the level of metatarsal heads
  - Abductor hallucis longus.
- ❖ *Instruction to the patient:*
  - *Warning:* Do not touch anything.
- ❖ *Current used:* Faradic current
  - *Feel:* Prickling sensation
  - *Purpose:* The muscles are innervated and one of the therapeutic effects of faradic current is reeducation of the muscle action.
- ❖ Regulating current.
- ❖ *Palpating tendon:* Abductor hallucis is palpable.
- ❖ Check the treatment part after treatment.
- ❖ *Home programs*:
  - Walking on medial and lateral border of foot
  - MCR slipper to be worn
  - Walking on beach, pebble board
  - Rolling the towel with toes
  - Spreading of toes
  - Picking up of marbles with toes.

Chapter 3: Low Frequency Currents

Common Motor Points (Figs. 3.23 to 3.28)

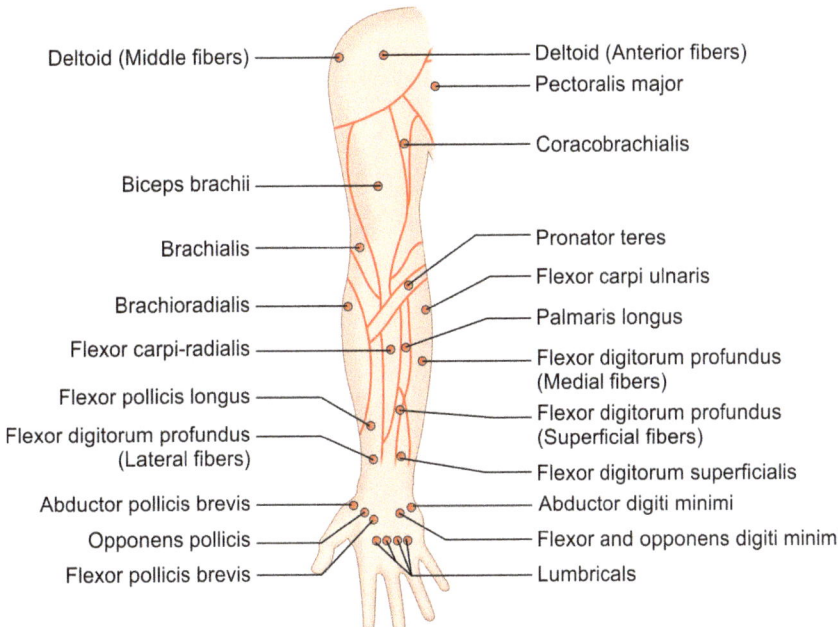

Fig. 3.23: Motor points of the anterior aspect of the right arm.

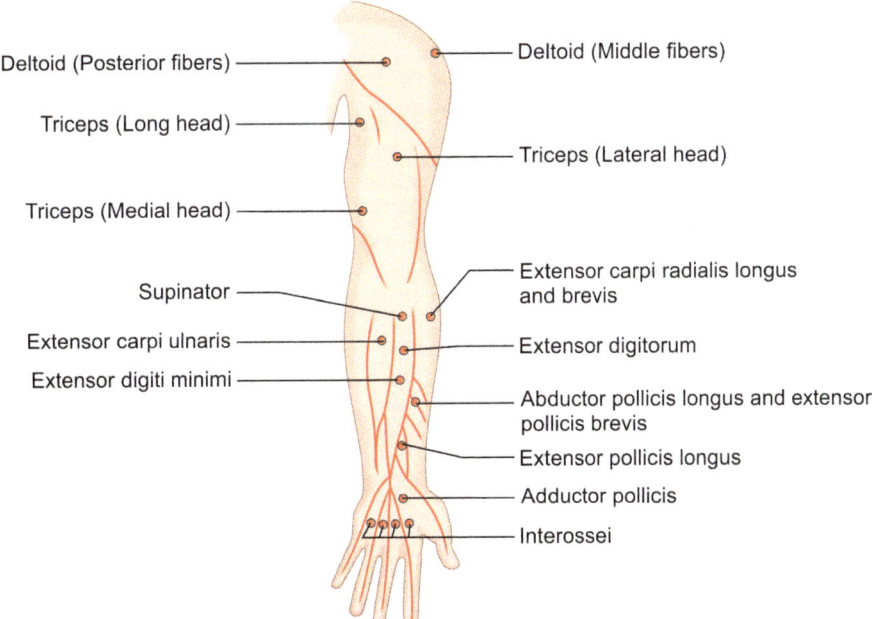

Fig. 3.24: Motor points of the posterior aspect of the right arm.

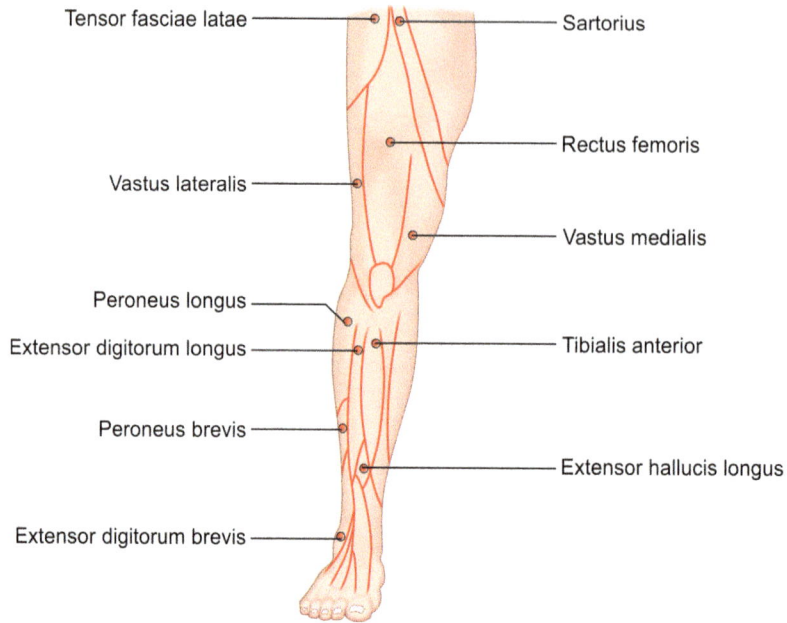

Fig. 3.25: Motor points of the anterior aspect of the right leg.

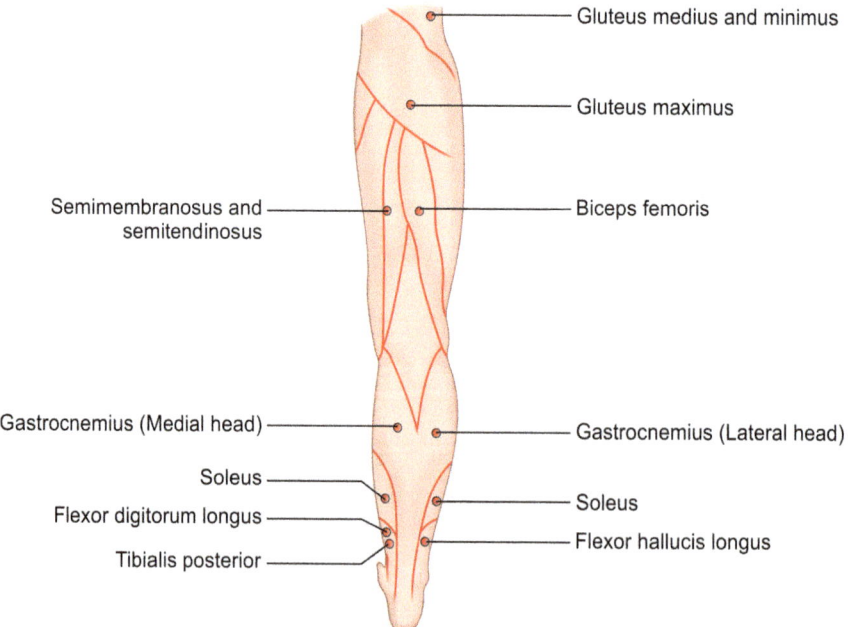

Fig. 3.26: Motor points of the posterior aspect of the right leg.

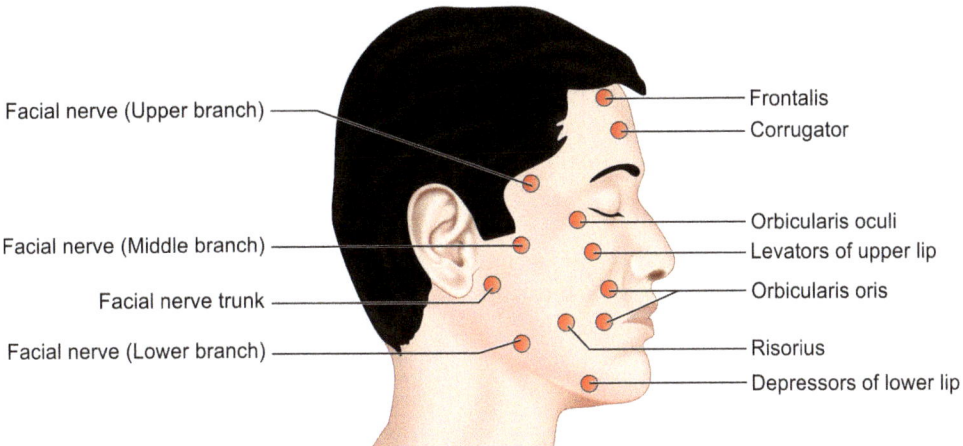

Fig. 3.27: Motor points of the muscles supplied by the facial nerve.

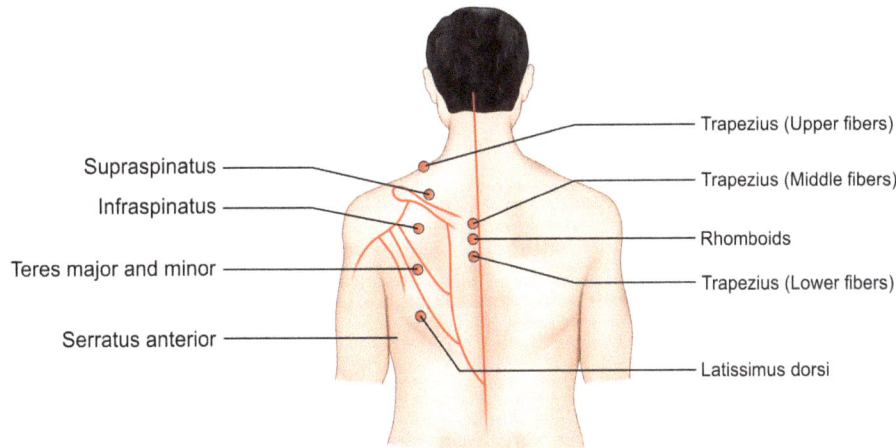

Fig. 3.28: Motor points of the back.

STRENGTH DURATION CURVE

Strength duration/intensity duration curve shows the relationship between the magnitude of the change of stimulus and the duration of the stimulus. The curve provides valuable information regarding the state of excitability of nerve lesion. It should be done only after 21 days following nerve injury.

Wallerian Degeneration

Nerve degenerates proximally to nearest node of Ranvier and distally throughout whole length. Debris is cleared by macrophagic activity. Process takes up to 21 days to complete and is a preparation for regeneration.

Nerve Regeneration

- Regeneration of axons send out many branches one of which becomes myelinated and continues to grow down the neural tube.
- Growth rate approximately 1 mm per day.
  It occurs unevenly throughout the regeneration period being initially faster.

Factor Influencing Rate of Regeneration

- *Age of the patient:* Faster in younger age group.
- *Site of lesion:* Faster when lesion is more proximal to spinal cord.
- *Nature of lesion:* Faster following spontaneous regeneration than following nerve suture.

Types of Injury

Seddon's Classification of Injury

Neuropraxia

- Loss of conduction without degeneration
- Nerve conduction possible below lesion
- Sensory part frequently least affected than motor.

Axonotmesis

- Disruption of axon, but nerve sheath intact
- Wallerian degeneration is followed by axons regrowing to own end organs.

Neurotmesis

- Disruption of axon and nerve sheath.
- Surgery required approximating nerve sheaths and enabling growing axon to reach correct end organ.

Part I

- Receiving the patient (as in proforma)
- Knowledge of condition
- Preparation of trays (as described earlier)
- *Preparation of apparatus:* Diagnostic electrical stimulator to be used.

Part II

- Positioning of the patient
- Position of physiotherapist
- Checking for local contraindications (as described earlier)
- Reducing skin resistance (as described earlier).

Part III

- Checking of apparatus
- Correct placing of pads and electrodes (depending upon the nerve).

Instructions to the Patient

- Feel of current

- ❖ Instruction to inform if any burning occurs
- ❖ *Warning:* Not to touch anything

Regulating current: Interrupted galvanic current
- ❖ Palpating tendon
- ❖ Winding up

Other Special Points

- ❖ Diagnostic stimulator to be used
- ❖ Interrupted galvanic current indicated
- ❖ Start with longer duration (from 100/300 ms)
- ❖ Select small muscle or select a muscle, which has distinguished action, compare with three muscles.
   - *For radial nerve:* Extensor indicis
   - *For median nerve:* Abductor pollicis brevis
   - *For ulnar nerve:* Abductor pollicis
   - *For lateral popliteal nerve:* Peroneus longus.

Shape of the Curve

Normal Innervation

When all the nerve fibers supplying the muscles are intact, the strength duration curve has a shape characteristic of normally innervated muscle **(Figs. 3.29A and B)**. The curve is of this typical shape because the same strength of stimulus is required to produce a response with all the impulses of longer duration, while those of shorter duration require an increase in the strengths of the stimulus each time the duration is reduced.

Complete Denervation

When all the nerve fibers supplying a muscle have degenerated, the strength duration produced is characteristic of complete denervation. For all impulses with duration of 100 ms or less the strength of the stimulus must be increased each time the duration is reduced and no response is obtained to impulses of very short duration. So that the curve rises steeply and is further to the right than that of a normally innervated muscle **(Figs. 3.30A and B)**.

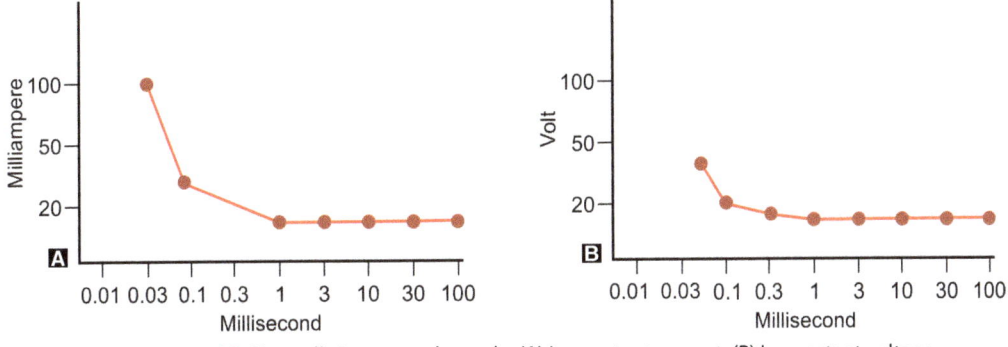

Figs. 3.29A and B: Normally innervated muscle. (A) In constant current; (B) In constant voltage.

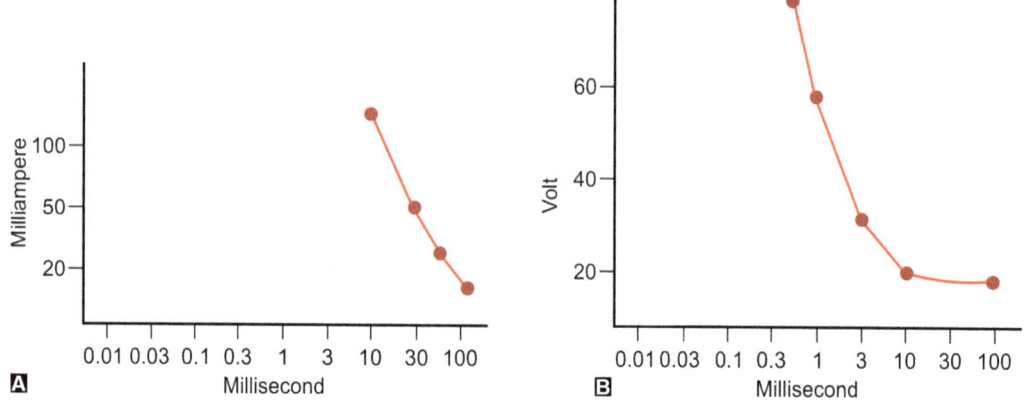

Figs. 3.30A and B: Complete denervated muscle. (A) In constant current; (B) In constant voltage.

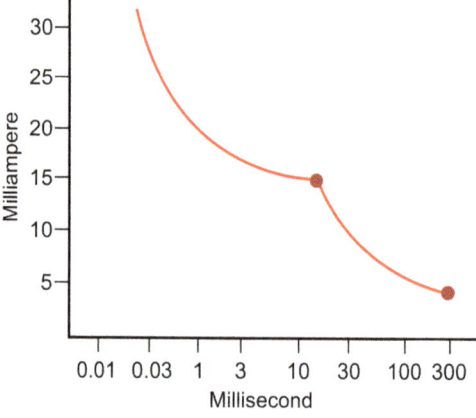

Fig. 3.31: Partially denervated muscle.

Partial Denervation
- As impulses shortened—denervated fibers respond less readily. So that a stronger stimulation is required.
- With impulse of shorter duration—innervated fibers responses **(Fig. 3.31)**.

When some of the nerve fibers supplying a muscle have degenerated while others are intact, the characteristic curve obtained clearly indicates partial denervation. The right hand part of the curve clearly resembles that of denervated muscle, the left hand part that of innervated muscle, and a kink is seen at the point where the two parts meet.

Rheobase
The rheobase is the smallest current that produces a muscle contraction if the stimulus is of infinite duration. In practice an impulse of 100 ms (0.1 s) is used. In denervation, the rheobase

may be less than that of innervated muscle and often rises as reinnervation commences. The rheobase varies considerably in various muscles and according to the skin resistance and temperature of the part. The rise of rheobase may be due to fibrosis of the muscle.

Chronaxie

The chronaxie is the duration of shortest impulse that will produce a response with a current of double the rheobase. The chronaxie of the innervated muscle is appreciably less than that of denervated muscle, the former being less and the latter more than 1 ms if the constant-voltage stimulator is used. With the constant-current stimulator the values are higher, but bear a similar relationship to each other. As practically seen the chronaxie of a muscle with 25% of its fibers innervated would be the same as that of a complete denervated muscle. Thus, chronaxie is not a satisfactory method of testing electrical reactions as partial denervation is not clearly shown.

Faradic and Interrupted Direct Current Tests

The faradic type current provides impulses with duration of 0.1–1 ms and a frequency of 50–100 Hz. These cause a tetanic contraction of innervated muscles, but with a faradic coil it is difficult or impossible to elicit a response from denervated muscle owing to the short duration of the stimuli. However, with modern stimulators a response can usually be obtained from denervated muscles with impulses of this duration because of greater output and more tolerable form of current being produced than that from older device.

Interrupted DC was used in impulses with duration of approximately 100 ms, repeated 20 times per minute. These usually produce a brisk contraction of innervated muscle fibers, but a sluggish contraction of denervated fibers. Innervated muscles may respond sluggishly if the temperature is below normal, while the contraction of denervated muscle becomes brisker as its temperature rises.

IONTOPHORESIS

Iontophoresis is a therapeutic technique, which involves the introduction of ions into the body tissue through the patient's skin. The basic principle is to place the ion under an electrode with the same charge, i.e., negative ion placed under cathode and positive ion placed under anode.

This technique is also known as "technique of ion transfer" into the body tissues by using electrical current as a driving force (*LeDuc*, 1903).

The electrode under which ions are placed, is therefore called "active electrode". A constant DC is used for propelling the ions into the patient's body tissues. DC ensures unidirectional flow of ions that is why only DC is used and alternative current cannot be used.

Iontophoresis has several advantages therapeutically such as being painless, sterile and noninvasive method to introduce specific ions into the body tissues. The common disadvantage associated with iontophoresis is chemical burn that usually occurs as a result of DC itself and not because of the ion being used in the treatment.

The quantity of the ions transferred into the tissues through iontophoresis is determined by the intensity of the current or current density at the active electrode, the duration of current flow and the concentration of ions at the active electrode or in the solution.

Type of Electrode

The size and shape of electrode can cause a variation in current density at the site of treatment. Less the size of electrode more will be the current density and more ions will be transferred. Increasing the size of electrode will decrease the current intensity thus reduces the concentration of ions at the electrode.

Current Intensity and Duration of Treatment

Low intensity currents are more effective for driving the ions into the body. The intensity may range from 5 to 12 mA. The treatment may last for about 15–20 minutes.

Methods of Treatment

- Skin should be cleaned preferably with soap, and hairy skin must be shaved.
- Electrodes must have proper contact with the skin surface. Proper straps must be used to keep the contact of electrodes.
- In case the ions are used in the form of ointment, a layer of it is applied at the site to be treated.
- In case the ions are in the form of a solution, lint pad of absorbent material is used and soaked in the ionic solution.
- Appropriate ions are used for specific conditions.
- The intensity of current and the duration of treatment must be regulated appropriately.
- Precaution must be taken to prevent any burning. Use talcum powder if erythema is seen after treatment.

Commonly Used Ions and their Indications for Use

Positive Ions

- *Hydrocortisone:* Used for its anti-inflammatory effects in conditions like rheumatoid arthritis, tendinitis, bursitis, etc.
- *Calcium chloride:* Calcium ions are used. It is found effective in stiff joint and post-traumatic pains.
- *Zinc oxide:* Used in cases of ulcers and open lesions, has property of healing.
- *Magnesium oxide:* Used in arthritis, is an excellent muscle relaxant, good vasodilator and mild analgesic.
- *Dexamethasone:* Used for treating musculoskeletal inflammatory conditions.

Negative Ions

- *Iodine:* It is an effective sclerolytic agent, an excellent bactericidal and a fair vasodilator. Effectively use for adherent scars, adhesive capsulitis.
- *Chlorine:* Also an effective sclerolytic agent, useful for scar tissue, keloids and burns.
- *Salicylic acid:* A general decongestant, sclerolytic and anti-inflammatory agent.
- *Sodium or potassium citrate:* Effective in rheumatoid arthritis.
- *Either ± tap water:* Used in the cases of hyperhidrosis (excessive sweating). Glycopyrronium bromide is also used along with tap water in the cases of hyperhidrosis.

Safety and precaution: Anticholinergic compounds have an atropine-like action, therefore, patients may feel drying of mouth and throat. The patient may feel restriction of general body sweating and therefore advised not to go for any strenuous activities, which may require sweating.

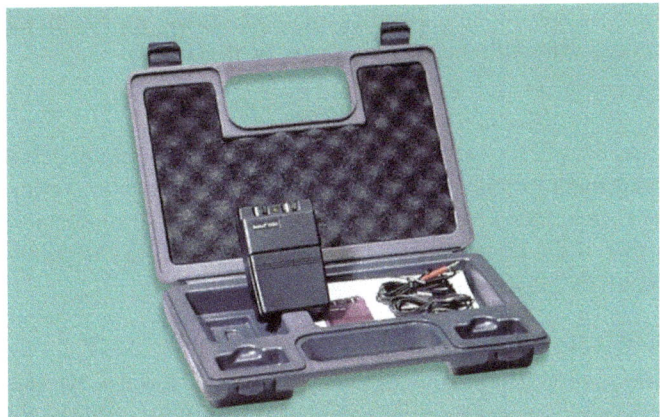

Fig. 3.32: Transcutaneous electrical nerve stimulation (TENS) apparatus.

TRANSCUTANEOUS ELECTRICAL NERVE STIMULATION

Transcutaneous electrical nerve stimulation (TENS) is the application of low frequency current in the form of pulsed rectangular currents through surface electrodes on the patient's skin to reduce pain. A small battery operated machine is generally used to generate current, which have specific stimulatory effect **(Fig. 3.32)**.

The effect and use of TENS depends upon gate control theory and pain modulation.

Pain is an unpleasant disturbed sensation, which accompanies the activation of nociceptors.

Pain is a subjective phenomenon with multiple dimensions.

Nociceptors are the sensory receptors, which carries pain stimulus. Any physical, chemical, thermal or mechanical stimulus like heat, cold or pressure activates these nociceptors. These are free nerve endings found in all body tissues. They carry pain stimulus to the higher centers. Once a nociceptor is stimulated, it releases a neuropeptide, which initiates the electrical impulses along the afferent fibers toward the spinal cord. These afferent fibers are of two types:

1. *A-delta fibers:* Fast conducting large diameter myelinated fibers, which conducts with a velocity of 5–30 m/s.
2. *C-fibers:* Slow conducting small diameter nonmyelinated fibers, which conducts with a velocity of 2–5 m/s.

First order or primary afferent fibers transmit impulses from the sensory receptors to the dorsal horn of the spinal cord. Second order afferent fibers carry sensory impulses from the dorsal horn of the spinal cord to the brain.

First order neurons include A-alpha, A-beta, A-delta and C-fibers. A-alpha and A-beta fibers are characterized by having large diameter afferents and A-delta and C-fibers are characterized by having small diameter afferents. The second order afferents are nociceptive specific. A nociceptive neuron transmits pain signals. Its cell body lies in the dorsal root ganglion. A-delta and C-fibers transmits the sensation of pain. Fast pain is transmitted over the larger, faster conducting A-delta afferent neurons and originates from receptors located in the skin. Slow pain is transmitted by the C afferent neurons and originates from both superficial (skin) and deeper (ligaments and muscle) tissue. Most nociceptive second order neurons ascend to higher centers along one of three tracts: (1) Lateral spinothalamic tract, (2) Spinoreticular tract, and (3) Spinomesencephalic tract, with the remainder ascending along the spinocervical tract or as projections to the cuneate and gracile nuclei of the medulla. Approximately 90% of the wide dynamic range second order afferents terminate in the thalamus.

Pain Gate Control

The pain gate theory was first postulated by *Ronald Melzack and Patrick Wall* in *1965*. This theory was later modified in *1982*. Afferent input is mainly through posterior root of the spinal cord and all afferent information must pass through synapses in the substantia gelatinosa (SG) and nucleus proprius of the posterior horn. It is at this level that the pain gate operates and presynaptic inhibition by TENS works.

Mechanism of Pain Gate Control

Nociceptive afferent enters the spinal cord via the dorsal root and make synapses either with interneuron or with second order neuron (called as transmission cells or T cells) in the SG in dorsal horn of spinal cord. The second order neuron crosses the midline of the spinal cord and transmits information to the higher centers via the lateral spinothalamic tract. These second order ascending neuron synapse with third order neuron in the nuclei of thalamus. The third order neuron carries the noxious stimulus to the cerebral cortex.

Modulation of transmission of pain can be achieved by altering the excitability of this pain pathway. The excitability of this pathway can be altered by other neurons (SG) in the dorsal horn. The SG cells have inhibitory influence on the T cells. This mechanism is called as presynaptic inhibition. Also the nociceptive afferent sends collaterals to the SG which inhibits the SG cells, when these nociceptive afferents are activated these causes inhibition of SG cell activity which will further inhibit the mechanism of presynaptic inhibition thus allowing the nociceptive stimuli to reach the higher centers.

Also low threshold large diameter mechanosensitive afferent have excitatory influence on SG cells. Their activation causes excitation of SG activity which in result causes increased presynaptic inhibition blocking the transmission at T cells thus closes the gate for nociceptive stimuli to travel up to the higher center. This is the site where the pain gate operates **(Fig. 3.33)**.

In addition to these input to SG cells from peripheral afferent there are descending influences on transmission cells (T cells) which came principally from higher center such as periaqueductal gray (PAG) matter (midbrain) and raphe nucleus (RN) (medulla). These both have excitatory influence on the SG cells activity thus have ability to reduce pain transmission. These pathways are thought to exert their effect on SG cells by release of neurotransmitters such as noradrenalin and 5-hydroxytryptamine.

Under normal conditions PAG matter and RN are inhibited by neurons from other areas of the brain. During pain the inhibition on PAG matter and RN is removed by influence of the limbic system thus allowing PAG and RN to exert its effect at SG of dorsal horn of the spinal cord.

The TENS stimulates the large diameter myelinated fibers as these are highly sensitive to electrical stimulation and quickly conduct the electrical impulse to the spinal cord. The A-delta and C-fibers are unable to pass the painful stimulus to spinal cord earlier than the large fibers.

This mechanism by which the nociceptor fibers are prevented from passing on their message to the spinal cord is called as presynaptic inhibition.

Types of Transcutaneous Electrical Nerve Stimulation

- *High transcutaneous electrical nerve stimulation:* In this high frequency and low-intensity electrical stimulation is applied. The stimulation will cause impulse to be carried along with

Chapter 3: Low Frequency Currents

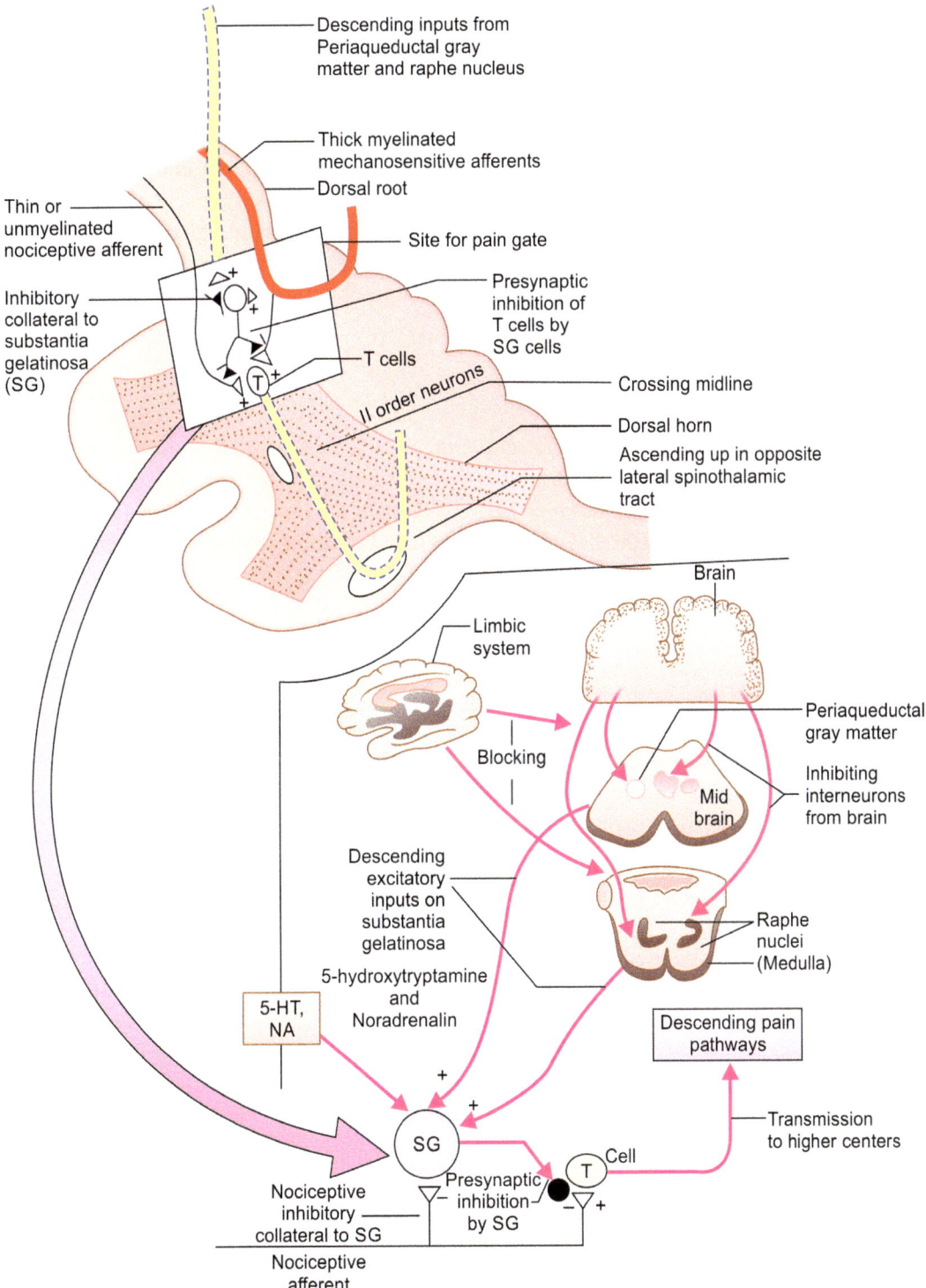

Fig. 3.33: Mechanism of pain gate control.

the large diameter afferent fibers and produces presynaptic inhibition of transmission of nociceptive A-delta and C-fibers at SG of the pain gate.
- *Frequency:* 100-150 Hz
- *Pulse width:* 100 and 500 ms
- *Intensity:* 12-30 mA.

❖ *Low transcutaneous electrical nerve stimulation:* In this low frequency and high-intensity electrical pulses are applied, it gives a sharp stimulus and like a muscle twitch. As the nociceptive stimulus is carried toward the cerebrum, its passage through the midbrain will cause the periaqueductal area of gray matter and RN to interact to release the opiate-like substances at cord level. The enkephalins and endorphins released have the effect of blocking forward transmission in the pain circuit.
- *Frequency:* 1-5 Hz
- *Pulse width:* 100 and 500 ms
- *Intensity:* 30 mA or more

❖ *Burst transcutaneous electrical nerve stimulation:* In this high frequency, short pulse, high-intensity electrical current is used.

Burst TENS is a series of impulse repeated for 1-5 times per second. Each train (burst) lasts for about 70 ms. The benefits for the burst TENS are that it combines both the conventional and acupuncture-like TENS and thus provide pain relief by the both routes.

Methods of Treatment

Electrode Placement

Transcutaneous electrical nerve stimulation electrode can be placed over:
❖ Area of greater intensity of pain.
❖ Superficial nerve proximal to the site of pain.
❖ To the appropriate dermatome.
❖ To the nerve trunk trigger point.

A number of treatment methods may be used depending upon the severity of the problem.
❖ Transcutaneous electrical nerve stimulation can be used for a single daily treatment of 40 minutes duration.
❖ Portable TENS can be used continuously for 24 hours.
❖ Transcutaneous electrical nerve stimulation can be used in night, e.g., for the treatment of phantom limb pain.

Indications for Use

Transcutaneous electrical nerve stimulation can be used for the treatment of:
❖ Chronic pain syndrome
❖ Phantom limb pain
❖ Reflex sympathetic dystrophy
❖ Postoperative pain
❖ Obstetric pain

Dangers and Contraindications

- Continuous application of high TENS may result in some electrolytic reaction below the skin surface.
- Transcutaneous electrical nerve stimulation is contraindicated in patients having cardiac pacemakers may be because of possible interference with the frequency of pacemaker.
- Transcutaneous electrical nerve stimulation should be avoided in first 3 months of pregnancy.
- Transcutaneous electrical nerve stimulation should be avoided in hemorrhagic conditions.
- Transcutaneous electrical nerve stimulation should be avoided over open wounds, carotid sinus, over the mouth, near eyes, etc.

MICROCURRENT ELECTRICAL NEUROMUSCULAR STIMULATION

Microcurrent electrical neuromuscular stimulation (MENS) commonly known as *microcurrent therapy* are extremely small pulsating currents (millionths of an ampere) used to relieve pain and to heal soft tissues of the body. These currents are so small that the patient rarely feels it. These currents are finely tuned to the level of the normal electrical potentials which occurs at body's own cellular level.

These electrical currents have a very close proximity of human body's own internal electrical potentials. Typically less than 600 microamperes, there is no patient discomfort or even sensation felt during application. These currents being more biologically compatible than any other electrical stimulation device, have the ability to penetrate the cell—as opposed to passing over the cell by other stimulation devices. It works on Arndt-Schultz Law which states that: "weak stimuli increases physiological activity and very strong stimuli inhibit or abolish activity". The human body has the equivalent of electrical circuits that play a very important role in healing.

Like TENS, microcurrents are capable of decreasing or eliminating pain. In addition to the treatment of pain, microcurrents also appear to have a capacity for stimulating the healing process. Clinical observation clearly shows that microcurrent therapy does more than just to block pain. Microcurrent therapy is often recommended in cases involving soft tissue inflammation or muscle spasm. The various modes of application, adjustable treatment variables and relatively few contraindications make this the modality of choice or wave of the future for a large variety of clinical problems.

This subsensory current normalizes the ordinary activity taking place within the cell if it has been injured or otherwise compromised. The external addition of microcurrent will increase the production of adenosine triphosphate (ATP), protein synthesis, oxygenation, ion exchange, absorption of nutrients, elimination of waste products and neutralizes the oscillating polarity of deficient cells thus restoring the homeostasis.

The biologically sensitive stimulation effect of microcurrent picks up where the body's own electrical current fails, as the human body must adhere to the natural law of electricity which is: "electricity must take path of least resistance". Therefore, its electrical current is destined to move around an injury or defect, rather than through it. By normalizing cell activity, inflammation is reduced while collagen producing cells are increased. Healthy cell metabolism creates a healthy, pain free internal environment.

The various effects produced by microcurrent electrical neuromuscular stimulation (MENS) are:
- Reduce acute and chronic pain
- Increase local blood circulation
- Reduce swelling and inflammation
- Improve soft tissue regeneration
- Decrease muscular spasm
- Prevent or retard the atrophy of muscular tissue
- Reeducate nerves and muscles
- Release muscle trigger points

CHAPTER 4

Medium Frequency Currents

INTRODUCTION

Medium frequency currents are the currents whose frequency falls between the range of 1,000 Hz and 10,000 Hz. They are being used therapeutically due to their advantage of greater penetration and with a higher tolerance and comfort over the low frequency current.

REBOX-TYPE CURRENTS

Rebox-type currents are derived from a device called Rebox. It was developed in Czechoslovakia in the 1970s. There is a point electrode and a handheld device. The point electrode is made the negative pole. The device consists of a microammeter and earphone. This system can be linked to a computer for display of graph of current. The current produced consists of unipolar rectangular pulses of between 50 µs and 250 µs at 3000 Hz.

RUSSIAN CURRENTS

Russian currents are evenly alternating currents with a frequency of 2,500 Hz (between 2,000 Hz and 10,000 Hz). These are applied with a series of separate bursts, i.e., polyphasic AC waveforms **(Fig. 4.1)**. There are thus 50 periods of 20 ms duration consisting of 10 ms burst and 10 ms interval. Each 10 ms burst contains 25 cycles of alternating current, i.e., 50 phases of 0.2 ms duration. These bursts reduces the total amount of current given to the patient thus increases patients tolerance. The other factor affecting patients' tolerance is the effect of frequency on the patients' tissue. Higher frequency current reduces the resistance to the current flow again making this type of waveform comfortable enough that the patient may tolerate with higher intensities. There are two basic waveforms which are used: A sine wave and a square waveform with a fixed intrapulse interval.

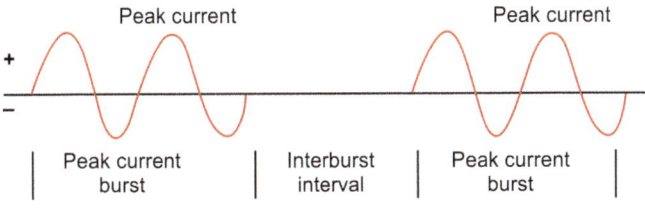

Fig. 4.1: Russian currents.

INTERFERENTIAL THERAPY

The principles of interferential therapy were first introduced by *Ho Nemec* (an Austrian scientist). Interferential currents are also known as *Nemec's currents*. In this two medium frequency currents are used to produce a low frequency effect. Since direct application of faradic current results in pain due to high impedance of tissues, so to have a low frequency effect two medium frequency currents are used. Out of these two medium frequency currents one current is always of 4,000 Hz because there is minimum impedance generated by the tissues against this frequency current. The other current can be varied accordingly.

Basic Principles of Interferential Therapy

The *interferential therapy* depends upon the principles of interferential effect of two medium frequency currents crossing in the patient's tissues. The interference produced by two currents in the tissues is called the *beat frequency*. For example, let us take two medium frequency currents, current in circuit A = 4,000 Hz and circuit B = 3,900 Hz. Where these two currents are applied to the tissues, at the point where the currents cross over, a new beat frequency current is set up whose amplitude is modulated and the frequency of new current is called beat frequency (interferential current) and that is 100 Hz **(Fig. 4.2)**.

By varying the frequency of the second channel relative to the constant frequency of the first, this is possible to produce a range of beat frequencies deep in the patient's tissues. Thus, it is possible to produce any desired frequency in the range of 1–250 Hz by varying the frequency difference of the carrier currents. One of the major advantages by the use of interferential therapy is that the effects are produced in the tissues where they are required, without unnecessary or uncomfortable skin stimulation. The advantage of interferential therapy is that, it can be used for pain relief as well as for muscle stimulation. The main advantage is that, patient cannot be given higher doses in low frequency therapy apparatus like faradic stimulator. The skin resistance offered to the 4,000 cycles/second is very much less than the resistance offered to the low frequency currents such as faradic currents. The principle of reduction in pain is because of gate control theory and stimulated release of pain reducing substances (endorphin and encephalin).

Definition and Terms Applied with Interferential Therapy

Interferential current is the resultant current produced when two or more alternating currents are applied simultaneously at the point of intersection in a given medium.

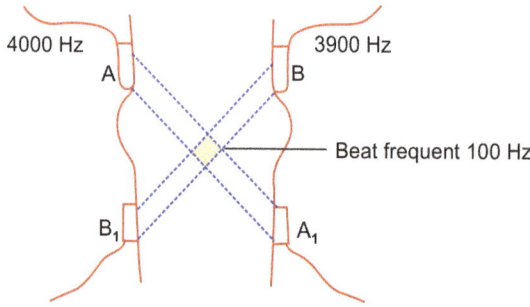

Fig. 4.2: Production of beat frequency by two medium frequency currents.

Impedance: Resistance, capacitance and inductance all these collectively form the impedance of the circuit. This impedance is a type of resistance produced by the tissues against any electrical stimulation of low frequency.

Impedance is denoted by "Z".

where, f = Frequency of current
          C = Capacitance
          Z = Impedance of tissues.

Phase: The current traveling from 0° to 180° is called to be in the same phase and the current traveling from 180° to 360° is called to be in opposite phase, i.e., if current A is traveling to B and C, then A to B it is called to be in same phase and from B to C it is called to be in opposite phase.

Wherever two waves of same frequency travel in same phase, then the peak of their crest and trough coincide and the resultant wave has amplitude more than the original amplitudes. But frequency will not change.

If two currents are traveling with little difference in their frequency then the amplitude of the resultant wave will increase or decrease in regular cycle. This is called amplitude modulation. This amplitude modulation is denoted by the difference of two original frequencies and is termed as beat frequency.

Modulation depth: Apart from frequency of modulation, the amplitude modulation is also characterized by depth of modulation. The modulation will be between 0% and 100%.

Sweep frequency: Sweep frequency is the frequency which can be directly fed to the beat frequency by the machine.

Electrodes: In interferential therapy, the flexible electrodes are used which are taped or bound to skin by vacuum electrodes which use suction to maintain contact. Usually four electrodes are used in interferential therapy, but two electrodes may be used in the treatment.

Balance: Electric current applied through the skin depends on the condition of electrode, sponge and the skin. Hence, when two currents are applied there may be unequal current passing through each circuit. This occurs due to the unequal resistance encountered. In order to compensate this situation the current in both the channels can be equalized.

Sweep: It is possible to change the frequency, between preset one and preset one plus additional frequency, continuously in a prefixed pattern and time, is the sweep.

Spectrum: Interferential therapy makes use of principle of Bernard of varying the frequency to prevent accommodation.

Spectrum denotes the range of frequency during the treatment. In this range, all frequencies are automatically transversed. The use of spectrum has the advantage that the tissue does not adapt to a certain frequency and thus a given treatment can be performed for a longer period and repeated more often.

Methods of Treatment

- Skin must be clean and clear before the start of the treatment.
- The part of the body to be treated should be washed and if there is any skin lesion it should be covered by applying petroleum jelly on it.

- The electrodes should be placed in such a way that the crossing point of two currents lie above or around the affected part.
- The suitable frequency current should be given for different conditions.
- Select the spectrum mode rectangular, triangular or trapezoidal as needed.
- Select the base frequency and upper frequency, the difference between upper frequency and base frequency would give the spectrum.
- Increase the power gently and cautiously until the patient starts feeling the current. It can be increased till the patient can tolerate.
- The current in channel-I and channel-II are independently measured.
- If there is difference in current in both the channels, this can be equalized by the balance control provided for this purpose. Usually, this difference is caused due to difference in resistance in the body where the two currents are passing.
- Remember that in case of two electrodes, there is current output available only in channel (I) by the superimposition of the two channels internally.
- After the treatment, adjust the intensity control to minimum.
- Switch "OFF" the mains and disconnect the electrodes.

Advantages of Interferential Currents

- The interferential currents do not produce any sensory nerve irritation, irrespective of amplitude. Their application is free of any burning sensation on the skin surface as is sometimes experienced with other low frequency currents which are disturbing to current sensitive patients.
- A medium frequency alternative current, it is high frequency and absence of direct current properties, are the most suitable for treating deeper layers of tissues. It is therefore most useful in treating tissues at a greater depth, e.g., in muscles, tendons, nerves, bursae and periosteum. Unlike galvanic, which has more reaction in the skin and subcutaneous tissues, interferential therapy is harmless.
- Resistance of skin is minimum while using frequencies in the range of 4,000 Hz, and therefore higher doses can be given to the body without any discomfort to the skin.
- The current can be localized more effectively in specific area. Extensive area can also be covered.

Physiological Effects of Interferential Therapy

The physiological effects of interferential therapy depend upon:
- Magnitude of the current
- Type of mode used—rhythmic or constant
- The frequency range used
- Accuracy of electrode positioning.

The effects are:
- *Relief of pain:* Relief of pain is an important physiological effect obtained by the use of interferential therapy. The increase in local blood circulation due to the local pumping effect of the stimulated muscles or the effect on autonomic nerves and thus the blood vessels help removing the chemicals from the local area. Short duration pulses at a frequency of 100 Hz may stimulate large diameter nerve fibers which will have an effect on the pain gate in the

posterior horn, and inhibit transmission of small diameter nociceptive traffic. A frequency of 80–100 Hz rhythmic is usually chosen for this effect, as the problem of accommodation is reduced. In order to selectively activate the descending pain suppression system, a frequency of 15 Hz is required and the stimulation of small diameter fibers produced will eventually cause the release of endogenous opiates (enkephalin and b endorphin) at a spinal level. A physiological blocking of nerve transmission is also postulated as a mechanism of pain modulation produced by interferential therapy. It is thought that the maximum frequency of transmission in C nerve fibers is 15 Hz and in Ad fibers is 40 Hz. The application of frequencies higher than this maximum could block transmission along these fibers altogether. Consideration should also be given to the effective aspects of pain modulation, and there is probably a strong placebo effect associated in many different countries claim good results in the modulation of both acute and chronic pain syndromes.

- *Motor stimulation:* Normal innervated muscles will be made to contract if interferential frequencies between 1 Hz and 100 Hz are used. The type of contraction depends on the frequency of stimulation, as the shape and length of each individual stimulus is of a muscle stimulating type. At low frequencies a twitch is produced, between 5 Hz and 20 Hz a partial tetany, and from 30 Hz to 100 Hz a tetanic contraction. A complete range of all these types of muscle contraction can be seen when a rhythmical frequency of 1–100 Hz is used. Muscle contraction is produced with little sensory stimulation, and can be of deeply placed muscles, e.g., pelvic floor. Unfortunately, the patient is unable to voluntarily contract with the current (unlike faradism), but this does not seem to adversely affect the results. It is claimed that the rapid return of tune to the pelvic floor when treated with interferential therapy is the result of stimulation of both the voluntary and smooth muscle fibers; faradism can only stimulate the voluntary component.
- *Absorption of exudates:* This is accelerated by a frequency of 1–10 Hz rhythmic, as a rhythmical pumping action is produced by muscle contraction, and there is possible an effect on the autonomic nerves which can affect the diameter of blood vessels, and therefore the circulation. Both of these factors will help absorb exudates and thus reduce swelling.

METHODS OF TREATMENT

TREATMENT OF PATIENT'S CONDITION

- *Relief of chronic pain:*
    - Low back pain
    - Periarthritis shoulder
    - Osteoarthritis knee
- Absorption of exudates
- Stress incontinence.

PROFORMA FOR PATIENT'S ASSESSMENT

- *Receiving the patient:* Good morning, a physiotherapist and I am going to treat you. Please, cooperate with me during the treatment and wait until I go through your case sheet.

- *History taking or going through the case sheet:*
  - Name
  - Father's and Mother's name
  - Age
  - Sex
  - Occupation
  - Address: Correspondence and permanent.

  Chief complaints:
  - History of present illness
  - History of past illness
  - Family history
  - Social and occupational history
  - Treatment history
  - Prognosis of the treatment
  - *Investigations:*
    - Hematological tests
    - Radiological tests—X-rays, MRI scan, etc.
    - Others.
- *Checking for general contraindications:*
  - Hyperpyrexia/fever
  - Hypertension
  - Anemia
  - Severe renal and cardiac failure
  - Deep X-ray and cobalt therapy
  - Epileptic patients
  - Non-cooperative patients
  - Mentally retarded patients
  - Very poor general condition of the patient.
- *Checking for local contraindications:*
  - Open wounds
  - Very recent fractures
  - Skin grafts
  - Severe edema
  - Hairy surface
  - Acute inflammation
  - Metal in the part
  - Malignant growth
  - Hypersensitive skin
  - Loss of sensation.
- *Preparation of trays:*
  - Treatment tray
  - Skin resistance lowering tray.

  Treatment tray:
  - Mackintosh

- Lint pads
- Pad or plate electrodes and pen electrodes
- Leads
- Straps
- Cotton
- Powder
- Gel, etc.

Skin resistance lowering tray:
- Saline water
- Soap
- Cotton
- Vaseline
- Towels, etc.

Preparation of Treatment Tray

- *Mackintosh:* The Mackintosh is to be kept under the patient's treatment part to prevent earth shock and to prevent dripping of water.
- *Lint pads:* The lint pad is made up of lint cloth, and it is used to prevent accumulation of chemicals in the tissues formed during the treatment which if not prevented leads to burn. It must be in 8 or 16 layers. More the layers of lint pad, less the chance of accumulation of chemicals, less the chance of burn.
- *Electrodes:* Electrodes could be of pad type or plate type. Pad or plate electrodes are kept in between the lint pads for even distribution of current. The edges of plate electrodes should be blunt. It should be smaller than the lint pad so that it cannot come in contact with the skin.
- *Leads:* Used to connect the electrodes with the stimulator.
- *Straps:* Usually, rubber straps are used. It should be placed over the pad. It should be fixed with the help of jaconet piece.
- *Cotton:* Used to prevent dripping of water and for cleaning the surface.
- *Powder:* Used to apply over the skin if there is any redness after the treatment. Redness occurs due to erythema. It gives soothing effect.
- *Gel:* Used for pad electrodes where lint pads are not used. Gel is used for proper contact of electrodes with the patient's surface.

Preparation of Skin Resistance Lowering Tray

- *Saline water:* Prepared by adding the pinch of salt to the bowl of water. The aim of preparing saline water is to prepare more ions so that minimum amount of current that is enough to get the desired effects. If we use more than 1% saline, there will be lowering of ions and less amount of current passes since there will be restriction of ions.
- *Soap:* It is used for cleaning the part to be treated to remove dirt, dust or sebum, etc. thus lowering the skin resistance **(Fig. 4.3)**.
- *Cotton:* It is used for cleaning the surface.
- *Vaseline:* It is applied over scar tissue. It prevents the concentration of more current on the scar tissue.

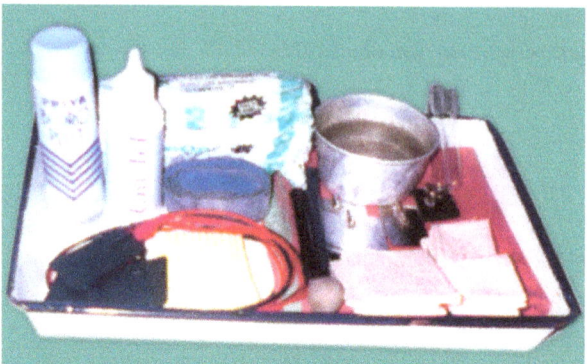

Fig. 4.3: Skin resistance lowering tray.

- *Towels:* Towels are used for covering the body part. Neat and clean towels should be used every time.
  Lowering skin resistance: By removing dust particles, sebum or sweat, skin resistance can be lowered. In the presence of all these dust particles, sebum or sweat greater intensity of current is required to get the contraction. It provides some resistance to the passage of current.
- *Preparation of apparatus:*
  - Check whether all the knobs are at *zero*.
  - Checking the pins of the plug and check whether the switch is turned off.
  - Check the insulation of the wire.
  - Check whether the switch in the stimulator is working.
  - Check whether fuse is present in the apparatus; see that it is not blown out.
  - Check whether hand switch for patients use is intact and is working.
- *Correct positioning of the patient:*
  - Position the patient in such a way that it is comfortable to the patient.
  - Part to be treated must be exposed and should be at adequate distance from the modality.
- *Correct positioning of Physiotherapist:*
  - Position of Physiotherapist should also be comfortable so that he/she may not get tired after the treatment.
  - Position should be such that it provides maximum accessibility to the treatment part and to the modality.
- Correct placing of pads and electrodes.
- *Instructions to the patient:* I am going to start the treatment:
  - Be relaxed
  - Do not touch anything around you
  - Do not pull the leads
  - Do not touch the walls or ground
  - If you feel uneasy switch off from the patients switch.
- *Regulating the current:*
  - Gradually increase the current
  - Keep talking with the patient about the feel of the current
  - Tell him to inform you immediately about any inconvenience, discomfort or burning.

- *Explanation to the patient:*
  - Explain the patient the advantages of the treatment
  - Explain the patient the course or duration of the treatment
  - Explain the patient the *dos and don'ts* in home and otherwise.

LOW BACK PAIN

Low back pain is characterized by pain which is present in the lower part of the back region. As much as 80% of the industrial population and 60% of the general population experience acute low back pain at some point of time in their life. Hence, low back pain is a cause of great economic and clinical significance.

Etiology

In the majority of the patients, the common causes of low back pain are:
- Idiopathic
- Diskogenic.

  However, LBA could result from various other causes. It is therefore necessary to identify and rule out the other causes of LBA before initiating physiotherapy.
- *Receiving the patient:* Good morning, I am a Physiotherapist and going to treat you. Please, cooperate with me during the treatment and wait until I go through your case sheet.
- *History taking or going through the case sheet*:
  - Name
  - Father's and Mother's name
  - Age
  - Sex
  - Occupation
  - Address: Correspondence and permanent.

  Chief complaints:
  - History of present illness
  - History of past illness
  - Social and occupational history
  - Treatment history
  - Prognosis of the treatment
  - *Investigations:*
    - Hematological tests
    - Radiological tests—X-rays, MRI scan, etc.
    - Others.
- *Checking for general contraindications*:
  - Hyperpyrexia/fever
  - Hypertension
  - Deep X-ray and cobalt therapy
  - Epileptic patients
  - Non-cooperative patients
  - Mentally retarded patients.

- *Checking for local contraindications*:
  - Open wounds
  - Hairy surface
  - Metal in the part
  - Malignant growth
  - Hypersensitive skin
  - Loss of sensation.
- *Preparation of trays*:
  - Treatment tray: Mackintosh, lint pads, pad or plate electrodes, leads, straps, cotton, powder, gel, etc.
  - Skin resistance lowering tray: Saline water, soap, cotton, Vaseline, towels, etc.
- *Preparation of apparatus*:
  - Check whether all the knobs are at zero
  - Checking the pins of the plug and check whether the switch is turned off
  - Check the insulation of the wire
  - Check whether the switch in the stimulator is working
  - Check whether fuse is present in the apparatus; see that it is not blown out
  - Check whether hand switch for patients use is intact and is working.
- *Correct positioning of the patient*:
  - Patient must be comfortably placed preferably in lying (prone) position.
  - Part to be treated must be exposed and should be at adequate distance from the modality.
- *Correct positioning of Physiotherapist:* Position of Physiotherapist should be in closed vicinity of the patient and at appropriate reachable distance from the modality.
- *Correct placing of pads and electrodes:* Four electrodes are placed in two pairs (sets) to be placed diagonal to each other **(Fig. 4.4)**.
- *Regulating the current:*
  - Gradually increase the current: For relief of pain, a frequency of 80-100 Hz rhythmic is used
  - Keep talking with the patient about the feel of the current
  - Tell him to inform you immediately about any inconvenience, discomfort or burning.

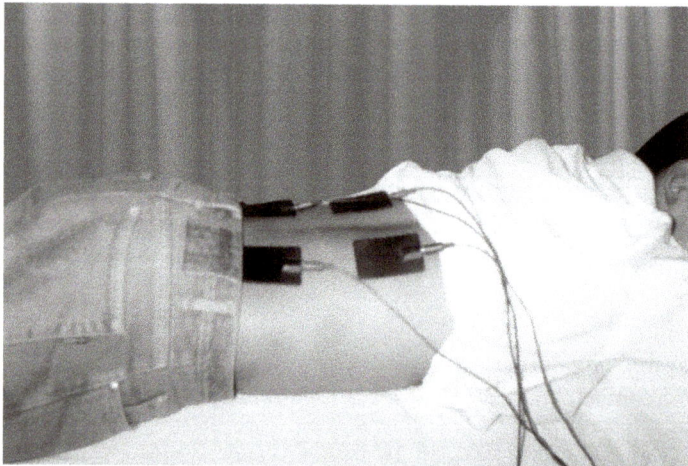

Fig. 4.4: Interferential therapy (low backache).

Treatment:
- Rest and analgesics
- Spinal extension exercises
- Postural correction.

PERIARTHRITIS SHOULDER

Periarthritis shoulder is a condition characterized by pain and progressive limitation of movements in the shoulder joint. In early stages, the pain is worst at night and the stiffness is limited to abduction and external rotation of the shoulder. Later, the pain is present at all times and all the movements of shoulder are severely limited. Often, there is a history of preceding trauma. The disease is common in diabetics.

- *Receiving the patient:* Good morning, I am a Physiotherapist and going to treat you. Please, cooperate with me during the treatment and wait until I go through your case sheet.
- *History taking or going through the case sheet:*
  - Name
  - Father's and Mother's name
  - Age
  - Sex
  - Occupation
  - Address: Correspondence and permanent.

  Chief complaints
  - History of present illness
  - History of past illness
  - Social and occupational history
  - Treatment history
  - Prognosis of the treatment
  - *Investigations:*
    - Hematological tests
    - Radiological tests—X-rays, MRI scan, etc.
    - Others.
- *Checking for general contraindications:*
  - Hyperpyrexia/fever
  - Hypertension
  - Deep X-ray and cobalt therapy
  - Epileptic patients
  - Noncooperative patients
  - Mentally retarded patients.
- *Checking for local contraindications:*
  - Open wounds
  - Hairy surface
  - Metal in the part
  - Malignant growth
  - Hypersensitive skin
  - Loss of sensation.

- *Preparation of trays:*
  - Treatment tray—mackintosh, lint pads, pad or plate electrodes, leads, straps, cotton, powder, gel, etc.
  - Skin resistance lowering tray—saline water, soap, cotton, Vaseline, towels, etc.
- *Preparation of apparatus:*
  - Check whether all the knobs are at Zero
  - Checking the pins of the plug and check whether the switch is turned off
  - Check the insulation of the wire
  - Check whether the switch in the stimulator is working
  - Check whether fuse is present in the apparatus; see that it is not blown out
  - Check whether hand switch for patients use is intact and is working.
- *Correct positioning of the patient:* Sitting with back support, forearm rests over the table with elbow flexed.
- *Correct positioning of Physiotherapist:* Position of Physiotherapist should be in closed vicinity of the patient and at appropriate reachable distance from the modality.
- *Correct placing of pads and electrodes:* Four electrodes are placed in two pairs, placed diagonal to each other.
- *Regulating the current:*
  - Gradually increase the current. For relief of pain, a frequency of 80-100 Hz rhythmic is used
  - Keep talking with the patient about the feel of the current
  - Tell him to inform you immediately about any inconvenience, discomfort or burning.
- *Explanation to the patient:*
  - Explain the patient the advantages of the treatment
  - Explain the patient the course or duration of the treatment
  - Explain the patient the *dos and don'ts* in home and otherwise.

Treatment:
- Make circle in air or against wall
- Pendular exercises or Codman's exercises
- Manipulation exercises.

OSTEOARTHRITIS KNEE

Osteoarthritis is a chronic degenerative disease of joints with exacerbations of acute inflammation.

Incidence: Old age people (over the age of 50 years).

Classification

- *Primary:* There is no obvious cause; primary osteoarthritis is due to wear and tear changes occurring in old age due to weight bearing.
- *Secondary:* There is a primary disease of the joint which leads to the degeneration of the joint.
  - Receiving the patient: Good morning, I am a Physiotherapist and going to treat you. Please, cooperate with me during the treatment and wait until I go through your case sheet.
  - History taking or going through the case sheet.

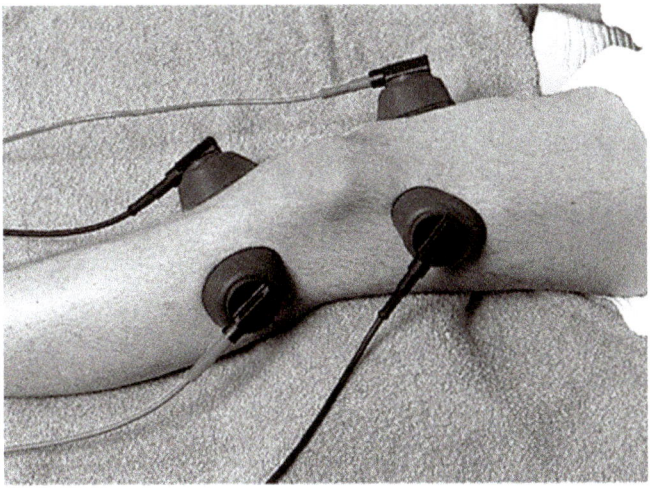

Fig. 4.5: Interferential therapy (osteoarthritis knee).

- *Checking for general and local contraindications:*
    - Hyperpyrexia/fever
    - Metal in the part
    - Hypersensitive skin.
- Loss of sensation.
- Preparation of trays and apparatus.
- *Correct positioning of the patient:*
    - Long sitting with back support and the affected leg is rest with a pillow below the knee.
    - Part to be treated must be exposed and should be at adequate distance from the modality.
- *Correct positioning of Physiotherapist:* Position of Physiotherapist should be in closed vicinity of the patient and at appropriate reachable distance from the modality.
- *Correct placing of pads and electrodes:* Four electrodes are placed in two pairs, placed diagonal to each other **(Fig. 4.5)**.
- Regulating the current:
    - Gradually increase the current. For relief of pain, a frequency of 80–100 Hz rhythmic is used
    - Keep talking with the patient about the feel of the current
    - Tell him to inform you immediately about any inconvenience, discomfort or burning.

Treatment:
- Static quadriceps exercises
- Avoid cross sitting and prolonged standing.

ABSORPTION OF EXUDATES

The accumulation of exudates in skin and subcutaneous tissues is known as edema. It could be due to heart failure, chronic venous inefficiency or due to nephrotic syndrome. In heart failure, excessive retention of salt and water leads to edema formation. In old age, there could be inferior vena cava obstruction or iliofemoral vein thrombosis leading to chronic venous inefficiency

and thus edema formation. In nephrotic syndrome, there is more generalized form of edema which often affects face and arms.
- Receiving the patient.
- *History taking or going through the case sheet:*
  - History of present illness
  - History of past illness
  - Social and occupational history
  - Treatment history
  - Prognosis of the treatment
  - *Investigations:*
    - Hematological tests
    - Other tests.
- Checking for general and local contraindications.
- Preparation of trays and apparatus.
- *Correct positioning of the patient:*
  - Patient must be comfortably placed preferably in supine lying position
  - Part to be treated must be exposed and should be at adequate distance from the modality.
- *Correct positioning of Physiotherapist:* Position of Physiotherapist should be in closed vicinity of the patient and at appropriate reachable distance from the modality.
- *Correct placing of pads and electrodes:* Two pairs (sets) of electrodes are placed diagonal to each other.
- *Regulating the current:* Frequency of 1–10 Hz rhythmic is used. The rhythmic mode helps to produce pumping action over muscles and effects autonomic nerves, which leads to improving circulation.
- *Explanation to the patient:*
  - Explain the patient the advantages of the treatment
  - Explain the patient the course or duration of the treatment
  - Explain the patient the do's and don'ts in home and otherwise.

STRESS INCONTINENCE

Incontinence is rather a symptom than a disease. A common neurological cause of incontinence is damage to cerebral cortex with damage to normal bladder inhibition. Stress incontinence is common in females due to weakness of pelvic floor muscles.
- Receiving the patient.
- *History taking or going through the case sheet:*
  - History of present illness
  - History of past illness
  - Social and occupational history
  - Treatment history
  - Prognosis of the treatment
  - Investigations.
- Checking for general and local contraindications.
- Preparation of trays and apparatus.

- *Correct positioning of the patient:*
  - Patient must be comfortably placed in supine lying position with hip and knee flexed.
  - Part to be treated must be exposed and should be at adequate distance from the modality.
- *Correct positioning of physiotherapist:* Position of Physiotherapist should be in closed vicinity of the patient and at appropriate reachable distance from the modality.
- *Correct placing of pads and electrodes:* The electrodes are placed over the lower abdomen and over the inner thighs so as to produce good strong contraction of the pelvic floor.
- *Regulating the current:* Frequency of 1–100 Hz rhythmic is used. At low frequencies a twitch is produced, between 5 Hz and 20 Hz a partial tetany and 30–100 Hz tetanic contraction occurs. Muscle contraction is produced with little sensory stimulation. It is claimed that the rapid return of the tone of pelvic floor muscles occurs when treated with interferential therapy due to stimulation of both voluntary and smooth muscle fibers. It has advantage over faradic current stimulation that faradic currents can only stimulate voluntary components. Also, feel of current is much reduced in interferential therapy.

CHAPTER 5

High Frequency Currents

DIATHERMY

Diathermy is a Greek word meaning *through heating.* Diathermies are of following types:
* Shortwave diathermy (SWD)
* Microwave diathermy
* Longwave diathermy (LWD)

SHORTWAVE DIATHERMY

Shortwave diathermy **(Fig. 5.1)** is the use of high frequency electromagnetic waves of the frequency between 10^7 and 10^8 Hz and a wavelength between 30 and 3 m to generate heat in the body tissues. It provides the deepest form of heat available to the physiotherapist.

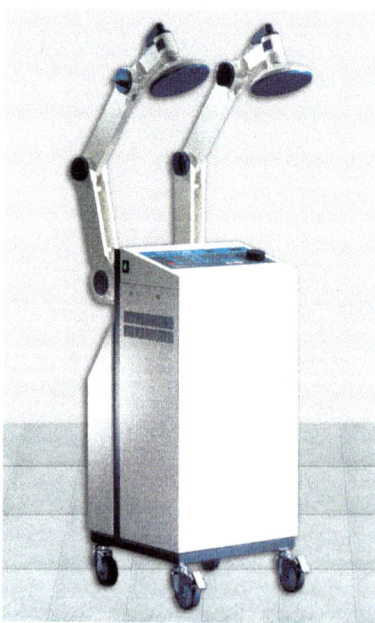

Fig. 5.1: Shortwave diathermy.

The therapeutically used frequencies and wavelengths are 27.12 MHz and 11 m (commonly). The less common frequencies and wavelengths are 40.68 MHz and 7.5 m and 13.56 MHz and 22 m.

Principles

It is not possible to produce high frequency currents by some mechanical device which produces sufficient rapid movements. This type of current can only be produced by discharging a condenser through an inductance of low-ohmic resistance. If a current of very high frequency is required, the capacitance and inductance should be small and if a current of low frequency is required the capacitance and inductance should be large. This is the mechanism of production of high frequency current.

Construction

The system consists of two circuits:
1. The machine circuit
2. The patient circuit.

The Machine Circuit

It consists of two transformers, whose primary coils are connected to source of AC. One is a step-down transformer and its secondary coil supplies current to the filament heating circuit of triode valve. The other is step-up transformer and connected to anode circuit. Anode circuit carries the current produced by valve. Here it consists of triode valve and oscillator circuit (**Fig. 5.2**). Oscillator circuit consists of condenser (XY) and inductor or oscillator coil (CD).

Current of different frequencies are obtained by selecting suitable condensers and inductances. To produce a current of high frequency the capacitance and inductance used must

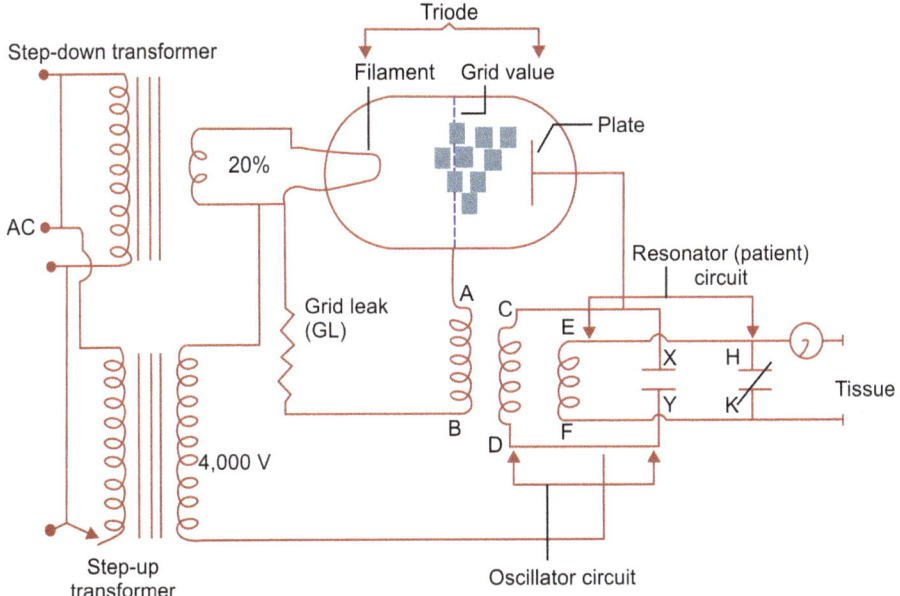

Fig. 5.2: Circuit for shortwave diathermy.

be small and is made to charge and discharge repeatedly and for obtaining this an oscillator is incorporated into machine circuit along with valve circuit.

Another coil AB lie close to oscillator coil (CD) and has one end connected to the grid of the valve and other through grid leak (GL) resistance to the filament.

The Patient Circuit

The patient or resonator circuit is coupled to machine circuit by a inductor coil (EF) lying close to oscillator coil (CD) and also consists variable condenser (HK) which is usually in parallel to patient terminal. A matching high frequency current is produced in the resonator circuit by electromagnetic induction. For this to happen the oscillator and resonator circuits must be in resonance with each other, which requires that the product of inductance and capacitance must be the same for both circuits.

Working

The AC from main passes through primary coils of the transformers and electromotive force (EMF) is induced in secondary coils. An EMF of 20–25 V is setup in secondary coil of step-down transformer and produces current through filament of the valve. The filament is heated and thermionic emission takes place and current flows through valve.

The EMF of about 4,000 V is induced in the secondary coil of step-up transformer and provided that anode of valve is positive and filament is negative, current flows in anode circuit. The electrons flows from filament to anode through valve, through oscillator coil in direction C to D and to transformer back to filament.

The electron form in CD will induce EMF in coil AB in direction that electrons will move to grid of valve making it negative thus blocking the flow of electrons from filament. This will lead to dying of current in anode circuit. This reduction in current will lead to self-induced EMF. According to Lenz law, this EMF will try to prevent fall in current by offering resistance to flow of current. This will charge condenser X (positive) and Y (negative) polarity opposite to earlier one. Now when self-induced EMF totally dies away, condensers again discharge through oscillator coil, but in opposite direction (D to C).

Flow of current from D to C induces an EMF in AB such that electrons move from A to B and grid loses its negative charge and anode current flows again. This sequence continues and each time condenser charges and discharges through oscillator circuit leading to production of high frequency current.

Grid leak: When the current flows across the valve some electrons are caught on the grid and GL is provided to enable these electrons to escape back to the filament.

The resonator coil (EF) lies within the varying magnetic field setup around the oscillatory coil, so provided that two circuits are in resonance high frequency current is induced in it. The current is similar to that in the oscillator circuit and is supplied to patient.

Methods of Applications

The transfer of electrical energy to the patient tissues occurs either by electrostatic field or by electromagnetic field. Therefore, two methods of applications are used:
- Condenser/capacitor field method
- Cable method

When SWD is applied by the condenser field method, the electrodes and the patient's tissues form a capacitor. The capacitance of such a capacitor depends upon:
- The size of electrodes
- The distance between the electrodes
- The tissue between the electrodes.

When SWD is applied by the cable method, the cable and the patient's tissue forms an inductance, the value of which varies according to its arrangement.

Consequently, either the capacitance or inductance of the patient's circuit is varied at each treatment, and so a variable condenser is incorporated in the patient's circuit to compensate for this.

Tuning of the circuit: When the electrodes are arranged in position with the patient's body, the capacitance of the variable capacity is adjusted until the product of inductance and capacitance of the resonator circuit is equal to that of the oscillator circuit. Thus, when the oscillator and the resonator circuits are in tune with each other, there is transfer of maximum energy into the patient's body parts.

Indications of tuning are:
- Indicator light on the equipment either comes "on" or changes its color, and attains a specific color on tuning, generally blue.
- An ammeter is used in the circuit to register the resonance between oscillator circuit and resonator circuit by showing maximum deflection on turning the tuning knob.
- A tube containing neon gas placed within the electric field between the electrodes or the ends of the cable glows at maximum intensity when the circuits are in resonance.

Nowadays, modern machines have automatic resonator or tuners in it which automatically searches for and selects the adjustment of the variable capacitor to ensure maximum energy transfer to the patient's body.

Capacitor Field Method

The electrodes are placed on each side of the part being treated. The electrodes are separated by the skin by means of an insulating material. The electrodes act as the plates of the capacitor, while the patient's tissues together with the insulating material which separates them from the electrodes for the dielectric.

When the current is applied, rapidly alternating charges are setup on the electrodes and gives rise to a rapidly alternating electric field between them. The electric field also influences the material which lies within it.

Effects of Electric Field on Conductors, Insulators and Electrolytes

As we know, conductors are the substances in which electrons can easily be displaced from their atoms. When such a material lies within a varying electric field, there is rapid oscillation of electrons and heat is produced.

An insulator is a substance in which the electrons are so firmly held by the central nuclei that they cannot be easily displaced and results in the distortion of molecules when varying electric field is applied.

An electrolyte is a substance which contains ions and when a varying electric field is applied, the ions tend to move from one direction to the other. Electrolytes also contain dipoles which contain two oppositely charged ions, when a varying electric field is applied, they rotate their

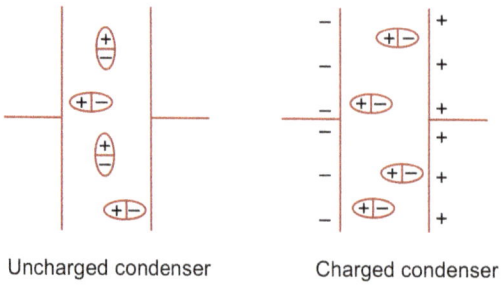

Uncharged condenser   Charged condenser

Fig. 5.3: Rotation of dipoles.

direction. These dipoles are electrically neutral, but one end bears positive and the other a negative charge. As a result of electric field they rotate themselves and come in an alignment with the electrodes **(Fig. 5.3)**.

Thus, the electric field influences the material that lies between the plates; this causes the oscillation of the ions, distortion of molecules and rotation of dipoles. This causes production of heat in the tissues by the electric field of SWD, which is the primary function of SWD. The heat production is in accordance with Joule's law, i.e., $Q = I^2RT$, but depends upon the distribution of the electric field.

Effects of Electric Field on Dielectric Constants of the Body Tissues

The dielectric constants of the various tissues differ considerably. The tissues of low impedance such as blood and muscles have higher dielectric constants. The tissues of high impedance such as fibrous tissues and fat have low dielectric constant.

The relative arrangement of the tissues in the body coming in the pathway of electric field affects the distribution of the lines of forces and the heat production. If the different body tissues lie parallel to the electric field, the density of the field and thus the heat production is greatest in the tissues of low impedance. Thus, when the field is passed longitudinally through the limb, blood is heated most because of low impedance.

If the different body tissues lie transversely to the electric field, the density of the field and thus the heat production is greatest in the tissues of high impedance. Thus, when the field is passed transversely through the limb, fat is heated most because of its high impedance.

Actually, the arrangement of the tissues in the body is such that they do not offer a true parallel or series (longitudinal or transverse) arrangement, but in fact the mixture of the two. As the deep tissues generally lie parallel to the field, heating is less in deep tissues. Also, the heating is more in the tissues of low impedance such as blood. Tissues in contact with those in which heat is produced, heats are transferred by means of conduction. For example, when muscles surrounding a deeply placed joint are heated some heat is transmitted to the joint. Also, when blood is heated in the part being treated, it provides the heat to other tissues like muscles, etc., and thus the heat is carried away. This helps in prevention of overheating in the part being treated. Also it helps in heating other tissues which are not in direct contact with the electric field. Therefore, intensity of electric field or any other form of heat needs to be gradually increased so as to allow vasodilatation of the vessels and to avoid overheating.

When SWD is applied by the capacitor field method the production of heat is determined by the distribution of electric field, and it tends to be greatest in the superficial tissues and the tissues of low impedance.

The aim is to achieve an even electric field as far as possible throughout the superficial and deep tissues so as to obtain even heating in the tissues. To obtain desirable therapeutic effects the selection and placement of electrodes should be proper. The selection or placement of electrodes should be based on:
- Type of electrodes
- Size of electrodes
- Spacing of electrodes
- Positioning of electrodes.

Type of Electrodes

There are various types of electrodes. Electrodes could be pad electrodes, plate electrodes and disk electrodes. Each electrode consists of a metal plate surrounded by some form of insulating material.

One type of electrode consists of a thin malleable metal plate covered with a rubber pad. This has an advantage to get moulded according to the body part. Electrodes of this type are separated from the skin by perforated felt pad and their position is maintained by the weight of the body. Undue pressure of the body part should be avoided as this may crack the plate inside and may hamper the blood supply. The insulating felt pad is perforated so that it contains a small quantity of air inside, which is preferably the best spacing material. Thus, it has a disadvantage of not having completely air spacing between the pad and the body.

Another type of electrode consists of a thick rigid metal plate coated with a thin layer of insulating material made up of rubber or plastic. The property of an electric charge is that it concentrates at the edges of a conductor than at anywhere else. Thus, these plates are frequently convex at the edges, which provide a more even electric field than a flat disk.

These plate electrodes are held at a distance from the skin by an adjusting device, thus provides air as an insulating material which is most preferable one **(Figs. 5.4A and B)**.

The third type of electrode is a disk type electrode. These are having a transparent plastic cover within which a metal plate is present. These electrodes are commonly circular in shape, but special shapes can be used for irregular areas. The position of metal plate inside the disk can be adjusted. It is advisable to leave small gap between the cover and the skin to allow for the better circulation of the air.

Size of Electrodes
- If the two electrodes are of different sizes, they will behave as a capacitor of different sized plates. The different quantities of electricity are required to charge them to the same potential. This puts an uneven load to the machine. The charge will concentrate on the part of larger electrode which lies opposite to the smaller electrode **(Fig. 5.5)**.
- If the electrodes are little larger than the area treated, the outer part where the spread is greatest is deliberately not utilized. The part of the body to be heated lies in the central part of the field, which is more even. For treatment of the limbs, the electrodes should be larger than the diameter of the limbs and for trunk and back electrodes should be as large as possible **(Fig. 5.6)**.

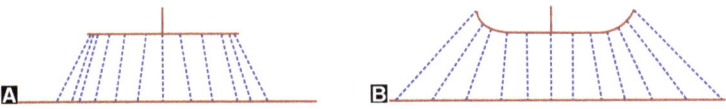

Figs. 5.4A and B: Electric fields produced by: (A) Flat; (B) Convex electrodes.

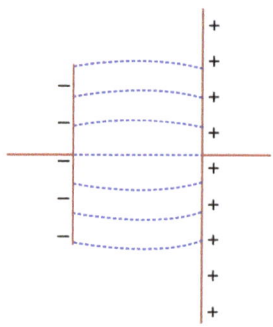

Fig. 5.5: Electrodes of different sizes.

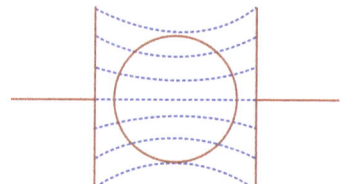

Fig. 5.6: Correct size of electrodes.

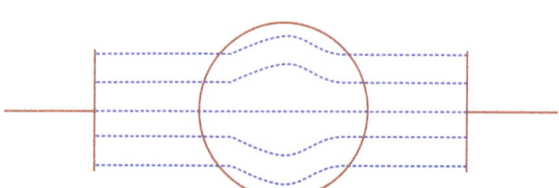

Fig. 5.7: Smaller electrodes.

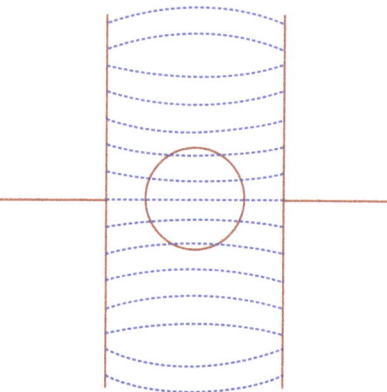

Fig. 5.8: Electrodes are too large.

- If the diameter of the electrodes is smaller than that of the limbs, the lines of forces spread in the tissues, causing more heating of the superficial than of deep structures **(Fig. 5.7)**.
- If the diameter of the electrodes is far larger than that of the diameter of the limb, some of the lines of force bypass it completely and thus results in wastage of energy **(Fig. 5.8)**.

Thus, as a general rule the electrodes should be equal in size and slightly larger than the area to be treated.

Spacing of Electrodes
- If the distance between the plates is small and the material between them is of high dielectric constant, the lines of forces spread as they pass between the plates of a charged condenser **(Fig. 5.9)**.
- When the distance between the electrodes is large, the spreading out of the electric field is minimal, while the use of spacing material of a low dielectric constant also limits the spread of the field **(Fig. 5.10)**.
- When the electrode spacing is narrow, the superficial tissue lies in the concentrated part of the field close to the electrode is thus heated more than the deep tissues, where density of the field is less **(Fig. 5.11)**.
- If the two electrodes are placed at an unequal distance from the body, the one electrode is placed nearer to the body than the other then there is a greater heating effect under the

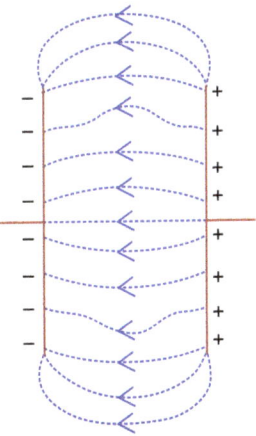

Fig. 5.9: The distance is too small.

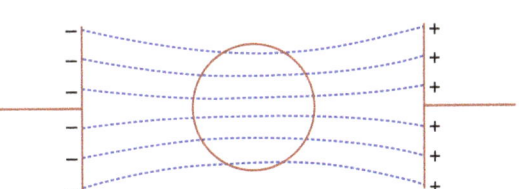

Fig. 5.10: Adequate distance.

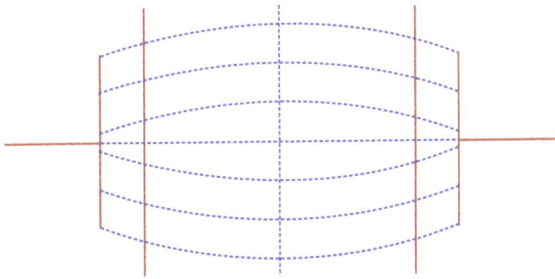

Fig. 5.11: Electrodes closer to the body.

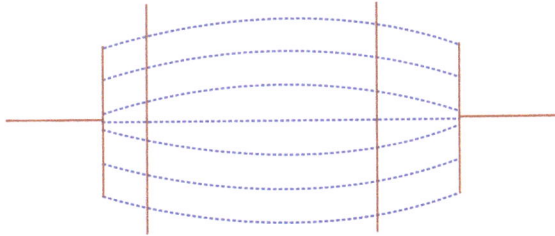

Fig. 5.12: Electrodes at uneven distance.

closer electrode than under the farther one. The lines of force under the farther electrode have a greater distance in which to spread before reaching the body than those under the nearer one. They therefore cover a greater area of skin and their density is less than under the nearer electrodes **(Fig. 5.12)**.

If the distance between two electrodes is less than the width of two pads, then the lines of force will travel through pads only and do not produce heat in the body tissues **(Fig. 5.13)**.

Thus, the spacing between the electrodes and the patient's body tissues should be as wide as possible as the machine allows and the material between the electrodes and skin should be of low dielectric constant, air being the most preferable one.

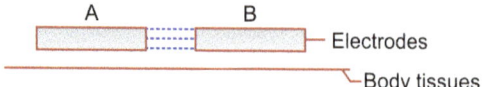

Fig. 5.13: Spacing between two electrodes.

Positioning of Electrodes
The positioning of electrodes is different for different structures to be treated. It depends upon the impedance of the structures and line of electric field. If the structures are of high impedance (fat and white fibrous tissue) the electrodes should be arranged in such a way that different tissues lies in series with each other, i.e., at right angles to electric field. If the structures are of low impedance (blood and muscles), the electrodes should be arranged in such a way that different tissues lies in parallel with each other and with the electric field.

When treatment is to be given to the ankle joint, the electrodes should be placed on the medial and lateral sides, so that tissues lie in series with each other and heating the joint is obtained. If the electrodes are placed longitudinally, tissues lie parallel to the field and heating of blood vessels and muscles is obtained. In injuries of soft tissues, longitudinal method may be used, where soft tissues need heating.

Common positioning of electrodes used are:
❖ Coplanar positioning of electrodes
❖ Contraplanar positioning of electrodes
❖ Monopolar method
❖ Crossfire technique.

Coplanar positioning of electrodes: This method is used over larger area of the body, e.g., spine and is also called parallel method of placement. It is important that the distance between the electrodes should be more than the total width of spacing otherwise electric field will not pass through the tissues at all and will pass directly between the electrodes **(Figs. 5.14A and B)**.

This method is particularly suitable for the superficial structures.

Contraplanar positioning of electrodes: This method is used for those structures where through and through heating is required, e.g., hip and shoulder joint. The electrodes are placed over the opposite aspects of the limb or joint, i.e., medial and lateral aspect or anterior or posterior aspect.

This method is particularly suitable for the deeper structures or tissues.

Monopolar method: Only one electrode is placed over the treatment area and other electrode is placed at a distance site or is not used at all. The electrode used produces a radial electric field **(Fig. 5.15)**.

The density of electric field becomes less as the distance from the electrode increases and thus the heating is superficial.

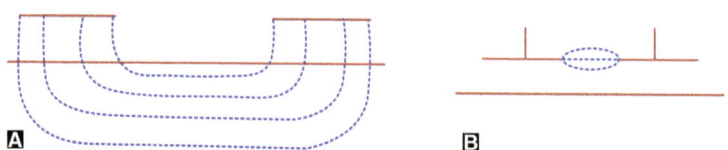

Figs. 5.14A and B: Coplanar arrangement of electrodes: (A) Correct spacing; (B) Incorrect spacing.

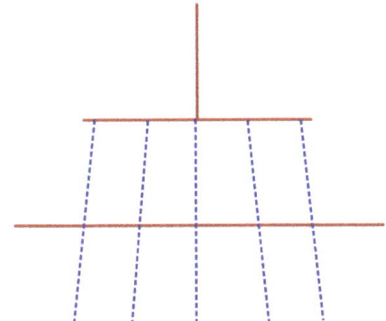

Fig. 5.15: Monopolar electrode with radial effect.

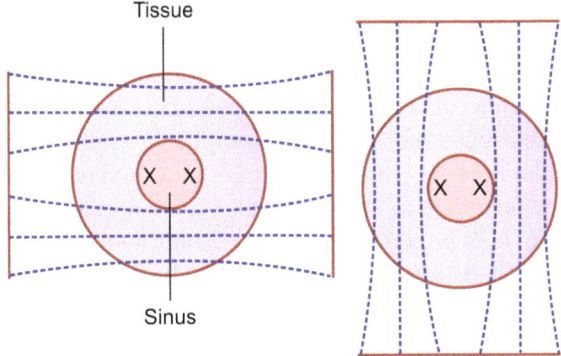

Fig. 5.16: Crossfire technique for sinus.

Crossfire technique: In this technique, half of the treatment is given with the placement of electrodes in one direction, i.e., medial or lateral aspect and another half is used with the placement of electrodes in other direction, i.e., anterior or posterior aspect. This method is commonly used for the treatment of the knee joint, sinuses (frontal, maxillary and ethmoidal) and for pelvic organs **(Fig. 5.16)**.

Cable Method or Inductothermy

In this method, a thick insulated cable is used for treatment purposes. Electric field or magnetic field or both are achieved by the use of cable method. When the high frequency current oscillates in the cable, a varying electrostatic field is set up between its ends and a varying magnetic field around its center. The cable is coiled around the patient's body and is separated from the patient's body by a layer of insulating material.

The electrostatic field: Electrostatic field is produced at the end of the cable and the effects are similar when the current is applied by a condenser method. The heating is more in superficial tissues and those of low impedance, also some heating is obtained in deeply placed structures of high impedance if suitable placing is done.

The magnetic field: The magnetic field varies as the current oscillates and an EMF is produced by electromagnetic induction. If the conductor is a solid piece of conducting material, the EMF gives rise to eddy currents. Such currents are produced especially in the tissues which lie close to the center of the cable. The eddy currents produce heat and their effect confines only to the tissues of low impedance, thus heating of fat and white fibrous tissue is avoided. The currents are produced primarily near the surface of the conductor, where the magnetic field is strongest and the superficial tissues are heated most. Some heat is transferred to adjacent tissues by conduction and by the circulation of blood, but the heating effect is primarily on superficial tissues of low impedance.

Effect of relative fields: If the cable is coiled around the material of high impedance the electric field predominates, while the current produced by the electromagnetic induction are strongest when the material around which the cable is of low impedance. Thus, when treating an area of high impedance, particularly if deep heating is required, the electric field between the ends of the cable is utilized in preference to the magnetic field at its center. When treating an area of low impedance, particularly if superficial heating is required, the eddy currents setup by the magnetic field at the center of the cable are utilized in preference to the electric field. Alternatively, both the effects can be utilized at the same time; if the whole cable is arranged in relationship to the patient's tissues, an electric field is setup between its ends and eddy currents near its center.

For treatment of the limbs, the cable is coiled around the part. If the area is large, e.g., the whole of a limb all the cable is used and both electrostatic and electromagnetic fields are utilized. When treating the smaller area the whole of the cable may not be required; either the ends or the center may be used, according to the depth of the heating required and the impedance of the tissues. If the area is of high impedance the electrostatic field between the ends of the cable is most effective, e.g., for the knee joint, two turns may be made with each end of the cable, which lies above and below the joint. When treating two joints both shoulders, a few turns may be made with one end of the cable round one joint and a similar arrangement of the other end around the other joint. If the area to be treated is of low impedance, e.g., muscles and blood the eddy currents produce satisfactory heating so the center of the cable is used.

To treat a flat "surface" like back, the cable can be arranged in a flat helix, two helices can also be made from its ends, or a grid arrangement may be used. With the grid the magnetic field is complex and does not penetrate deeply into the tissues, so heating is mainly by the electric field, but with the other two methods the tissues are heated with eddy currents. This flow at right angles to the magnetic lines of forces and the heating produced by a single helix is therefore in the form of a hollow ring in the tissues lying under the coil.

Advantages of Cable Method

The cable method is useful:
- For the treatment of an extensive area which could not be included between the condenser electrodes
- When the area is irregular
- When it is desirable to avoid heating of the subcutaneous fat.

Disadvantage of Cable Method

The impossibility of using air spacing:

Monode electrode: The main benefit of using a monode electrode is that it uses air spacing. The monode works on the principle of a cable. It consists of a flat helix of a thick wire mounted on a rigid support, a condenser is lying parallel with the coil making it possible to use shorter length of wire than that required for the cable. Heating is produced by the eddy currents.

Dosage

The treatment dosage should have an intensity that causes sufficient warmth (thermal dosage) of the tissues and the duration of the treatment should be 20-30 minutes. The treatment may be given daily or on an alternate day.

As a general rule, for the treatment of acute inflammation or any recent injury the intensity of the treatment should be less but it should be carried out more frequently, i.e., twice daily. The current used may be that which produces mild warmth (midthermal) and may be reduced to the point at which no warmth is felt (subthermal or athermal). The duration of treatment is reduced to 5-10 minutes.

Physiological Effects of Heating the Tissues

The principal effect of SWD to the body is heating of tissues. This is the modality which provides deepest heating of the tissues. The main physiological effects due to heating of the body tissues are:
- Effects on metabolism of the body
- Effects due to increased blood supply
- Effects of heat on the nervous tissues
- Effects of heat on the muscular tissue
- Effects of heat on the sweat glands.

Effects on Metabolism of the Body

As the van't Hoff's statement states that "any chemical change which is capable of being accelerated is accelerated by the rise in temperature". Therefore, all the chemical changes of the body that can be accelerated are accelerated by heat. The metabolism of the body itself is accelerated. Both the anabolism as well as catabolism is enhanced. The oxygen supply to the tissues is increased, removal of waste products is enhanced, the nutritional supply to the tissues is increased and thus the healing of damaged tissues is accelerated.

Effects Due to Increased Blood Supply

The heat has a direct effect on the blood vessels. It causes vasodilatation of the vessels in the area of heating. Stimulation of the superficial nerve endings can also cause reflex dilatation of the arterioles. As a result of vasodilatation, there is an increased flow of blood through the area, so that the necessary oxygen and nutritive materials are supplied and the waste products are removed. Also, there is increased filtration and diffusion through different membranes and faster transport of some enzymes. Thus, this results in faster healing of the damaged tissues and early recovery from the injury.

When there is generalized vasodilatation, the peripheral resistance is reduced. Heat also reduces viscosity of the blood and thus there is generalized fall in the blood pressure.

Effects of Heat on the Nervous Tissues

Heat alters conduction in the nervous tissues. It produces a sense of sedation. Perception of pain is also reduced as it enhances the pain threshold.

A high frequency current does not stimulate motor or sensory nerves. The shorter the impulse of the current, the less is the effect on the nervous tissue. Thus, when a current of high frequency is used, there is no discomfort in the body and also no contraction of muscle is produced.

Effects of Heat on the Muscular Tissue

Increased blood supply provides optimal environment for the muscles to contract. It provides fresh nutrients, oxygen and removes the waste products faster. Thus, efficacy of muscles to contract is increased. Rise in temperature also induces muscle relaxation due to faster removal of the waste products.

Effects of Heat on the Sweat Glands

The heat has an effect on the sweat glands as well. As the heated blood is circulated throughout the body, it stimulates the centers for the regulation of the sweat. The production of sweat is increased and thus there is increased elimination of waste products.

Therapeutic Effects of Shortwave Diathermy

Effects on Inflammation

The dilatation of arterioles and capillaries results in an increased flow of blood to the area which increases supply of oxygen and nutritive material. This increased flow of blood enhances the supply of more antibodies and white blood cells. The dilatation of capillaries increases the exudation of fluid into the tissues and this is followed by increased absorption which along with the increased flow of blood through the area assists in the removal of waste products. These effects help to bring about the resolution of inflammation. Additional effects are obtained when the inflammation is associated with bacterial infection which is discussed in the next point.

In the acute stages of inflammation, treatment should be given with a caution, where there is already marked vasodilatation and exudation of fluid, as an increase in these processes may aggravate the symptoms. In the subacute stages, stronger doses may be applied with considerable benefit. When the inflammation is chronic, a thermal dose of fairly long duration must be used to have effective.

Shortwave diathermy is particularly valuable for lesions of deeply placed structure such as the hip joint, which cannot easily be affected by other forms of electrotherapy and radiation. It is of valuable use, in conjunction with other forms of physiotherapy, the use of various inflammatory conditions (e.g., rheumatoid arthritis, capsulitis and tendonitis) and for the inflammatory changes which frequently occur in the ligaments surrounding osteoarthritic joints.

Effects in Bacterial Infections

Inflammation is the normal response of the tissues to the presence of bacteria, the principal features being vasodilatation, exudation of fluid into the tissues and an increase in the concentration of white blood cells and antibodies in the area. Heating the tissues augments these changes and so reinforces the body's normal mechanism of body dealing with the infecting organisms; therefore SWD is of value in the treatment of bacterial infections like boils, carbuncles and abscesses. Treatment in the early stages may occasionally bring about resolution of the inflammation without pus formation occurring; failing this, the development of the inflammatory response is accelerated. Until there is free drainage, the treatment should be given cautiously, as in all cases of acute inflammation. When the abscess is draining freely, stronger doses may be applied, the increased blood supply assisting the healing processes once the infection has been overcome.

In some cases, SWD appears to aggravate the condition, but increased discharge for a few days is an indication of acceleration of the changes occurring in the tissues, and not a contraindication to treatment. However, should be increased discharge persist it may be an indication that the body's defense mechanism is already taxed to its uttermost, so that it is impossible to reinforce its action. This is most liable to occur in cases of long-standing infection and under these circumstances no benefit is derived from the application of SWD.

Bacteria can be destroyed by heat, but it would be impossible to raise the body tissues to the necessary temperature without causing damage to the tissues themselves.

Relief of Pain

Mild degree of heating is found to be effective in relieving pain, presumably as a result of a sedative effect. It has been suggested that pain may be due to the accumulation of waste products in the tissues due to metabolism and that the increased flow of blood through the area assists in removing these substances. Strong superficial heating probably relieves pain by counter-irritation, but it is unlikely that the heating of the skin produced by SWD is great enough to have this effect. When pain is due to inflammatory processes, resolution of the inflammation is accompanied by relief of pain. SWD assists in bringing about the resolution of inflammation, and so indirectly helps in relieving the pain. However, strong heating in these cases may cause an increase of pain, especially in acute inflammation, if the increased blood flow and exudation of fluid cause an increase of tension in the tissues.

Thus, when SWD is used in the treatment of inflammatory conditions and in post-traumatic lesions, it brings about relief of pain in addition to its other beneficial effects. This is particularly valuable when the treatment forms a preliminary to active exercise, which can then be performed more efficiently.

Effects on Muscle Tissue

The heating of the tissues induces muscle relaxation, so SWD may be used for the relief of muscle spasm associated with inflammation and trauma, usually as a preliminary in conduction with the movements. Increased efficiency of muscle action should also aid the satisfactory performance of active exercises.

Traumatic Conditions

The beneficial effects of SWD on traumatic lesions are similar to those produced in inflammation. The exudation of fluid (followed by increased absorption) and the increased flow of blood through the area assist in the removal of waste products, while the improved blood supply makes available more nutritive materials, so assisting the healing processes.

Recent injuries should be treated with the same caution as acute inflammation, as excessive heating is liable to increase the exudation of fluid from the damaged vessels. Stiff joints and other after-effects of injury require stronger doses, the treatment being a preliminary to the exercise which is usually the essential part of the treatment.

Reducing Healing Time

To promote the healing of a wound or injured tissue, an increased blood supply to the tissues may be of benefit, provided that the vascular responses to heat to the tissues are normal.

Dangers of Shortwave Diathermy

Burns

Shortwave diathermy can cause burn therefore, the word "burn" must be used to warn the patient of this possible danger. In milder cases, tissue is not destroyed but a bright red patch, i.e., erythema is seen and blistering is liable to occur. In severe cases, there is coagulation and therefore destruction the tissues, and then burn appears as a white patch surrounded by a reddened area.

Burns may arise from various causes: Concentration of the electric field, use of excess current, impaired blood flow, hypersensitivity of the skin, or leads touching the skin.

Concentration of the electric field: Burn is caused due to concentration of the electric field in the tissues. This causes overheating of the tissues in the affected area. It may be due to the presence of a small area of material of high dielectric constant within the field, such as metal or moisture on the tissue, also due to inadequate spacing over a prominent area of tissue, or to an electrode being badly placed so that one part of it lies nearer to the tissues than the rest.

In some cases, metal may be embedded in the tissues, e.g., in internal fixation of fractures, and the danger of causing burns then varies with the position in which the metal lies. It is the concentration of the electric field, not overheating of the metal, which is dangerous. If a narrow strip of metal lies parallel to the lines of force, it provides a pathway of low impedance for a considerable distance and is liable to cause serious concentration of the field. If, however, it lies across the field, the easier pathway is provided only for a short distance, and being wide is much less likely to cause concentration of the lines of force. In these cases, there is considerable danger of burn, so heating such an area should be avoided.

Excess current: The patient's sensation is the only indication of the intensity of the application in SWD. If excess current is applied due to any of these causes such as: Patient does not understand the sensations that he should experience, or cutaneous sensation is defective or if he fall asleep during treatment, burn could result. Also, if the intensity of the current is increased quickly at the beginning of the treatment a dangerous level may be reached, and failure to reduce the current immediately if the heat becomes intense may result in a burn. The patient should be told that he should feel mild, comfortable warmth such as if blowing on the dorsum of hand with the mouth and not more than that, otherwise a burn could result.

Impaired blood flow: The blood circulating through the tissues normally dissipates the heat and thus prevents excessive rise of temperature in the area being treated. If the blood flow is impaired due to any of the causes such as by pressure on a bony point, tight garments, impaired vascularity or arterial disease, etc., a burn may occur.

Hypersensitive skin: If the skin has become hypersensitive, e.g., by X-ray therapy or cobalt therapy or due to recent use of liniment, a dose of diathermy which would normally be safe may cause damage.

Leads touching to the skin: If a lead approaches close to the patient's tissues and touches the skin, heat may be produced in the area and it may be sufficient to cause burn.

If a burn does occur, in any case it must be reported immediately to the head of the physiotherapy department. Efforts should be made to minimize the effects of burn. Medical advice should be taken. As far as possible the burn must be kept clean and dry, usually being protected with a dry sterile dressing. Legal advice from a lawyer to protect oneself may also be taken, otherwise patient may take the concerned staff to the consumer forum.

Scalds

A scald is caused by moist heat. It may occur if the area being treated is damp or moist, e.g., due to perspiration, or if damp towels are used for treatment. If the moisture is not localized it does not cause concentration of the field. But if it is localized, it may become overheated and may cause scalding of the skin.

Electric Shock

An electric shock can occur if contact is made with the apparatus circuit with the current switched on. It is less possible in modern systems to come in contact with the apparatus circuit. An electric shock could result from contact with the casing of the apparatus if casing is not proper or plastic coating is not made on the apparatus.

Overdose

Overdose of application of treatment may cause an increase in symptoms, especially pain and is most liable to occur when there is an acute inflammation within a confined space. It can occur under other circumstances as well and any increase in pain following treatment is an indication to reduce the intensity of subsequent applications.

Precipitation of Gangrene

Heat accelerates chemical changes, including metabolic processes in the tissues, so increasing the demand for oxygen. Normally, this is supplied by the increased blood flow, but should there be some impedance of the flow of arterial blood to the tissues the demand of oxygen is not met and gangrene is liable to develop. Consequently, heat should never be applied directly to an area with an impaired arterial blood supply.

Faintness

Faintness is produced by hypoxia of the brain following a fall in blood pressure. It is particularly liable to occur if, after an extensive treatment, the patient rises suddenly from the reclining to the erect position from the bed. So, patient should not be allowed to rise up suddenly from the bed after the treatment. Patient should be allowed to drink water after treatment.

Giddiness

Any electrical current applied to the head may cause giddiness due to its effects on the contents of the semicircular canals. All diathermic treatments to the head should be given with the patient fully supported and, if possible, with the head in a horizontal or an erect position. Also, it is wiser to avoid concentration of diathermy currents to the eyes because of poor dissipation of heat from the eyes.

Dangers to Hearing Aids or Cardiac Pacemakers

As the SWD produces substantial amount of radiofrequency energy, it may cause interference with the electrical implants such as hearing aids or cardiac pacemakers. Such patients those who are using hearing aids or cardiac pacemakers should not be treated with SWD and should not be allowed to come in close proximity of the apparatus for at least 2 m.

Dangers to Other Equipments

Low frequency stimulators or interferential therapy apparatus are also at risk with the SWD. There are also chances of interference and damage to these low frequency stimulators or interferential therapy apparatus. Therefore, these apparatus must not be kept in the close proximity of the SWD and at least a distance of 2 m must be maintained.

Contraindications of Shortwave Diathermy

- *Open wound or hemorrhage:* Diathermy should never be applied to the open wounds. It should also be not applied where hemorrhage has recently occurred, because diathermy causes further dilatation of the blood vessels.
- *Metal in the tissue:* Diathermy should also be not applied in cases of metals in the tissues because diathermy currents may get concentrated in the metals and excessive heating may cause burn.
- *Disturbed skin sensation:* Skin should always be checked for its sensation. Diathermy may cause burn in cases of disturbed skin sensation.
- *Venous thrombosis or thrombophlebitis:* Diathermy is contraindicated in the cases of venous thrombosis or thrombophlebitis around the area drained by the vessel because the increased flow of blood may dislodge the clot or aggravates the inflammation.
- *Arterial disease:* Diathermy should never be applied to the area having defective arterial supply. The inability of the circulation to disperse the heat could result in an increase of temperature in the area, which could lead to burn. Also, if demand of nutrients cannot be fulfilled with its supply then gangrene can precipitate.
- *Menstruation:* Diathermy should never be applied to the abdomen during menstruation because hemorrhage may further increase.
- *Pregnancy:* Diathermy should never be applied to the abdomen or pelvis during pregnancy.
- *Tumors:* Diathermy should not be applied to the area of tumor growth because the temperature could accelerate the growth of the tumor. Further, due to increased circulation metastasis, i.e., spreading of tumor may occur.
- *Deep X-ray or cobalt therapy:* Due to deep X-ray or cobalt therapy the devitalization of tissues occurs, which could lead to further damage due to the application of SWD.
- *Children:* SWD should also be avoided in children.
- *Mentally-retarded patient:* It is unsafe to give SWD to mentally retarded patients who are unable to understand the degree of heating required and the necessity to report excessive heating.
- *Unconscious patient:* Diathermy should never be given to an unconscious patient.
- *Epileptic patients:* Diathermy should also be avoided in epileptic patients.
- *Uncooperative patient:* SWD should also be avoided in uncooperative patient.

Pulsed Shortwave Diathermy

Pulsed SWD is referred to as pulsed electromagnetic energy or field, diapulse, etc., which is created by simply interrupting the output of continuous SWD at regular intervals. It was invented in 1930s, but became popular only after 1950s. The frequency of pulsed SWD is same as that of continuous SWD, i.e., 27.12 MHz but interpulse interval or off-time is added to it. Pulse frequency is between 25 and 600 pps, pulse width is between 20 and 40 ms (65 ms is most commonly used). By adding rest period to the treatment, the average power is considerably reduced. The heat developed in the tissues is dispersed by the circulation and treatment is thus referred to as *nonthermal treatment.* Pulsed SWD increases the cellular activity, increases the reabsorption of hematoma, reduces inflammation, reduces swelling and increases the repair process. The treatment duration varies from 15 to 60 minutes and indications and contraindications are almost similar to that of SWD.

MICROWAVE DIATHERMY

Microwave diathermy can be defined as the use of microwaves for various therapeutic purposes. Microwave diathermy has a much higher frequency and a shorter wavelength than shortwave diathermy. The frequency and wavelength ranges from 300 MHz to 300 GHz and 1 cm to 1 m. The commonly used frequencies are 2,456 MHz, 915 MHz and 433.92 MHz with wavelengths of 12.24 cm, 32.79 cm and 69 cm, respectively. Therefore, it ranges between infrared and SWD. The microwave diathermy can directly penetrate into the tissues to some extent and can be strongly absorbed by water and high vascular tissues.

Production of Microwave

The microwave diathermy apparatus is connected to main AC which provides it a current of 50 Hz and a voltage of 220 V **(Fig. 5.17)**. It is not possible to produce microwaves by mechanical means and hence a special type of thermionic valve is used which is called a *magnetron*. The primary function of a magnetron is to produce high frequency current required for the production of microwaves. Magnetron is a special type of thermionic valve characterized by centrally placed cathode and a surrounding circular metal anode. Coaxial cable carries these high frequency currents from the magnetron and passes it to the antenna of the emitter. Emitter is also known as director or applicator. Emitter consists of antenna and reflector. Antenna is mounted in front of a metal reflector. Reflector is a metal plate which directs the microwaves in only one direction. Emitters are of various size and shapes. Basically emitters are either circular in shape or rectangular shape. The circular emitter produces microwaves which are circular in cross-section and denser in periphery than in the center. Rectangular emitter produces waves which are oval at the cross-section and denser at the center than at the periphery **(Figs. 5.18A and B)**.

The distance between the emitter and the skin should be about 10–20 cm from the body. However, this can vary according to the size of the emitter, the part to be treated and the condition of the patient. If a small area is to be treated, emitter should be closer to the skin (around 2–5 cm). If the area to be treated is larger, the distance can be increased to around 10–15 cm.

Physiological and Therapeutic Effects

Physiological and therapeutic effects of microwave diathermy are same as that of SWD. Microwave diathermy is useful more in local conditions rather than in the generalized conditions. The amount of heat production is more in muscles as compared to SWD since the heat production by the microwaves depends on the watery content of the tissues. The depth of penetration of microwaves in the tissues is less and is ranges between 3 mm and 3 cm, while short

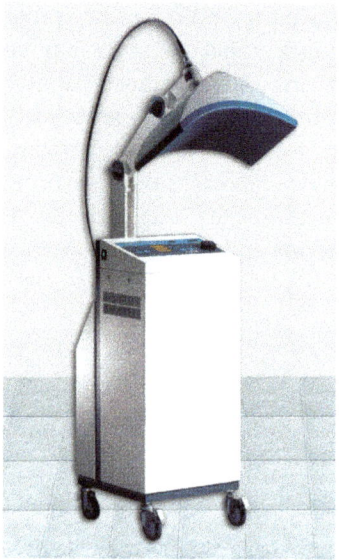

Fig. 5.17: Microwave diathermy.

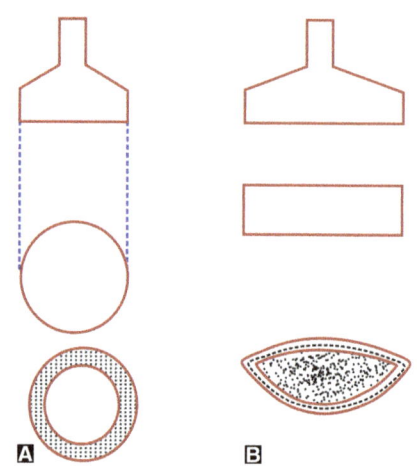

Figs. 5.18A and B: Different emitters: (A) Circular; (B) Rectangular.

wave can penetrate as deep as 6 cm. Other therapeutic effects are the same as of SWD. It can be used in traumatic and inflammatory conditions, degenerative arthropathies, enthesopathies, arthritis of joints, etc. It is useful in the treatment of soft tissues and superficial joints because it is generally possible to irradiate only one aspect of the body at a time. Microwave diathermy is more useful in the treatment of superficial tissues those with high fluid content.

Dosage: In acute conditions—5-10 minutes and in chronic conditions 15-30 minutes, depending upon the condition of the patient and the type of applicator used. The patient should feel comfortable warmth as observed while blowing from the mouth on the dorsum of the hand. Power output can be around 200 W so as to raise the body temperature in the therapeutic range of 40-45°C. Treatment may be given daily or on alternate days.

Dangers and Contraindications

- *Burns:* Microwave diathermy can cause burn on the superficial tissues. Skin must be kept dry to avoid burns. Water is heated more rapidly by microwaves because of high degree of absorptive power of these waves. The patient's perception of heat is the only guide of the treatment. The patient must be asked for comfortable warmth. In all cases of diminished sensations, microwave diathermy should be avoided.
- *Metal in the tissue:* Microwave diathermy should not be applied in cases of metals in the tissues because diathermy currents may get concentrated in the metals.
- *Dangers to hearing aids or cardiac pacemakers:* Such patients those who are using hearing aids or cardiac pacemakers should not be treated with microwave diathermy and should not be allowed to come in close proximity of the apparatus.
- *Eyes:* Treatment on eyes should be avoided. There may be concentration of heat in the intraocular fluid.

- *Circulatory defects:* Patients with hemorrhage, vascular disease, thrombosis or thrombophlebitis must not receive microwave diathermy.
- *Menstruation:* Diathermy should never be applied to the abdomen during menstruation because hemorrhage may further increase.
- *Pregnancy:* Diathermy should never be applied to the abdomen or pelvis during pregnancy.
- *Tumors:* Diathermy should not be applied to the area of tumor growth because the temperature could accelerate the growth of the tumor. Further, due to increased circulation metastasis, i.e., spreading of tumor may occur.
- *Deep X-ray or cobalt therapy:* Due to deep X-ray or cobalt therapy the devitalization of tissues occurs, which could lead to further damage due to the application of microwave diathermy.
- *Patient at particular risk:* Treatment should be avoided in children, mentally retarded patients, uncooperative patient or epileptic patient because these patients cannot appreciate the amount of heat required for the treatment and thus cannot report for the overheating.

LONGWAVE DIATHERMY

Longwave diathermy is the use of high frequency electromagnetic waves of the frequency 1 MHz and wavelength 300 m.

It has advantage over shortwave diathermy in that:
- Longwave diathermy has less frequency (1 MHz) than SWD (27.12 MHz), so there is minimal loss of energy. The power output required for LWD is 25–75 W only, whereas SWD generates 250–1,000 W of power.
- Unlike SWD, LWD does not produce any interference with other equipments. It is said that LWD can be used even with patients having metal implants.
- Also, the portability and affordability of equipment is good in LWD as compared to SWD.

METHODS OF TREATMENT

TREATMENT OF THE PATIENT'S CONDITION
- Cervical spondylosis
- Periarthritis shoulder
- Low backache (LBA)
- Lumbar spondylosis
- Shortwave diathermy to hip joint
- Sciatica
- Osteoarthritis knee
- Ligament injuries
  - Medial collateral ligament injuries of knee
  - Lateral collateral ligament injuries of knee
  - Lateral ligament of ankle
  - Medial ligament of ankle
- Plantar fasciitis
- Salpingitis

PROFORMA FOR PATIENT'S ASSESSMENT

- *Receiving the patient:*
  - Good morning, I am a Physiotherapist and going to treat you. Please, cooperate with me during the treatment and wait until I go through your case sheet.
- *History taking or going through the case sheet:*
  - Name
  - Father's and mother's name
  - Age
  - Sex
  - Occupation
  - Address: Correspondence and permanent
  - Chief complaints
  - History of present illness
  - History of past illness
  - Family history
  - Social and occupational history
  - Treatment history
  - Prognosis of the treatment
  - Investigations
    - Hematological tests
    - Radiological tests: X-rays, MRI scan, etc.
    - Others: Vertebrobasilar insufficiency (VBI) syndrome—for cervical spondylosis
- *Checking for general contraindications:*
  - Hyperpyrexia
  - Hypertension
  - Severe renal and cardiac failure
  - Deep X-ray and cobalt therapy
  - Epileptic patients
  - Noncooperative patients
  - Mentally retarded patients
  - Anemia
  - Very poor general condition of the patient
  - Menstruation
- *Checking for local contraindications:*
  - Skin condition
  - Wound
  - Tumor
  - Any metal in the treatment area
  - Pregnant uterus
  - *Preparation of trays:*
    - Two test tubes:
      - One with hot water
      - One with cold water
        - Neon tube
        - Towels

- Pillows
- Sandbags
- *Preparation of the apparatus:*
  - Switching on
  - Tuning
  - Regulation of amplitude
  - Electrodes (selection of size)
  - Checking the insulation
  - Checking the plugs
  - Checking the socket
  - Checking the main wire whether it is properly fitted in the main machine.
- Gaining the confidence of the patient
- *Positioning the patient:* Comfortable with good support.
- *Preparation of the patient:*
  - Explain (remove the clothing where the area to be treated)
  - Testing the skin sensation
  - Inspection of the part to be treated
  - Palpation of the part to be treated
- *Positioning of the electrodes:*
  - Spacing of electrodes
  - Do's and don'ts about the cable. Keep the cables wide apart, do not allow the patient to touch the cables
  - Instruction to the patient
  - Warning to the patient: Not to move, not to sleep.
- *Application to the patient:*
  - Development of appropriate heat level
  - Duration
  - Safety
- *Termination:*
  - Switch off
  - Removal of the apparatus
  - Inspection of the part (erythema)
  - Palpating the part (pain).
- *Record about the patient condition:*
  - Dosage given
  - Space (narrow and wide)
  - Duration of the treatment
  - Name
  - Address
- *Knowledge of dangers:* If erythema presents, apply powder
- *Knowledge of contraindications*
- *Knowledge of effects of spacing*
- *Home instructions*

- *General informations:*

Power	–	230 V AC
Frequency	–	50 Hz
	Disk electrodes	Pad electrodes
Narrow	1 inch	2 to 4 folds
Medium	2 inches	4 to 6 folds
Wide	3 inches	6 to 8 folds

CERVICAL SPONDYLOSIS

Cervical spondylosis is the condition in which there are degenerative changes in the intervertebral joints between the bodies and disk in the cervical spine.

In early stage, it is localized in 2-3 cervical vertebrae region due to degeneration of the inter vertebral disk and there is narrowing, osteophytes formation of the anterior and posterior margins of the spine and these osteophytes causes narrowing of intervertebral foramen resulting in nerve root irritation (in later stage). It occurs early in persons involved in "white collar jobs" or those susceptible to neck strain because of keeping the neck constantly in one position while reading or writing.

Incidence
Middle-aged and elderly (30-45 years of age) women and men.
Particularly, in those occupations which involves a posture of prolonged neck flexion.

Etiology
Poor posture associated with anxiety habit occupation stress (involves) a posture of prolonged neck flexion. Typists of poorly positioned desks, writer, drivers, holding telephone on one shoulder, sleeping in awkward conditions.

Pathogenesis
Degeneration of disk results in reduction of disk space and peripheral osteophyte formation. The posterior intervertebral joints get secondarily involved and generate pain in the neck. The osteophytes impinging on the nerve roots give rise to radicular pain in the upper limb.

Clinical Features
- *Pain:*
  - Headaches due to upper cervical pathology
  - Neckache due to middle cervical pathology
  - Shoulder girdle, shoulder and arm pain due to pathology from C4 to T2 (radiating pain)
- Neck postural muscles are often weak
- Tenderness in the cervical spine present
- Limitation of all movements of cervical spine.

Investigations
- *X-rays:*
  - Osteophytes formation (new growth)
  - Narrowing of joint space
  - Narrowing of intervertebral foramen.

- ❖ *Treatment:* Physiotherapy
- ❖ *Relief of pain:*
  - Analgesics, SWD to neck and intermittent cervical traction
  - Shoulder bracing and neck exercise
  - Use of cervical collar (in acute and extremely painful conditions).

Local Contraindications
- ❖ Pulmonary tuberculosis (TB)
- ❖ Hearing aids
- ❖ *VBI:* For giddiness
- ❖ Any skin diseases
- ❖ Abscess
- ❖ Recent injury

Positioning of the Patient
Arm lean sitting (neck and shoulder should be in neutral position).

Placement of Electrodes
- ❖ *Monoplanar technique:* For localized pain
- ❖ *Coplanar technique:* For radiating pain
- ❖ *Spacing:* Narrow
- ❖ *Dosage:*
  - Acute: Subthermal
  - Subacute: Mildthermal
  - Chronic: Thermal
- ❖ *Duration:*
  - Acute: 10–15 minutes
  - Subacute: 15–20 minutes
  - Chronic: 20–30 minutes

Home Instructions
- ❖ Isometric neck exercise
- ❖ Shoulder bracing exercise
- ❖ Advise not to use pillows
- ❖ Advise not to flex the head
- ❖ Teach how to read the books
- ❖ Cervical collar should be used daily
- ❖ Cervical collar should not worn during sleeping, bathing
- ❖ Cervical pillow (made of resin, like roll of towel) can be used
- ❖ Contour pillows can be used
- ❖ Advise not to take cold water bath only hot water bath can be taken
- ❖ Advise not to carry weight over the head
- ❖ Advise not to take frequent head bath
- ❖ While traveling, advise to sit in middle and on front seats

- While climbing or getting down, ask the patient to keep the neck in neutral position
- Advise not to use two wheelers on rough roads.

Effect: Relief of pain.

PERIARTHRITIS SHOULDER

Periarthritis shoulder is a condition characterized by pain and progressive limitation of some movements in the shoulder joint. In early stages, the pain is worst at night and the stiffness is limited to abduction and internal rotation of the shoulder. Later, the pain is present at all times and all the movements of shoulder are severely limited. Often, there is a history of preceding trauma. The disease is more common in diabetic patients.

Incidence: Elderly.

Clinical Features

- Pain in the shoulder joint may radiate usually to the upper and middle of the upper arm.
- Limitation of abduction and external rotation of the shoulder with forced flexion and extension movements.
- Tenderness is present in the subacromial region and in the anterior joint line.

When the condition involves the whole rotator cuff it results in total restriction of all movement of the joint. The condition is then termed as *frozen shoulder (or) adhesive capsulitis*.

Types

- *Primary idiopathic type:* Cause is unknown.
- *Secondary type:* Occurs in patients with diabetes.
  - Tuberculosis, cardiac ischemia and hemiplegia.

Investigations

X-rays are usually normal.

Treatment

- *For pain:* Analgesics, SWD and wax bath
- Mobilization is done to increase external rotation and abduction movements.
- Local infiltration of hydrocortisone and manipulation under anesthesia can also be given by orthopedic surgeon.

Local Contraindications

- Open wounds
- Abscess
- Hemorrhage
- Vascular impairment
- Metal inside the area
- *VBI:* Giddiness result
- Metal tooth
- Hearing aids
- Mastoiditis
- Hypertension

Positioning of the Patient

Sitting with back support, one pillow between the arm and trunk, and forearm rest over the thigh or table, i.e., in slight abduction of arm and flexion of forearm.

Placement of the Electrodes

Contraplanar technique [anteroposterior (AP) view].
- *Spacing:* Medium
- *Dosage:*
  - Acute: Subthermal
  - Subacute: Mildthermal
  - Chronic: Thermal
- *Duration:*
  - Acute: 10-15 minutes
  - Subacute: 15-20 minutes
  - Chronic: 20-30 minutes

Home Instructions

- Do not lift heavy weight
- Do not sleep on affected side
- Pendulum exercises or Codman's exercises
- Ask the patient to do manipulation exercise
- Do not expose the affected part to cold.

Effects: Relief of pain and increasing joint range of motion.

LOW BACKACHE

Low backache is characterized by pain which is present in the lower part of the back region. As much as 80% of the industrial population and 60% of the general population experience acute LBA at some point of time in their life.

Etiology

In the majority of the patients, the common causes of low back pain are:
- Idiopathic
- Discogenic

However, LBA could result from various other causes. It is therefore, necessary to identify and rule out the other causes of LBA before initiating physiotherapy.

Other common are:
- *Congenital:* Congenital bony malformations of vertebra, sacralization of lumbar vertebra, lumbarization of the sacral vertebra, spondylolisthesis, etc.
- *Traumatic:* Injudicious sudden lifting, fall with indirect or direct injury to the back, compression fracture of the vertebral body or transverse process, subluxation or partial dislocation of lumbar vertebral facet joints, spondylosis and spondylolisthesis.
- *Degenerative diseases:* These include annular tears, herniated nucleus pulposus, spinal stenosis, osteoarthritis, spondylosis and spondylolisthesis.

- *Inflammatory diseases:* Rheumatoid arthritis, ankylosing spondylitis, and various types of sacroiliitis.
- *Infectious diseases:* Tuberculosis, pyogenic infections of the spine, pelvic or sacroiliac joint infections.
- *Neoplastic diseases:* Benign and malignant tumors involving nerve roots, meninges and pelvic tumors.
- *Metabolic diseases:* Osteoporosis and other metabolic diseases.
- *Circulatory disorders:* Vascular insufficiency like varicose veins, abdominal aortic aneurysm.
- *Toxicity:* Chronic radium poisoning may cause aseptic necrosis of bones and pathological fractures of vertebral bodies.
- *Psychoneurotic problems:* Psychoneurotic pain also occurs due to anxiety, tension or trouble at work.

The disk lesion: If the lesion is due to the disk pathology, it is important to identify the type, extent and the site of the lesion.

The commonly affected disks in the lumbar region are the fourth and fifth disks.

The physical examination: Detailed physical examination is necessary to diagnose the exact site, extent and cause of lesion. It may consist of the following:
- Detailed history of the episode
- Examination of the posture
- Evaluation of pain characteristics
- Palpation
- Range of spinal movements
- Neurological examination
- Diagnostic physical tests
- Evaluation of the functional status

Neurological Examination

- *L4 and L5:* Prolapse of the disk between L4 and L5 will compress the L5 nerve root. There will be diminished sensation in the dorsum of the foot and anterolateral aspect of the leg, weakness of the extensor hallucis longus—ankle jerk will be normal.
- *L5 and S1:* Prolapse of the L5 and S1 disk compress the S1 nerve root. There will be diminished sensation over the lateral aspect of the leg and foot, weakness of plantar flexion of big toe and foot. Ankle jerk will be absent.

Investigations

X-ray of the spine should be done in all cases of LBA.

There are a number of advance techniques of investigations like CT scan, MRI, bone scan, etc.

Treatment

Most back pain falls in the nonspecific category of classification and has almost a set program of treatment. The following things single or in combination are generally employed in the conservative management of low back pain **(Fig. 5.19)**:
- Rest and analgesics
- Spinal extension exercises

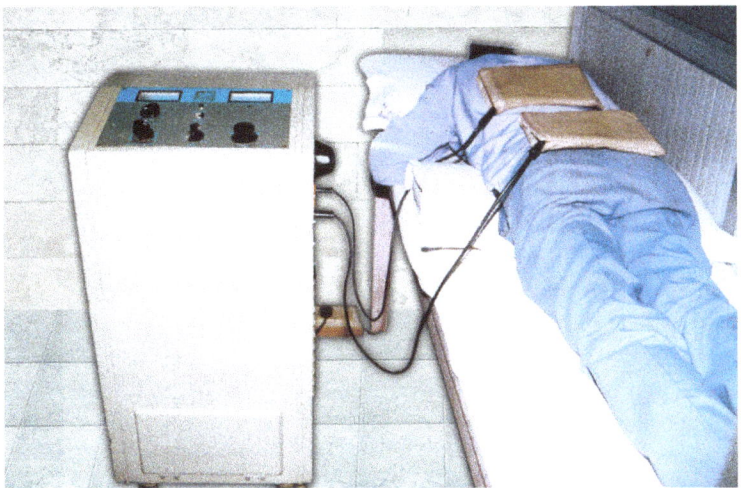

Fig. 5.19: Coplanar method.

- Physical agents—moist heat, SWD, ultrasonic therapy, infrared therapy, etc.
- Spinal traction
- Spinal support or brace
- Postural correction

Application of Shortwave Diathermy

Local Contraindications

- *Peptic ulcer:* An ulceration of the mucous membrane of the esophagus, stomach, duodenum, due to action of the acid gastric juice.
- *Duodenal ulcer:* Peptic ulcer in the duodenum
- Pelvic floor infections
- Tuberculosis
- Metal inside the tissues.

Positioning of the Patient

- *Prone lying:*
    - One pillow: Under ankle
    - Other: Under abdomen
    - Another: Under head

Placement of Electrodes

- *Monoplanar technique:* If there is localized pain pad is kept in L5 region.
- *Coplanar technique:* If there is radiating pain one over lumbar, another over thigh/calf- ankle.
- *Spacing:* Medium
- *Dosage:*
    - Acute: Subthermal
    - Subacute: Mildthermal
    - Chronic: Thermal

- *Duration:*
    - Acute: 10–15 minutes
    - Subacute: 15–20 minutes
    - Chronic: 20–30 minutes.

Home Instructions
- Patient is advised to avoid flexion strains
- Advised to avoid weight lifting
- Advised to sleep on a firm mattress and not on saggy mattress
- Advised to do spinal extension exercises
- Ask to avoid using two wheelers
- While traveling in bus sit in the middle or front seat
- Avoid prolonged standing.

LUMBAR SPONDYLOSIS

Acute degenerative disorder of the lumbar spine is characterized clinically by an insidious onset of pain and stiffness along with radiological finding of osteophyte formation.

Cause
Bad posture and chronic back strain is the most common cause, other cause includes any previous injury to the spine or an old intervertebral disk prolapse.

Pathology
Primary degeneration begins in the intervertebral joints. This is followed by a reduction in the disk space and there is formation of osteophytes in the margins. Degenerative changes develop in the posterior facet joints. The osteophytes around the intervertebral foramen may encroach upon the nerve root canal and thus interfering with the functioning of the passing nerve.

Clinical Features
The symptoms begin as LBA, initially worst during activity, but later present almost all the time. There may be a feeling of "a catch" while getting up from a sitting position, which improves as one walks a few steps. The pain may radiate down the limb up to the calf (sciatica) because of irritation of one of the nerve root. There may be complaint of transient numbness and paresthesia in the dermatome of a nerve root, commonly on the lateral side of leg or foot (L5, S1 roots) respectively.

Treatment: The principles of treatment are similar to that described under low back pain.

Application of Shortwave Diathermy

Position of the patient: Prone lying with adequate support posteriorly.
- *Methods:* Monoplanar
- *Spacing:* Narrow
- *Dosage:*
    - Acute: Subthermal
    - Subacute: Mildthermal
    - Chronic: Thermal

SHORTWAVE DIATHERMY TO HIP JOINT

Indications

- *Rheumatoid arthritis:* This is a nonsuppurative systemic inflammatory disease of acute immune response of unknown cause characterized by a symmetrical polyarthritis affecting peripheral joints and extra-articular structure.
- *Osteoarthritis, rheumatoid arthritis, fracture in neck of femur:* Inflammation of the synovial membrane which becomes edematous and thickened with inflammatory exudates. In later stages, synovium is vascular and throws fibrous exudates, which gets organized into granulation tissues and spreads over the articular cartilage, the pannus.

The articular cartilage gets loosened from the surface. A similar lytic process occurs on the deeper surface of the articular cartilage from the granulation. Lesion in the subchondral region causes the inflammation process to spread into the capsule and into the surrounding tissue.

Clinical Features

There is symmetrical peripheral polyarthritis with early involvement of small joint of the hands and wrists. The cervical spine, elbows, knee, ankles, and metatarsophalangeal joints are often affected.

Treatment

- Rest
- Splinting
- Exercise

During recovery, ice towels or cold packs (paraffin wax, SWD, hot/cold packs and hydrotherapy).

Local Contraindications

- Acute appendicitis
- Nephritis
- Menstruation
- Pregnancy
- Pelvic floor infections
- Metal inside the joint
- Infected wounds

Position of the patient: Supine lying
- *Method:* Crossfire technique
  - First half: Anterior and posterior
  - Second half: Anterior and lateral
- *Dosage:*
  - Acute: Subthermal
  - Subacute: Mild thermal
  - Chronic: Thermal
- *Spacing:* Wider

Home Instructions

- Advise the patient to walk (not long distance)
- Advise the patient to take hot water bath
- Advise the patient to avoid weight lifting
- Advise the patient to bear the weight

Sinus: A cavity or channel that permits the escape of pus or fluid.
- *Narrow:*
  - Cervical spondylosis
  - Ligament injuries
  - Hip joint, plantar fasciitis

Medium:
  - Posteroanterior shoulder
  - Sciatica

Wider:
- Osteoarthritis knee
- Salpingitis

SCIATICA

Sciatica is the condition in which there is a shooting pain along the course of the great sciatic nerve on the back of the thigh due to a pressure or irritation of the nerve roots of the sciatic nerve.
- Herniation of nucleus pulposus into the annulus fibrosis compresses the sciatic nerve root.
- Sciatica is manifested commonly in intervertebral disk prolapse. The prolapse is usually posteriorly.
  Common levels are the L4–L5 or L5–S1 level.

Causes

- Lumbar disk prolapse (LDP)
- Osteoarthrosis of lumbar spine
- Sacroiliac strain
- Osteoarthrosis or other bone diseases of hip
- Lordosis and scoliosis of lumbar spine
- Rectal tumor or chronic constipation

Neuralgia: Due to some compression force on the nerve.

Neuritis: Inflammation of the nerve sheet or connective tissues surrounding the axon.

Clinical Features

Patient is usually a young man complaining of backache and sciatica which come on after some exertion like lifting a weight.
- Pain is increased on coughing or sneezing
- *On examination:* Sciatic scoliosis is present
- In acute case, spine is rigid with very acute pain and muscle spasm
- Limitation of the movements of the spine with muscle spasm

- Straight leg raising (SLR) is limited on the side with sciatica 25°
  - Normal—45°
❖ Tenderness at the L-S junction
❖ Burning pain is severe at night
❖ Worse on any position that cause pressure on the nerve, e.g., sitting or with stretching, i.e., the heel on the ground, when in bed patient with hip and knee fixed with ankle plantar flexed.

Gait: To avoid stretching of the nerve, the patient walks on toes to the foot of the affected side with plantar flexed ankle. The hip and knee being kept bend, this produces pain while walking.
❖ Advise the patient not to walk or stand for longtime
❖ Advise to take complete rest.
   (If there is radiating pain usually in the region of leg, diagnosis should be proper).
❖ *Differential diagnosis:* Lumbar spondylosis
❖ *Positioning of the patient:* Prone lying
❖ *Placement of electrodes:*
  - Coplanar technique
  - One pad on the lumbosacral region
  - One pad on the hamstring region (also in the thigh region—if the pain is present on the anterior aspect).

Duration

10–15 minutes for all stages.

OSTEOARTHRITIS OF KNEE

Osteoarthritis is a chronic degenerative disease of joints with exacerbations of acute inflammation.
❖ *Synonyms:* Degenerative arthritis, degenerative joint disease and arthritis deformans.
❖ *Incidence:* Old age people (over the age of 50 years).

Classification

❖ *Primary:* There is no obvious cause; primary osteoarthritis is due to wear and tear changes occurring in old age due to weight bearing.
❖ *Secondary:* There is a primary disease of the joint which leads to the degeneration of the joint. Secondary osteoarthritis arises as a consequence of other conditions, such as:
  - Trauma after injury resulting in fracture of the joint surfaces
  - Dislocation—repeated minor trauma, occupational (tailors)
  - Infection
  - Deformity
  - Obesity
  - Hemophilia
  - Acromegaly
  - Hyperthyroidism

Clinical Features

❖ Pain
❖ Swelling

- Restricted movement
- Stiffness (maximum at the end of long rest)
- Muscle spasm (usually in hamstrings)
- Deformity from prolonged hamstring spasm is flexion and there is deformation of the tibia with valgus deformity.
- The joint is enlarged and there is quadriceps atrophy especially vastus medialis.
- Inability to squat in Indian toilet.

On Examination

The following findings may be present:
- Tenderness of the joint line
- Crepitus on moving the joint
- Irregular and enlarged-looking joint due to formation of osteophytes
- *Deformity:* Varus of the knee and flex-add-external rotation of the hip
- *Effusion:* Rare and transient
- Terminal limitation of joint movement
- Subluxation detected on ligament testing
- Wasting of quadriceps femoris muscle.

Investigations

Radiological Examination

The diagnosis of osteoarthritis is mainly radiological. X-rays are usually done to find changes in the joint.

The following are some of the radiological features:
- Narrowing of joint space, often limited to a part of the joint, e.g., may be limited to medial compartment of tibiofemoral component of the knee.
- *Subchondral sclerosis:* Dense bone under the articular surface
- Subchondral cysts
- Osteophyte formation
- Loose bodies
- Deformity of the joint.

SECONDARY OSTEOARTHRITIS

Alteration in the congruency of the articular surfaces of tibia, femur, and patella.

Treatment

- Rest and analgesics
- Static quadriceps exercises
- Shortwave diathermy
- Intra-articular hydrocortisone (if required).

Local Contraindications

- Hemorrhage
- Abscess

- Ulcer
- Thrombosis
- Vascular impairment
- Metal around the area
- Loss sensation
- Recent injury
- Fracture
- Recent scars
- Varicose veins
- Hemophilic arthritis

Positioning of the Patient

Long sitting with back support and the affected leg is rest on a stool with a pillow.

Placement of Electrodes

- Contraplanar technique (medial and lateral view).
- Crossfire technique (medial × lateral side; superior × inferior side).
- Duration:
  - *Acute:* 1st day to 10th day
  - *Subacute:* 2nd weeks to 6th month
  - *Chronic:* More than 6th month.

Duration of Treatment

- *Acute:* 10–15 minutes
- *Subacute:* 15–20 minutes
- *Chronic:* 20–30 minutes

Dosage

- *Acute:* Mild thermal
- *Subacute:* Subthermal
- *Chronic:* Thermal

Home Instructions

- Advise hot bath fomentation
- Teach static quadriceps exercises
- Avoid prolonged standing
- Avoid weight lifting.

LIGAMENT INJURIES

Ligaments are comprised of white connective tissue which form bands either inside or outside capsule of a synovial joint. They are tough, inelastic but flexible. So that they limit and control normal movement.

Medial Collateral Ligament Injuries of Knee

Medial collateral ligament is more commonly injured than the lateral.

Anatomy

Attachments are the medial femoral condyle and the medial tibial condyle. The deep fibers are attached to the medial meniscus. It stabilizes the knee against valgus strain.

Etiology

Cause is usually an abduction force where the foot and tibia are fixed, and the femur is forced medially.

A rotation force of the femur on the fixed tibia will also injure the ligament. A combination of these two forces produces a severe injury.

It is common in sports activities such as football, high jumping and skiing. Sometimes happens in swimming during an excessively forceful kick in breast stroke.

Sprain of Ligament

Clinical Features

- Pain over medial side of the knee
- Tenderness over the upper and lower attachment of the ligament
- Pain is increased on applying abduction stress at the knee
- No abnormal motility
- Swelling in severe stage.

Position: Patient is positioned with a leg on the table in high sitting with pillow under thigh and leg and a pad under tendo Achilles **(Fig. 5.20)**.

Treatment

- Rest (by applying posterior toe splint)
- Compression bandage for a week.

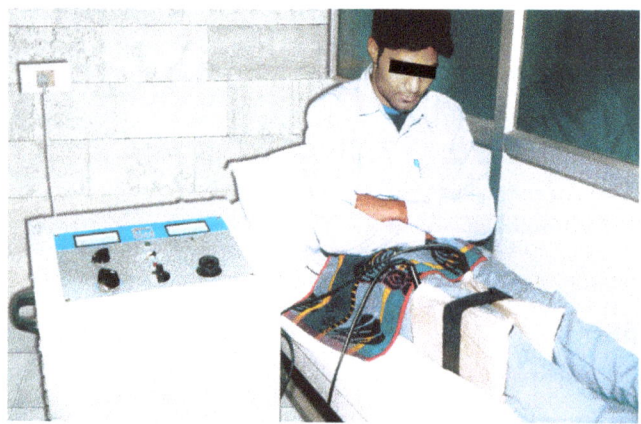

Fig. 5.20: Contraplanar method.

Partial Rupture of the Ligament

Clinical Features
- Hemarthrosis
- On applying abduction force at the knee, there will be severe pain and abnormal mobility.
- Tenderness at the attachment.

Treatment
- The knee is aspirated under aseptic precautions
- Compression bandage
- Posterior plaster slab for 3 weeks
- Quadriceps exercises.

Complete Rupture of the Ligament

This is caused by a very severe valgus strain at the knee. This may be associated with fracture of the femoral condyle of the tibia.

There is abnormal mobility, where the knee is flexed to 10°.

Clinical Features
In addition to marked swelling of the knee due to hemarthrosis, there will be abnormal abduction mobility at knee when knee is held at 10° flexion.

Investigation
X-ray: Anteroposterior view shows widening of the medial joint space.

Treatment
- Early repair should be done.
- Reconstruction of the ligament is sometimes necessary.

Lateral Collateral Ligament Injuries of Knee

Anatomy
Attachments are the lateral femoral condyle and the head of the fibula. It has no connection to the lateral meniscus. It stabilizes the knee against varus strain.

Lateral ligament injury is less common than the injury to medial ligament injury.

Etiology
It is caused by a varus stress. It may happen when there is a sideway fall for, e.g., off a motor cycle or bicycle. Severe twisting may tear this ligament.

The same types of injuries, sprain, partial rupture and complete rupture of the ligament occur due to hit on knee aspect of the weight.

Treatment is also based on the same principles as above.

Local Contraindications
- Hemorrhage
- Abscess

- Thrombosis
- Injuries
- Ulcers
- Metal around the area
- Loss of sensation
- Hemophilic arthritis
- Varicose vein
- Recent fracture
- Recent scars

Positioning of the Patient

Long sitting with back support.

Placement of the Electrodes

Contraplanar technique (medial and lateral aspect).
- *Spacing:* Uneven spacing
  - For medial ligament injury:
    - Medial aspect: Narrow
    - Lateral aspect: Wider
  - For lateral ligament injury:
    - Medial aspect: Wider
    - Lateral aspect: Narrow
- *Dosage:*
  - Acute: Mildthermal
  - Subacute: Subthermal
  - Chronic: Thermal
- *Duration:*
  - Acute: 10–15 minutes
  - Subacute: 15–20 minutes
  - Chronic: 20–30 minutes.

Home Instructions

- Avoid prolonged standing
- Avoid prolonged walking.

Lateral Ligament Injuries of Ankle

The ligaments of the ankle are injured when the plantar flexed foot is forced suddenly into inversion (lateral ligament) or eversion (medial ligament) injury of the lateral ligaments is the most common.

Anatomy

Lateral ligament of the ankle consists of three segments—(1) anterior talofibular, (2) posterior talofibular, and (3) the middle calcaneofibular.

Etiology

Acute: This injury is common in sports activities such as cross country running and hiking. It is also quite common in general terms when a person slips off a pavement or walks on uneven surfaces.

Chronic: Poor reflex coordination of peroneal to prevent twisting during walking over uneven ground.
- Poor support from footwear, torn heels or old shoes which have become too large.
  - Prolonged sitting with feet turned in (causes lengthening).

Clinical Features
- Pain
- Swelling in the lateral aspect of the ankle
- Loss of function.

Investigations

X-rays: Widening of lateral half of the joint spaces.

Treatment

First aid: Ice, compression bandage, elevation of the part, strapping (everted).

Complications

Chronic pain, instability at the ankle.

Medial Ligament Injuries of Ankle

Less common, sudden eversion violence causes injury to medial ligament.
Tenderness is at the upper attachment of the medial ligament to the medial malleolus.
- *Spacing:* Uneven spacing
  - For medial ligament injury:
    - Medial aspect: Narrow
    - Lateral aspect: Wider
  - For lateral ligament injury:
    - Medial aspect: Wider
    - Lateral aspect: Narrow

Treatment

Strapping (inverted position)

PLANTAR FASCIITIS

Plantar fasciitis is an aseptic inflammation of the plantar fascia occurs in persons who do a great deal of standing and walking. It causes severe pain and tenderness over the sole of foot.

Incidence

Middle-aged adults on injury or a pulling on plantar aponeurosis. Repeating attack during physical training produces ossification in the postattachment of the plantar aponeurosis forming a calcaneal spur.

Clinical Features
- Pain is present in one or both heels.
- Pain is worse in early morning and patient is unable to bear weight on the foot while getting up from bed.
- Tenderness on pressure over the medial tuberosity of calcaneum.

Procedures
- Receiving the patient
- Case sheet reading
- Preparation of trays
- Preparation of apparatus
- Position of the patient
- Preparation of the patient
- Position of the electrodes
- Application of the modality.

Investigations
X-rays: In the lateral view, heel show calcaneal spur (spur occurs as a reaction to the local inflammation of the plantar fascia and ligaments with deposition of calcium at the side of ligamentous attachments).

The severity of the pain is not proportionate to the size of the spur.

Treatment
Hot water fomentation: Shortwave diathermy, footwear with microcellular rubber (MCR).
- Pain is relieved by addition of soft foam pad in the heel of the footwear
- Ultrasound therapy
- Hydrocortisone injection
- Surgical removal of spur.

Plantar fasciitis is the formation of bony spur due to continuous pull of plantar aponeurosis leads to periosteal ossification.

Position of the Patient
Long sitting with back support, heels supported over a stool with a pillow.

Local Contraindications
- Hemophilia
- Recent injury
- Open wounds over foot
- Ulcer
- Cracks over heels
- Recent fracture of foot
- Trophic ulcers (plantar ulcer)
- Fissures
- Gangrene
- Thorn prick

Dosage

Thermal dose for all three stages (blow of air can be felt).

Duration

- *Acute:* 10–15 minutes
- *Subacute:* 15–25 minutes
- *Chronic:* 20–30 minutes
- *Spacing:* Narrow
  - Size of the electrodes: 2 inches
  - Placement of the electrodes: Monoplanar (close of the heel).

Home Instructions

Hot water fomentation:
- Ask the patient to avoid prolonged standing
- Ask the patient to wear MCR
- Ask the patient not to walk for prolonged duration
- Ask the patient not to walk on the improper road without MCR
- Ask the patient to avoid high-heel shoes
- Ask the patient to bear the weight.

Effects: Effect on inflammation, relief of pain.

SALPINGITIS (PELVIC INFLAMMATORY DISEASE)

It is the infection of the female reproductive organs (infection acute or chronic in the fallopian tubes).

- Salpingitis may be caused by any of pyogenic organisms that is *Streptococcus, Staphylococcus,* gonococci—suppurative salpingitis.
- Tuberculous salpingitis—(extrapulmonary tuberculosis).
- Physiologic salpingitis—pelvic inflammatory changes at the time of menstrual cycle cause pelvic pain (edema in tubes).

If salpingitis is not treated, it may lead to sterility.

Local Contraindications

- Pelvic floor infection—gonorrhea
- Epilepsy
- Hyperpyrexia
- Hypersensitive skin
- Intrauterine devices like Copper-T
- Pelvic tumors
- Pregnancy
- Infection
- Hemorrhage
- Any abscess
- Open wounds
- Deep X-ray therapy
- Cobalt therapy

Positioning of the Patient

Half lying: One pillow under head and back and other pillow under the leg.

Placement of Electrodes

Crossfire technique*:*
- *First half:* Lower abdomen × L3–L5 region
- *Second half:* L3–L5 region × gluteal sides region
- *Spacing:* Wider
- *Dosage:* Thermal dose for all three stages
- *Duration:* 10–15 minutes for all stages.

Home Instructions

Advise the patient to look for any erythema formation or burns. If there are burns, apply powder until erythema subsides.

CHAPTER 6

Radiation Therapy

INTRODUCTION

Radiation therapy may be defined as treatment by means of radiations. The term actinotherapy is also used for this.

Radiation therapy may include:
- Infrared radiations
- Ultraviolet radiations.

INFRARED RADIATIONS

The infrared rays are electromagnetic waves with the wavelengths of 750–400,000 nm and frequency 4×10^{14} Hz and 7.5×10^{11} Hz. It lies beyond the red boundary of visible spectrum. Any hot body can produce infrared rays such as the sun, electric bulb, coal fire, gas fire, etc. Sun is the natural source of infrared radiations. Infrared radiations can be produced by artificial generators. In the physiotherapy departments infrared rays are produced by two types of generators:
1. Nonluminous generators
2. Luminous generators.

Nonluminous generators provide infrared rays only whereas luminous generators emit infrared rays, visible as well as ultraviolet rays. Therefore, nonluminous generators are termed as infrared radiation generators because they emit only infrared rays. *The heat produced by luminous generator is called the "radiant heat".*

Nonluminous Generators

Nonluminous generator consists of a simple type of element or coil wound on a cylinder of some insulating material such as fireclay or porcelain. An electric current is passed through the wire, which results in the production of heat. This heat produces infrared rays which are transmitted through the porcelain. Porcelain gets heated by the method of conduction but the radiations generated in this way also include some of the visible rays. Therefore to avoid this, the coil is embedded in fireclay or porcelain or placed behind fireclay. Now the emission of rays is entirely from the fireclay which is commonly painted black and thus very few visible rays are produced. The element or the coil is thus placed at the focal point of a parabolic or spherical reflector. The reflector is mounted on a stand and its position can be adjusted as required **(Fig. 6.1)**.

In another type of nonluminous generator, a steel tube within which an electric coil is embedded on some material which is electric insulator but good conductor of heat is used. Electric current is passed through the central coil and thus heat is produced. The steel tube thus emits infrared rays.

The construction of the outer part of the apparatus should be such that the reflectors and other parts do not become excessive hot and there should be wire mesh surrounding the element.

All of these nonluminous generators take some time to get heated up for the production of infrared radiations, so they should be switched on before 5-7 minutes of the treatment.

Luminous Generators

Luminous generators emit infrared, visible and a few ultraviolet rays. These generators are in the form of incandescent lamps or bulbs. An incandescent lamp consists of a wire filament enclosed in a glass bulb, which may contain an inert gas at low pressure. The filament is a coil of fine wire which is usually made up of tungsten. Tungsten is a metal which is used because it can tolerate repeated heating and cooling. The exclusion of air prevents oxidation of the filament, which would cause an opaque deposit to form on the inside of the bulb. Incandescent bulb is usually mounted at the center of the parabolic reflector and the reflector is mounted on an adjustable stand. These luminous generators emit the electromagnetic waves with the wavelength in between 350 nm and 4,000 nm, the maximum proportion of the rays having wavelength in the region of 1,000 nm. The front of the bulb is usually red so as to filter out the shorter visible and the ultraviolet rays.

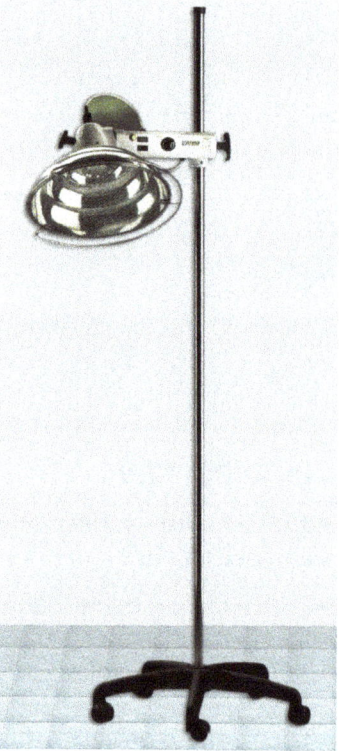

Fig. 6.1: Nonluminous infrared lamp with counter-balanced height adjustment and a wire mesh guard.

Depth of Penetration of Rays

Luminous generator produces infrared rays having wavelength between 350 nm and 4,000 nm. It can penetrate into dermis and epidermis of the subcutaneous tissue. Nonluminous generator produces infrared rays of wavelength 750-15,000 nm which can penetrate the superficial dermis only. The depth of the penetration depends upon the wavelength and the nature of the material **(Fig. 6.2)**. Thus, infrared rays produced from a luminous generator have more penetration power than that produced from nonluminous generator.

Techniques of the Treatment

The Choice of Apparatus

In most cases luminous and nonluminous generators are equally suitable, but in some instances one proves more satisfactory than the other. When there is acute inflammation or recent injury, the sedative effect of rays obtained from nonluminous generator may prove more effective for relieving pain than the counter-irritant effect of those from the luminous source. For lesions of

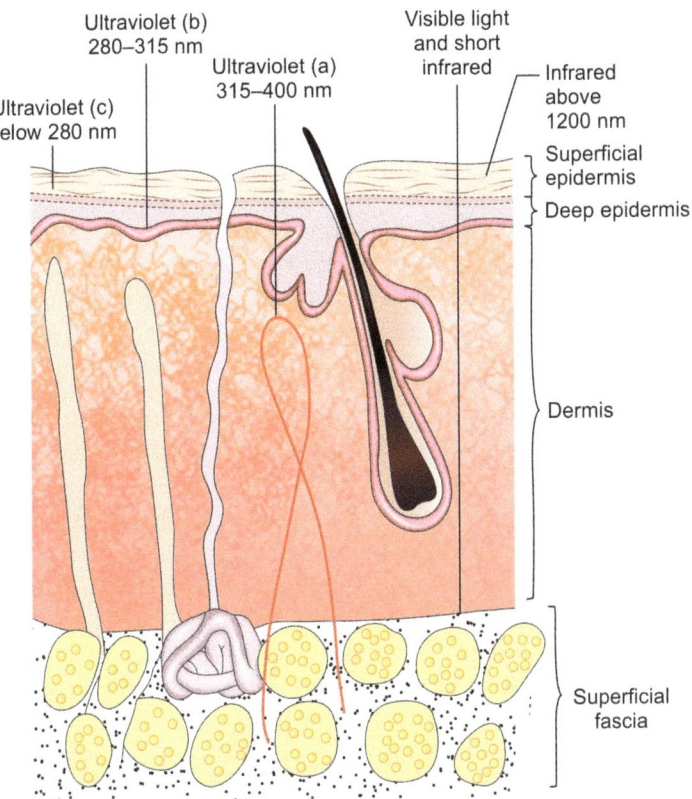

Fig. 6.2: Cross-section of the skin, showing the extent of penetration of radiations of different frequencies.

a more chronic type, the counter-irritant effect of the shorter rays may prove to be of value, and under these circumstances a luminous generator is chosen.

Selection of the generator according to the area to be treated is done. If only one surface is to be treated, a lamp of a single element mounted on a reflector is used. If several aspects are required to be irradiated, a tunnel bath is more effective. The temperature reached in a tunnel bath is higher than produced by other lamps and this may be advantage if chronic lesions are to be treated.

Before application the lamp must be checked to ensure that it is working correctly. Nonluminous generators must be switched on an adequate time before application.

Preparation of the Patient

The clothes must be removed from the area to be treated and skin is checked for its sensation against heat and cold. It is unwise to give treatment if the skin sensation is found defective. The patient should be comfortable and fully supported so that he does not move unduly during treatment. The patient is warned that he should experience comfortable warmth and he should report immediately if the heating become excessive as undue heat may cause burn. He should be instructed not to touch the apparatus and nor to move nearer to the apparatus.

Arrangement of the lamp and patient: The lamp is positioned so that it is opposite to the center of the area to be treated and the rays strike the skin at the right angle thus ensuring maximum absorption. The distance of the lamp from the patient should be measured. Optimum distance is around 50–75 cm depending upon the output of the generator.

Care must be taken that the patient's face is not exposed to infrared rays, eyes must be shielded to avoid this.

Laws Governing the Effects of Electromagnetic Radiations

When electromagnetic radiations strike or come in contact with other objects they may be reflected, refracted or absorbed. As a general rule, those radiations that have a longest wavelengths tend to have greatest depth of penetration, regardless of the frequency. It should also be noted that a number of other factors can also contribute to the depth of penetration.

Various laws regulating the depth of penetration are:
- *Arndt-Schultz principle:* It states that no reaction or changes can occur in the body tissues if the amount of energy absorbed is insufficient to stimulate the absorbing tissues. Addition of threshold energy and above quantity of energy will stimulate the absorbing tissue to normal function and if too great a quantity of energy is absorbed then added energy will prevent normal function or will destroy tissue.
- *Law of Grothus-Drapper:* It states that the rays must be absorbed to produce the effect and the effects will be produced at that point at which the rays are absorbed.
- *Cosine law:* It is also known as Lambert-Cosine law. Cosine law explains the effect of angle at which the rays strike. It states that the proportion of rays absorbed varies as per the cosine of the angle between the incident and the normal. Thus, the larger angle at which the rays strike at the body surface, lesser will be the absorption and vice versa. If the rays strike at 90° to the body part, then angle between the incident and normal are perpendicular will be zero and the cosine of 0° is maximum, i.e., 1. Thus, there will be maximum absorption if the rays that will strike the body part at 90° as per this law.
- *Law of inverse square:* Law of inverse square explains the effect of distance on the intensity of infrared rays. It states that the intensity of a beam of rays from a point source is inversely proportional to the square of the distance from the source.

Application of Infrared Treatment

At the start of the treatment exposure the intensity of the radiation should be low, but after 5–10 minutes when vasodilatation has taken place and the increased blood flow has become established, the strength of the radiation may be increased. This can be achieved by moving the lamp closer to the patient or by adjusting the variable resistance.

The Physiotherapist should be near the patient throughout the treatment session and should reduce the intensity of radiation if the heat becomes excessive. If the irradiation is extensive, it is desirable that sweating should occur to counteract any excess rise in body temperature. Sweating is encouraged if the patient is provided water to drink during treatment.

At the end of the treatment the skin should be mild red, not excessively red. After extensive irradiation the patient should not rise suddenly from the recumbent position or go out into the cold immediately.

Duration and frequency of treatment: In cases of acute inflammation or recent injuries and for the treatment of wounds, an exposure of 10–15 minutes is adequate, but it may be applied several times during the day. In cases of chronic conditions longer exposures may be used.

Physiological Effects

Infrared treatment produces heating effect in the superficial epidermis and dermis, thus resulting in vasodilatation which increases blood circulation in that area. This will lead to more oxygen supply and nutrient supply in that area leading to draining of waste products resulting in the relief of pain. The sedative effects on nerve endings lead to reduction in the muscle spasm.

Therapeutic Effects

- *In relieving pain:* Infrared radiations are effective in relieving pain. Mild heating on the superficial tissues by infrared radiations causes sedative effects on the superficial sensory nerve endings. Pain may be due to accumulation of waste products of metabolism, an increased flow of blood through the part removes these substances and thus relieves the pain.
  The pain due to acute inflammation or recent injury is relieved most effectively by mild heating. When pain is due to chronic injury or inflammation, stronger heating is required. The treatment may last up to 30 minutes.
- *In muscle relaxation:* Relaxation of muscles is achieved by heating the tissues. Mild heating by infrared causes relaxation of muscles and thus relieves spasm. Relief of pain also induces relaxation in muscles and helps relieving muscle spasm associated with injury or inflammation. Relaxation of muscles provides greater range of motion to the exercising part as it relieves muscular spasm.
- *In increasing blood supply:* Infrared radiations increase the temperature in the superficial tissues, causing vasodilatation in the superficial tissues. It provides more white blood cells and fresh nutrients to the area being treated. It also accelerates removal of waste products and helps bring about resolution of inflammation. It is most beneficial in the treatment of various arthritic conditions of joints which leads to inflammation and stiffness. Cases of postimmobilization stiffness, open wound and infections can also be effectively treated. Fresh supply of blood rejuvenates the tissues, removes waste products of metabolism and also relieves muscular spasm.

DANGERS OF INFRARED RADIATIONS

- *Burn:* Excessive heating of superficial tissues causes burn. Sensation must be checked before starting the treatment. If sensation is not proper, the patient may not appreciate the extent of heating. The burn may be caused due to the following reasons:
  - If intensity of radiation is too high
  - If sensation is not proper
  - Patient fails to report overheating
  - Unconscious patient
  - Patient moves closer to the lamp
  - Falls asleep during the treatment.

  The patient must be warned to inform undue heating immediately. The spacing must be reduced gradually in order to increase the heating. Impaired blood flow through the part, which may be due to some circulatory defect or due tight garments reduces circulation and thus causes burn.
- *Electric shock:* Electric shock can occur if some exposed part of the circuit is touched by the patient. Due to heating of the wires in the circuit, insulation of wires may go off and thus regular checking of wires is necessary to avoid electric shock.

- ❖ *Faintness or giddiness:* Extensive irradiation may cause fall in blood pressure which may result in faintness or giddiness due to hypoxia of the brain. This is particularly common when the patient rises up suddenly from the recumbent position after extensive treatment.
- ❖ *Headache:* Irradiation of the back of the head may cause headache. Headache may also occur when treatment is given during hot weather. Lots of fluid goes off the body in the form of sweating during treatment. Plenty of water needs to be replenished during or after the treatment especially in hot weather.
- ❖ *Gangrene:* Gangrene may be caused in the areas of defective arterial blood supply following prolonged irradiation by infrared radiation. Arterial supply to the area being treated needs to be proper to avoid gangrene.
- ❖ *Injury to the eyes:* Direct heating over the eyes causes drying up and thus leads to corneal or retinal burns. Eyes need to be protected following treatment to avoid injury.

Contraindications

Infrared radiations should not be applied to the areas of:
- ❖ Defective arterial blood supply
- ❖ Areas where there is danger of hemorrhage
- ❖ Defective skin sensation
- ❖ Directly over the eyes
- ❖ After deep X-ray or cobalt therapy
- ❖ Known cases of tumors.

METHODS OF TREATMENT

TREATMENT OF PATIENT'S CONDITION

- ❖ Low backache
- ❖ Postimmobilization stiffness
- ❖ Edema.

INFRARED RADIATIONS PROFORMA FOR PATIENT'S ASSESSMENT

- ❖ *Receiving the patient:* Good morning, I am a Physiotherapist and going to treat you. Please, cooperate with me during the treatment and wait until I go through your case sheet.
- ❖ *History taking or going through the case sheet*:
  - Name
  - Father's and Mother's name
  - Age
  - Sex
  - Occupation
  - Address: Correspondence and permanent

  Chief complaints:
  - History of present illness
  - History of past illness
  - Family history

- Social and occupational history
- Treatment history
- Prognosis of the treatment
- Investigations:
  - Hematological tests: Urine—albumin, sugar, etc.
  - Radiological tests—X-rays, etc.
- Any allergic reaction (e.g., hypersensitivity to sunlight)

❖ *General contraindications:*
  - Hyperpyrexia
  - Hyperesthesia
  - Dermatitis
  - Tuberculosis
  - Inflammation and injury
  - Deep X-ray therapy or cobalt therapy
  - Photosensitivity
  - Epilepsy
  - Renal or cardiac problems
  - Vascular impairment
  - Mental retardation
  - Use of sensitizers like insulin, etc.

❖ *Local contraindications:*
  - Skin conditions
  - Ulcers
  - Tumor
  - Neoplastic tissue.

❖ *Preparation of trays:* Two test tubes
  - One with hot water
  - One with cold water.

❖ *Preparation of apparatus:* The infrared lamp is conveniently positioned. Points to keep in mind are:
  - Selection of lamp
  - Switching on
  - Regulation of power
  - Checking the plugs
  - Checking the socket
  - Checking the main wire whether it is properly fitted in the main machine

❖ Gaining the confidence of the patient.

❖ *Positioning the patient:* Comfortable with good support.

❖ *Treatment:*
  - Checking of apparatus
  - Placing the lamp
  - Instructions to the patient:
    - Not to move
    - Not to touch the machine
    - Not to sleep

- *Application:* Maintain the lamp so that rays are at right angles in order to achieve maximal penetration. Record the distance between the lamp and the treatment area.
- *Termination:* Record the time duration for which lamp was applied. Switch off the lamp. Check the skin condition. Immediate increase or decrease of pain needs to be recorded.
- *Other points:*
  - Knowledge of condition
  - Record of treatment.

LOW BACKACHE

Low backache is characterized by pain which is present in the lower part of the back region. As much as 80% of the industrial population and 60% of the general population experience acute low backache at some point of time in their life.

Etiology

In the majority of the patients the common causes of low back pain are:
- Idiopathic
- Diskogenic.

However, low backache could result from various other causes. It is therefore necessary to identify and rule out the other causes of low backache before initiating physiotherapy.

Other common causes are:
- *Congenital:* Congenital bony malformations of vertebra, sacralization of lumbar vertebra, lumbarization of the sacral vertebra, spondylolisthesis, etc.
- *Traumatic:* Injudicious sudden lifting, fall with indirect or direct injury to the back, compression fracture of the vertebral body or transverse process, subluxation or partial dislocation of lumbar vertebral facet joints, spondylosis and spondylolisthesis.
- *Degenerative diseases:* These include annular tears, herniated nucleus pulposus, spinal stenosis, osteoarthritis, spondylosis and spondylolisthesis.
- *Inflammatory diseases:* Rheumatoid arthritis, ankylosing spondylitis, and various types of sacroiliitis.
- *Infectious diseases:* Tuberculosis, pyogenic infections of the spine, pelvic or sacroiliac joint infections.
- *Neoplastic diseases:* Benign and malignant tumors involving nerve roots, meninges and pelvic tumors.
- *Metabolic diseases:* Osteoporosis and other metabolic diseases.
- *Circulatory disorders:* Vascular insufficiency like varicose veins, abdominal aortic aneurysm.
- *Toxicity:* Chronic radium poisoning may cause aseptic necrosis of bones and pathological fractures of vertebral bodies.
- *Psychoneurotic problems:* Psychoneurotic pain also occurs due to anxiety, tension or trouble at work.

The disk lesion: If the lesion is due to the disk pathology it is important to identify the type, extent and the site of the lesion.

The commonly affected disks in the lumbar region are the fourth and fifth disks.

The physical examination: Detailed physical examination is necessary to diagnose the exact site, extent and cause of lesion. It may consist of the following:
- Detailed history of the episode
- Examination of the posture
- Evaluation of pain characteristics
- Palpation
- Range of spinal movements
- Neurological examination
- Diagnostic physical tests
- Evaluation of the functional status.

Neurological Examination
- *L4 and L5:* Prolapse of the disk between L4 and L5 will compress the L5 nerve root. There will be diminished sensation in the dorsum of the foot and anterolateral aspect of the leg, weakness of the extensor hallucis longus. Ankle jerk will be normal.
- *L5 and S1:* Prolapse of the L5 and S1 disk compress the S1 nerve root. There will be diminished sensation over the lateral aspect of the leg and foot, weakness of plantar flexion of big toe and foot. Ankle jerk will be absent.

Investigations
X-ray of the spine should be done in all cases of low backache. There are a number of advance techniques of investigations such as computed tomography (CT) scan, magnetic resonance imaging (MRI), bone scan, etc.

Treatment
Most back pains fall in the nonspecific category of classification and have almost a set program of treatment. The following things single or in combination are generally employed in the conservative management of low back pain:
- Rest and analgesics
- Spinal extension exercises
- Physical agents—moist heat, short wave diathermy (SWD), ultrasonic therapy, infrared therapy, etc.
- Spinal traction
- Spinal support or brace
- Postural correction.

Applications of Infrared Therapy
General Contraindications
- Hyperpyrexia
- Tuberculosis
- Inflammation
- Deep X-ray therapy or cobalt therapy
- Photosensitivity
- Epilepsy
- Renal or cardiac problems.

Local Contraindications
- Skin conditions: allergy, ulcer, etc.
- Tumor, etc.
- Abnormal skin sensation.

Checking skin sensation

Preparation of Trays
Two test tubes:
1. One with hot water
2. One with cold water.

Positioning of the Patient
Sitting position: With back unsupported and exposed toward the lamp.

Side lying position: Comfortable with support of pillows and back exposed toward the lamp.

Placement of Infrared Lamp
Place the lamp at about 1–2 feet away from the treatment area so that rays are at right angles in order to achieve maximal penetration. Record the distance between the lamp and the treatment area.

Duration
- *Acute condition:* 10–15 minutes
- *Subacute condition:* 15–20 minutes
- *Chronic condition:* 20–30 minutes.

Home Instructions
- Patient is advised to avoid flexion strains
- Advise to avoid weightlifting
- Advise to sleep on a firm mattress and not on saggy mattress
- Advise to do spinal extension exercises
- Ask to avoid two wheelers
- While traveling in bus sit in the middle or front seat
- Avoid prolong standing.

POSTIMMOBILIZATION STIFFNESS

Postimmobilization stiffness could occur due to immobilization under plaster cast or due to some arthritic conditions such as rheumatoid arthritis, gouty arthritis or infective arthritis, etc.

Aim of treatment with infrared lamp is to increase vascularity and to reduce pain.
- Receiving the patient
- History taking:
    - History of present illness
    - History of past illness
    - Family history
    - Social and occupational history

- Treatment history
- Investigations:
  - Hematological tests: Hb, TLC, DLC, ESR, etc.
    Urine—albumin, sugar, etc.
    Rheumatoid arthritis factor
  - Radiological tests—X-rays, etc.

❖ *General contraindications:*
  - Hyperpyrexia
  - Dermatitis
  - Tuberculosis
  - Inflammation
  - Deep X-ray therapy or cobalt therapy
  - Photosensitivity
  - Epilepsy, etc.

❖ *Local contraindications:*
  - Skin conditions: Hyperesthesia, etc.
  - Ulcers, tumors, etc.
  - Neoplastic tissue.

❖ *Preparation of trays:* Two test tubes:
  - One with hot water
  - One with cold water.

❖ *Preparation of apparatus:* The infrared lamp is conveniently positioned at about 1–2 feet away from the treatment area.

❖ *Positioning the patient:* Comfortable with good support and exposing the part to be treated toward the lamp.

❖ *Application:* Maintain the lamp so that rays are at right angles in order to achieve maximal penetration. Duration: 10–15 minutes and later duration can be gradually increased up to 20–30 minutes.

❖ *Check for excessive redness:* Immediate increase or decrease of pain needs to be recorded. Check for any headache, faintness or giddiness. Advise the patient not to rise suddenly from the recumbent position.

ABSORPTION OF EXUDATES OR EDEMA

The accumulation of exudates in skin and subcutaneous tissues is known as edema. It could be due to heart failure, chronic venous inefficiency or due to nephrotic syndrome. In heart failure, excessive retention of salt and water leads to edema formation. In old age there could be inferior vena cava obstruction or iliofemoral vein thrombosis leading to chronic venous inefficiency and thus edema formation. In nephrotic syndrome there is more generalized form of edema which often affects face and arms.

Aim of treatment with infrared lamp is to increase vascularity and to reduce exudates.
❖ Receiving the patient
❖ *History taking or going through the case sheet:*
  - History of present illness
  - History of past illness

- Social and occupational history
- Treatment history
- Investigations:
  - Hematological tests: Urine—albumin, sugar, etc.
- *General contraindications:*
  - Hyperpyrexia
  - Hyperesthesia
  - Dermatitis
  - Tuberculosis
  - Inflammation and injury
  - Deep X-ray therapy or cobalt therapy
  - Photosensitivity
  - Epilepsy
  - Mental retardation.
- *Local contraindications:*
  - Skin conditions
  - Ulcers
  - Tumor
  - Neoplastic tissue.
- *Preparation of trays:* Two test tubes
  - One with hot water
  - One with cold water.
- *Positioning of the patient:* Comfortable with good support.
- *Correct positioning of Physiotherapist:* Position of Physiotherapist should be in closed vicinity of the patient and at appropriate reachable distance from the lamp.
- *Placing of infrared lamp:* The infrared lamp is conveniently placed at about 1-2 feet away from the treatment area. Maintain the lamp so that rays are at right angles in order to achieve maximal penetration.
  Duration: 10-15 minutes and later duration can be gradually increased up to 20-30 minutes.
- Check for any redness or excessive rise in skin temperature. If there is excessive rise in skin temperature which could lead to burn, treatment can be discontinued. Check for any headache, faintness or giddiness. Advise the patient not to rise suddenly from the recumbent position.

THE ULTRAVIOLET RADIATIONS

Ultraviolet radiations are the electromagnetic energy which falls between visible rays and X-rays and have wavelength between 10 nm and 400 nm. Ultraviolet radiations are invisible to the human eye. Ultraviolet radiations can cause sunburn and tanning on exposure to the sunlight. Ultraviolet radiations transmit much more energy than the visible radiations. For descriptive purposes, the therapeutic part of the ultraviolet spectrum may be divided into:

- *UVA:* Wavelength 315-400 nm
- *UVB:* Wavelength 280-315 nm
- *UVC:* Wavelength below 280 nm.

PRODUCTION OF ULTRAVIOLET RADIATIONS

Although ultraviolet rays are emitted by the sun but for therapeutic purposes, some form of generator is used. Most of these generators produce ultraviolet rays from mercury. Various types of generators are used such as high pressure mercury vapor lamp, Kromayer's lamp, fluorescent tubes, theraktin tunnel, PUVA apparatus, etc. for the production of ultraviolet rays.

High Pressure Mercury Vapor Lamp

It consists of a U-shaped glass tube, filled with argon gas at a low pressure. Small amount of mercury is enclosed in the tube and the tube is sealed at both the ends **(Fig. 6.3)**.

U-shaped glass tube is used so as to act as a point source. The burner is made up of quartz as this material allows the passage of ultraviolet rays and can withstand very high temperatures with low coefficient of expansion. At the ends of the glass tube, electrodes are placed, enclosed in metal caps across which a high potential difference is applied.

Step-up transformer is used to apply high potential difference, i.e., 400 volts across the two metal caps surrounding ends of tube to ionize the argon gas.

Once the argon has been ionized, normal mains voltage between the electrodes causes the positive and negative particles to move through burner, constituting an electric current. The electrons move toward the positive terminal and positive ions move toward the negative terminal, collision between moving ions and neutral argon atom causes further ionization and a glow of discharge is produced. Also, sufficient heat is produced to vaporize the liquid mercury inside the tube and further ionization of mercury.

Thus, ultraviolet rays are produced by the process of argon ionization, mercury vaporization and mercury ionization which takes about 5 minutes to reach its peak.

When the lamp is turned off, the ions of argon and mercury recombine so that within the tube everything returns to its neutral state.

The tridymite formation: Some of the quartz changes to one another form of silica called tridymite due to very high temperature in the burner. It is harmful to the total output of ultraviolet rays as it is opaque to the rays and total output of the lamp gradually decreases as the proportion

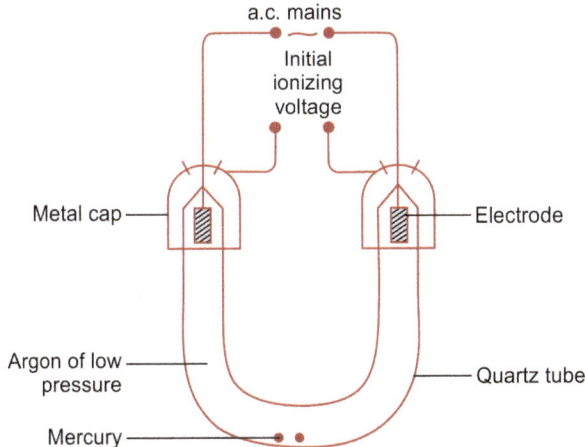

Fig. 6.3: High pressure mercury vapor tube.

of tridymite increases at around 1,000 hours of ultraviolet rays production that much tridymite can form that the whole burner tube needs to be replaced.

A variable resistance is included in the burner circuit as a method of compensation and resistance is reduced in order to increase the current intensity so as to produce adequate ultraviolet rays.

The Kromayer's Lamp

It has advantage over high-pressure mercury lamp that it can be used in contact with the body tissues as the harmful infrared rays are absorbed by the circulating water so there is no danger of burns.

Construction of Kromayer's Lamp

The Kromayer's lamp is a water-cooled mercury vapor lamp which eliminates the danger of burn and absorbs infrared rays. The high pressure mercury vapor lamp is surrounded by circulating distilled water so as to absorb infrared rays **(Fig. 6.4)**.

Kromayer's lamp can also be used to treat sinuses or deep body cavities. Direct contact method can also be used as it minimizes the danger of burn.

Fluorescent Tubes

Mercury vapor lamp has disadvantage that it produces a certain proportion of short ultraviolet rays. Modern treatment methods often require the use of long waves ultraviolet rays only without having short waves. In order to achieve this, fluorescent tubes are used. Each tube is about 120 cm long and is made up of a glass which allows long ultraviolet rays to pass. The inside of tube is coated with special phosphor. The spectrum of each tube depends upon the type of phosphor coating.

A low pressure arc is set up inside the tube by the process of ionization. Phosphor is used to absorb short wave ultraviolet rays and these are reemitted at longer wavelengths. Accurate control of emitted wavelength is possible depending upon the type of phosphor used.

Theraktin Tunnel

The Theraktin tunnel is a semicylindrical framework in which four fluorescent tubes are mounted in its own reflector in such a way that an even irradiation of a patient is achieved **(Fig. 6.5)**. Normally, fluorescent tubes with a spectrum of 280–400 nm are used.

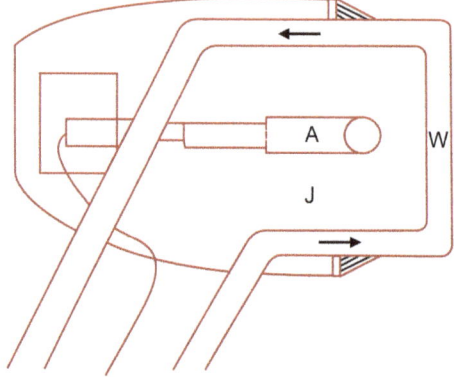

Fig. 6.4: Section through the Kromayer's lamp.

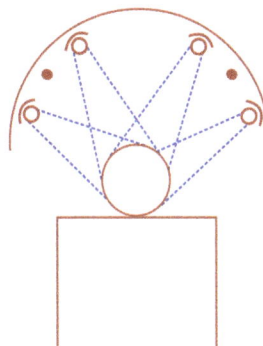

Fig. 6.5: Theraktin tunnel arrangement of fluorescent tubes.

PUVA Apparatus

Irradiation with UVA only, may be performed with special fluorescent tubes which may be mounted in a vertical battery on a wall or on four sides of a box totally surrounding the patient. This form of ultraviolet rays are usually given for two hours after the patient has taken a photoactive drug such as Psoralen, hence the term *PUVA (Psoralen-Ultraviolet-A)* is used.

TECHNIQUES OF APPLICATION

Test Dose

Individual patient's reaction to the ultraviolet radiations is used to assess the test dose. The technique of administering the test dose is very similar whether the Kromayer's lamp, fluorescent tube or theraktin tunnel is used. The only difference is of distance and timings.

Calculation of Test Dose by Air-cooled Lamp

A suitable area of skin such as flexor aspect of forearm is used for calculation of test dose. The skin is washed to remove any dust or grease. Three differently shaped holes are cut with a material which is resistant to the passage of ultraviolet rays such as card board, paper or lint. The size of the middle hole is about 2 cm × 2 cm with the hole on one side larger and on the other side smaller.

A number of people are tested to find out average E1 time and distance by seeing an erythema reaction. By knowing the average E1 (time and distance) for a particular lamp, the duration of E2, E3 and E4 doses can be calculated.

E2 time = E1 time × 2½
E3 time = E1 time × 5
E4 time = E1 time × 10

Also, by inverse square law half the distance requires quarter the time for having the same effect.

The cut out test paper or lint is applied to the patient's forearm and the body is screened. The middle hole receives the calculated E2 dose. The small hole receives an exposure slightly longer than E2 and the larger hole receives an exposure slightly shorter. The procedure is carefully recorded on the patient's treatment card and all the three holes are given to the patient to record when the erythema appears, how severe it is and how long it lasts. The patient's reaction will determine further dosages.

Calculation of Test Dose by Theraktin Tunnel

Same procedure is used to calculate the test dose as discussed above, however larger holes of about 4 cm × 4 cm are used and are placed on the abdomen. The rest of the body is screened.

Calculation of Test Dose by Kromayer's Lamp

Since the Kromayer's lamp is used in contact with the skin, the test dose is calculated by using very small holes, i.e., 0.25 cm × 0.25 cm and the exposure time needs to be very short. Ultraviolet radiations can cause severe damage to the skin; the only indication seen is the erythema reaction on the skin. The E1 dosage needs to be carefully recorded and clearly marked on the treatment lamps.

TECHNIQUES OF GENERAL IRRADIATION

- The patient's body part is washed to remove any dust or grease by soap and soaked with a towel to remove any moisture.
- The patient is explained about what is going on and how it will occur.
- The patient is positioned in comfortable posture so as to allow the maximum exposure of the part being treated and to avoid undue exposure of other parts.
- A thin film of petroleum jelly (an effective screening agent) is used for soft structures such as lips, ear lobes, eyelids, nipples, navel, etc. A thick blanket is used to cover rest of the body which does not need exposure. Eyes need to be protected by cotton wool or goggles to avoid exposure.

PHYSIOLOGICAL EFFECTS OF ULTRAVIOLET RADIATIONS

Ultraviolet rays are absorbed by the skin which acts as protective layer. UVB and UVC are absorbed by the epidermis whereas UVA may penetrate as far as capillary loops in the dermis. The skin protects the underlined cells and intracellular structures from most ultraviolet rays because the energy these rays release is sufficient to cause damage to the cells and the intracellular structures.

- *Carcinogenesis:* Sun can be called as a universal carcinogen. Prolonged exposure of UVB or UVC can lead to carcinogenesis as these rays may affect DNA and thus cell replication. The extent of carcinogenesis depends upon the wavelength of the ultraviolet radiations and amount of ultraviolet rays absorbed. So, prolonged exposure of patient's skin to ultraviolet rays should be avoided and the course of treatment should not exceed beyond four weeks.
- *Erythema:* Damage to cells causes release of histamine-like substance from the epidermis and the superficial dermis. A gradual diffusion of this chemical takes place until sufficient chemical has accumulated around the blood vessels in the skin to make them dilate. The greater the quantity of histamine-like substance, the sooner and fiercer is the reaction. The erythema reaction is used to classify doses of ultraviolet rays given to the patients. The erythema is produced by wavelengths shorter than 315 nm.
- *Pigmentation:* Pigmentation develops within 2 days of irradiation. Ultraviolet rays stimulate melanocytes in the skin so as to produce melanin. The melanin covers the nucleus of the cell to protect it from ultraviolet rays and forms an umbrella over the nucleus of the cell. Pigmentation substantially reduces the penetration of UVB. The extent of pigmentation varies from individual-to-individual and it is more in the dark skin than in the fair skin.

- *Thickening of the epidermis:* Sudden over-activity of the basal layer of the epidermis causes a marked thickening, particularly of the stratum corneum (the outermost layer). The thickening may occur to the extent that as much as three times its normal thickness. The therapeutic doses may be required to increase until desquamation has not taken place.
- *Desquamation:* The increased thickness of the epidermis is eventually lost by the process of desquamation or peeling. When desquamation has taken place, the resistance of the skin to the ultraviolet rays is substantially reduced.
- *Production of vitamin D:* Vitamin D is necessary for the absorption of calcium and is essential for the formation of bones and teeth. When ultraviolet rays are absorbed in the skin, it converts 7-dehydrocholesterol into vitamin D. It helps reducing osteoporosis and thus reducing fractures.
- *Effects on eyes:* Strong doses of ultraviolet rays to the eyes can lead to irritation and watering. Strong doses of UVB and UVC to the eyes can lead to conjunctivitis or slow blindness.
- *Aging:* The normal process of aging is accelerated if there is continuous exposure to the ultraviolet rays. There is thinness of epidermis, loss of epidermal ridges, dryness, loss of melanocytes and wrinkling due to lack of dermal connective tissue. Fair skin races are at more danger than others. Persons taking sun-bath regularly should be aware of harmful effects of ultraviolet rays.
- *Antibiotic effect:* The increased body resistance to infection as a result of ultraviolet rays is due to its action on reticuloendothelial system. Short ultraviolet rays can destroy bacteria and some other small organisms such as fungi commonly found in wounds. E4 dose effectively destroys such microorganisms.

INDICATIONS OF ULTRAVIOLET IRRADIATIONS

- *Wounds:* The ultraviolet radiations are used for the treatment of infected and noninfected wounds. *For infected wounds,* the effects of ultraviolet radiations are to destroy bacteria, to remove infected dead material, to promote repair and to increase healing. UVB rays are generally used by using Kromayer's lamp with E3 or E4 doses. *For noninfected wounds,* the effects of ultraviolet radiations are to stimulate the growth of granulation tissue and to promote repair and to increase healing. UVA rays are generally used by using some filter such as cellophane, etc.
- *Acne vulgaris:* Acne is a chronic inflammatory condition of the skin which presents with pustules, papules and comedones. It blocks the hair follicles and sebaceous glands on the face, back and chest. An E2 dose of ultraviolet radiation may be given with the following aims:
  - An erythema will bring more blood to the skin and so improves the condition of the skin.
  - Desquamation will remove comedones and allow free drainage of sebum, thus reducing the number of lesions.

  Also, it has a sterilizing effect on the skin. The intensity of dose needed, i.e., E2 + is often painful and cosmetically not acceptable to the patient. Treatment is only palliative and the condition usually returns within a few weeks of UVR. Unfortunately, it may even appear to be worse a few weeks after UVR, as all the lesions in the skin reach their peak at the same time, whereas in the normal course of acne some will be resolving and others develop. Irregular rates of desquamation may restrict the frequency of treatment and possibly produce a mottled erythema.

- *Pressure sores:* Ultraviolet radiations are used for the treatment of pressure sores. Pressure sores occurs due to any pressure injury which may vary from an area of erythema to a deep seated ulcer exposing the underlying bone. Ultraviolet rays are used to treat the pressure sores as described in wounds.
- *Psoriasis:* Psoriasis is a skin condition in which there are localized patches on the skin. It affects about 2% of population and the cause is unknown but thought to be inherited. Formation of thick pink or red plaques sharply demarcated and covered with silver scales are common features. The aim of the UVR treatment is to decrease the proliferation by reducing the DNA synthesis. Treatment is given by using the Goeckerman regimen, Leeds regimen or PUVA.

    Goeckerman regimen: This consists of coal tar application 2–3 times a day with general (total body) UVB radiation given once a day as a subthermal or E1 dose.

    Leeds or Ingram regimen: In this the sensitivity of the patient's skin is increased by the local application of coal tar, added to the bath prior to the treatment. The psoriatic lesions are covered with dithranol cream, which inhibits DNA synthesis. Next day the dithranol is cleaned off, and the process is repeated. A suberythemal dose E1 is given to the patient, using a Theraktin tunnel or an aircooled lamp at 100 cm. The dose is repeated daily and is increased daily at a rate of 12.5%.

    PUVA: Psoriasis is treated with ultraviolet radiations along with a sensitizer. Sensitizing drug psoralen is given 2 hours before the exposure of UVA rays. This inhibits the DNA synthesis and thus cell replication. Dosage of PUVA regimen needs to be measured regularly. Dosage depends upon the patients' skin type. Using psoralen along with ultraviolet rays gives its name PUVA (psoralen ultraviolet A). Long-term use can lead to skin damage and increases the risk of squamous cell carcinoma.
- *Alopecia:* Alopecia is premature falling of hairs leading to baldness. Alopecia is a relatively common condition in which hairs falls out in patches. Suberythemal doses of E1 are usually given for around 10 minutes daily. Individual patches can be treated by E2 or E3 doses by Kromayer's lamp twice a day.
- *Rickets:* When ultraviolet rays are absorbed in the skin, it converts 7-dehydrocholesterol into vitamin D. Vitamin D is necessary for the absorption of calcium and is essential for the formation of bones and teeth. It helps reducing osteoporosis and thus reducing fractures. It is beneficial in bed-ridden, elderly patients or chronic debilitating patients where chance of osteoporosis is more.
- *Counter-irritation effect:* Ultraviolet rays are used to produce strong counter-irritation effects over the site of deep rooted pain. An E3 or E4 dose is given to the area and is then covered with dry dressing. Superficial pain produced by the erythema, mask the deeper pain and also the modern pain gate theory also justifies this.
- *Psychological effects:* UVR therapy also gives the patient a sense of general well-being.

Dangers of Ultraviolet Radiations

- *Eyes:* Eyes of the patient or the Physiotherapist need to be protected by goggles from ultraviolet radiations otherwise there is a danger of conjunctivitis formation or cataract to occur. UVB and UVC are absorbed by the cornea, but UVA is absorbed by the lens and is implicated in the formation of cataract. Thus, wearing suitable goggle is necessary from preventing any injury to the eyes.

- *Overdose:* There are a number of factors due to which the patient can receive overdose during treatment.
  - Too long the exposure: The duration of exposure needs to be accurate. A proper timer with suitable audible sound and autocut device should be used.
  - Moving the lamp closure to the patient: This leads to exposure of larger doses to the patient. Patient needs to be instructed not to move during treatment. Therapist himself must calculate the distance by the application of inverse-square law.
  - Changing the lamp: It can also lead to overdose. Average E1 must be carefully recorded and marked on every lamp. Care must be taken while using any new lamp.
  - Use of sensitizers: Sensitizers must be administered and used carefully to avoid any harmful effect.

CONTRAINDICATIONS

- *Acute skin conditions:* Certain skin conditions such as acute eczema, dermatitis, lupus erythematosus, or herpes simplex must be avoided irradiation.
- *Hypersensitivity to sunlight:* Certain patients those who are hypersensitive to the sunlight are also avoided irradiation.
- *Deep X-ray or cobalt therapy:* Patients those who have taken deep X-ray or cobalt therapy can have devitalization of the tissues. Hypersensitivity of the skin can occur.
- *Skin grafting:* Recent cases of skin grafting should not be given UVR.

METHODS OF TREATMENT

TREATMENT OF PATIENT'S CONDITION

- Ulcers
- Acne vulgaris
- Pressure sores
- Psoriasis
- Rickets
- General debilitating condition
- Vitiligo
- Alopecia
- Sensitizers.

ULTRAVIOLET RADIATIONS

PROFORMA FOR PATIENT'S ASSESSMENT

- *Receiving the patient:* Good morning, I am a Physiotherapist and going to treat you. Please, cooperate with me during the treatment and wait until I go through your case sheet.
- *History taking or going through the case sheet:*
  - Name
  - Father's and Mother's name

- Age
- Sex
- Occupation
- Address: Correspondence and permanent
- Chief complaints
- History of present illness
- History of past illness
- Family history
- Social and occupational history
- Treatment history
- Prognosis of the treatment
- Investigations:
  - Hematological tests: Urine—albumin, sugar, etc.
  - Radiological tests—X-rays, etc.
- Use of sensitizer—egg, fish, alcohol, strawberry, insulin, coal tar
- Any allergic reaction (e.g., hypersensitivity to sunlight).

❖ *General contraindications:*
- Hyperpyrexia
- Hyperesthesia
- Dermatitis
- TB
- Inflammation and injury
- Deep X-ray therapy or cobalt therapy
- Photosensitivity
- Epilepsy
- Renal or cardiac problems
- Vascular impairment
- Mental retardation
- Use of sensitizers like insulin, etc.

❖ Local contraindications.

❖ *General instructions to the patient:*
- Do not expose the area to sunlight
- Do not use soap or water
- Do not wash
- Do not apply any cream or powder.

Laws of Radiations

$$\text{New dose} = \frac{\text{Old dose} \times (\text{New distance})^2}{(\text{Old distance})^2}$$

Inverse square law: It states that the intensity of a beam of rays from a point source is inversely proportional to the square of the distance from the source.

Cosine law: It states that the proportion of rays absorbed varies as per the cosine of the angle between the incident and the normal. Thus, larger the angle at which the rays strike at the body surface, lesser will be the absorption and vice versa.

Grothus law: It states that the rays must be absorbed to produce the effect and the effects will be produced at that point at which the rays are absorbed.

Calculation of UVR dosage:
Suberythemal dose = 1/2
E1 time E2 dose = 2.5 × E1 time
E3 dose = 5 × E1 time
E4 dose = 10 × E1 time

Degree of erythema: The degree of erythema is given in **Table 6.1**.

Table 6.1: Degree of erythema.		
Disappears	*Appearance*	*Duration*
E1	6–12 hours	24 hours
E2	4–6 hours	48 hours (2 days)
E3	2–4 hours	72 hours (3–5 days)
E4	2 hours	1 week

ULCERS

An ulcer is a loss of epithelial cells causing exposure of the underlying tissue.

Types
- Venous
- Arterial (ischemic)
- Pressure sores.

Venous Ulcers
- *Sex:* Women > men
- *Age:* 50–70 years
- *Site:* Lower two-thirds of the lower leg and on parts of the foot not supported by the shoe.

Predisposing Factors
- Venous congestion associated with varicose veins or deep vein thrombosis (DVT)
- Occupations demanding prolonged standing
- Poor personal hygiene and malnutrition.

Components of an Ulcer
- Floor (E4)
- Wall (E3)
- Base (E2).

Clinical Features
- Floor of the ulcer (Part showing loss of tissue, exposing underlying tissues may be:
  - Pale and anemic with watery discharge—indolent ulcer
  - Green or yellow discharge—infected ulcer
  - Pink, purple with red spots—granulating ulcer.

- The wall of ulcer (boundary between the floor and surrounding skin) may be:
  - Well-defined, straight, red and shiny—ulcer spreading
  - Hard, edematous, over banging floor—ulcer chronic
  - Shallow, sloping out from floor with bluish tinge—ulcer healing.
- The base of the ulcer (zone of the tissue immediately surrounding and underlying the ulcer) may show:
  - Hardening, the extent varies according to severity and duration of the ulcer.
  - Pigmentation due to breakdown of red blood cells.
  - Poor circulation.
  - Coarse skin texture with heavy heading or papery thin and eczematous tissue.
- Edema of the base of the ulcer of foot and ankle to the shoe line.
- Considerable pain around the ulcer, especially if infected, pain increased on walking.
- Limited movement of the feet and ankle.
- Muscle weakness and atrophy—mainly calf muscles with loss of pumping action.
- Walking pattern poor with no push off.

Treatment

Conservative: Aims to relieve pain, relieve congestion and reduce edema, improve general circulation to lower limb, mobilize the joints and strengthens lower limb muscles (especially—calf), improve condition of skin of lower leg.
- Soft tissue techniques
- UV rays.

For Infected Ulcer

Base of the ulcer: E2; edges are screened with clamp. Sterile gauze, this is repeated two or three times a week. If the edges are clear of infection, a E1 may be given to edges and surrounding skin to promote healing.

Effect: To promote granulating tissue.

For indolent: E4 is given to the floor with ulcer-screened and to the edges of the surrounding skin.

Effect: To stimulate the circulation
- Ultrasound (contraindicated in DVT)
- 0.25–0.5 W/cm² for 5–10 minutes
  - For small area: Pulsed beam
  - For large area: Continuous.

  Ultrasound is given with coupling cream to the surrounding skin or in a sterile saline. Both to the ulcer as well as to the surrounding area. Also,
- Pulsed electromagnetic energy (PEME)
- Laser
- Support and pressure (compression bandage)
- *Active exercise:*
  - Complications: Superficial and deep VT
  - Arterial (ischemic ulcer)
  - Sex: Men and Women
  - Age: Elderly

- Site: On toes, foot and heel (may be on lower leg)
- Cause: Lack of nutrition to the skin due to inadequate arterial blood supply.

Clinical Features

Floor is pale, anemic and liable to infection, surrounding skin may be normal or ischemic.

- *Distance:* 36"
- *Dosage:*
  - Base—E2
  - Wall—E3
  - Floor—E4

ACNE VULGARIS

This is a chronic inflammatory disease of the sebaceous glands:
- *Age:* It starts between 9 years and 17 years, is associated with puberty, and is generally clear by 30 years.
- *Sex:* Males > females.
- *Site:* Face, chest and upper back.

Predisposing Factors

- Puberty
- Lack of fitness, exercise without fresh air
- Poor health, constipation
- Diet high in butter, cream, sugar, chocolates or alcohol
- Sweating
- Endocrine abnormalities involving testosterone
- Anxiety
- Skin type—dark complexion, heredity.

Etiology: Propionibacterium acnes.

Pathology

Sebum production and keratin blocks the pilosebaceous duct and hair follicle. The exposed surface becomes oxidized and blackened the walls of the follicle and inflammation takes place. This causes swelling and distension of the follicle and duct by bacteria causing pus formation (pustule). Once the pus is discharged the duct and follicle shrink and healing takes place. But repeated attacks can result in scar tissue formation.

Clinical Features

Comedones, papules (reddened round raised areas), pustules (yellow raised areas surrounded by reddish purple area), cysts scars can occur.

Management

Topical: Sulfur-based ointment, salicylic acid-based ointments, benzoyl peroxide gel.
General: Antibiotics
Patients positioning:

Sitting position: Two pillows
- Back of the head
- Neck line and head line maintenance
- Remaining part must be covered
- Wearing cotton wool on the eyes.

Physiotherapy
- *UVR:* Spectrum 190–390 nm
  - Distance: 18"
  - Dose: E2 dose
- *Position of the patient:* Sitting on stool with back supported on wall. Wash the affected areas at least twice a day with oil-free soap and rinse with cool water.
- *Focusing point:* Tip of the nose.

Dosages depend upon the patient's weight and patient skin type.

PRESSURE SORES

Pressure sore is a term used to describe any pressure injury which may vary from an area of erythema to a deep seated ulcer exposing the underlying bone.
- *Age:* At any stage
- *Sex:* Equal
- *Site:* Heels, buttock, hips, elbows—pressure area
- *Cause:*
  - External factors: Postoperative pain, immobility, unconsciousness, prolonged bed rest.
  - Internal factors: Muscle tone, incontinence, diabetes, trophic ulcer.

Clinical Features
- *Floor of sore:* Pink, vascular or filled with infected exudates, cavity may be shallow or deep with loss of subcutaneous tissue and exposure of bone.
- *Around the cavity:* Skin is red or blue. If sensory nerve endings are not destroyed—pain will be there.

UVR Treatment
- *Positioning of the patient:* Oblique side lying (45°)
- *Dosage:*
  - Floor—E4 dose
  - Wall—E3 dose
  - Base—E2 dose
- *Distance:* 36".

PSORIASIS

Psoriasis is a chronic inflammatory disease of the skin characterized by clearly defined dry rounded red patches with silvery scales on the surface.
- *Age:* Common age is 15–30 years
- *Sex:* Equal
- *Climate:* The condition is worse in damp, cold climate.

Predisposing Factors
- Heredity
- Infection (after upper respiratory tract infection)
- Trauma (mechanical friction, cuts, stings)
- Anxiety (often appear in relation to mental stings, e.g., bereavement, exams)
- Drugs (e.g., chloroquine precipitates this)
- Arthropathy.

Cause
Cause is unknown, in normal skin the maturing of epidermal cells takes 21–29 days in psoriasis; this is accelerated to 4 days.

Distribution: Elbows, knees, back and sacrum.

Clinical Features
- Sharply defined red and pink areas
- Plaques
- Silvery scales.

Treatment
Psoriasis can be treated with UVR. Two sources are used—the theraktin and PUVA:
- *The theraktin:* This is usually in the form of a tunnel with four fluorescent tubes. The patient is generally naked and lies supine for half the treatment session and prone for other half. It may be used alone or in conjunction with coal tar on diathermal.
  Suberythema dose is given daily or 3 times a week. Prominent parts have a mild erythema, but fades before the next treatment.
- *PUVA:* This is psoralens plus UVA. Psoralens are photosensitizing substances, which occur in plants such as parsley, parsnips and celery. The one used for psoriasis is 8-methoxypsoralen (8-MOP).

Methods: Patient takes 8–6 tablets of psoralens with milk two hours before exposure.
- *Posture upper trunk:* Midpoint of line joining the inferior angles of the scapula
- *Post lower trunk:* Midpoint of line joining the 2 popliteal fossa
- *Right side:* Right greater trochanter
- *Left side:* Left greater trochanter

UVA doses in PUVA treatment:
- Always burns, never tan
- Always burns, then slight tan
- Sometimes burn, always tan
- Never burn, always tan
- Lightly pigmented
- Black.

Precaution: To patient on PUVA
- Do not take psoralens on empty stomach.
- Protective goggles are essential polaroid sunglasses must be worn from the time of taking the psoralen to at least 12 hours after treatment.

- Stop using all ointments during PUVA.
- If the skin is dry, simple oil or lubricating lotions may be used.
- During the treatment, if the patient feels pain, the Physiotherapist must be called immediately.

Aims of Ultraviolet Radiations

- To decrease the rate of DNA synthesis in the cells of the skin and thus slow down their proliferation.
- *Dosage:* Suberythemal dose (half E1)
- *Distance:* 36"
- *Positioning of the patient:* Oblique side lying.

Methods of Treatment

- *General: Focusing point*
  - Umbilicus (supine lying)
  - Midpoint between the posterior SI spines prone lying
- *Fractional: Edibase tech.*
  - Body is divided into 6 parts
  - Focusing points:
    - Anterior upper trunk—xiphisternum
    - Anterior lower trunk—midpoint of line joining two patella.

RICKETS

Rickets is a disease of disordered calcium metabolism occurring in infants and young children. The most characteristic changes taking place in the bones.

Type of Rickets

- *Nutritional rickets:* This is due to deficiency in the diet and occurs in children below 4 years.
- *Celiac rickets (intestinal diminished):* This is due to diminished absorption of calcium from the intestines in celiac disease and other malabsorption disorders.
- *Renal rickets:* This is due to various types of defects in the renal function in children above 5 years.

Positioning of the patient: Oblique side lying (45° inclination).

Dosage: Suberythemal dose.

GENERAL DEBILITATING CONDITION

- *Positioning of the patient:* Oblique side lying.
- *Dose:* Suberythemal dose.

VITILIGO

Vitiligo is a condition in which the areas of the skin are depigmented owing to the loss of normal melanocyte function.

Treatment: Aim is to produce pigmenting of the abnormal areas. PUVA is very successful. The psoralens may be taken by mouth or painted on to the affected areas. The psoralens used may be trimethyl psoralens (TMP).

If UVA source is not available, UVB from the theraktin can be successful. Suberythemal dose should be tried one or two times per week for 6–8 weeks.

ALOPECIA

It is the absence or premature loss of hair.

Classification

- *Alopecia areata:* Loss of scalp hair
- *Alopecia totalis:* Loss of all scalp hair and eyebrows
- *Alopecia universalis:* Total loss of body hair.

Etiology

- *Age:* Under 30 years
- *Sex:* Equal
- Predisposing factors—general anxiety, fatigue, poor health, heredity.

Treatment

- Aims are to improve general health.
- To improve nutrition to the hair follicles.

General Health

Suberythema or E1 dosage is given daily for 6–8 treatments.

Promotion of nutrition (Kromayer)*:* E2 or E3 dosage
Dose for alopecia*:* E2 dose.

SENSITIZERS

- *Thiazide diuretics:* Doburil, Aldoril, Enduron
- *Sulfonamides:* Thalazole, Furadantin, Gantrisin
- *Tetracycline:* Terramycin, Achromycin, Panmycin
- *Antifungal agents:* Griseofulvin
- *Hypnotic drugs:* Veronal, Sulfonal, Benzodiazepines
- *Barbiturates:* Phenobarbital, Allobarbital, Barbital

- *Phenothiazine:* Tranquilizer, Melleul, Stelazine
- Gold therapy
- Various hormones—insulin, thyroid extracts
- Aspirin and derivatives
- Psoralens (8-methoxypsoralens)
- Coal tar
- Dithranol
- Eosine
- Strawberry, lobster.

CHAPTER 7

Laser Therapy

INTRODUCTION

The word "laser" is an acronym for *light amplification of stimulated emission of radiation*. It refers to the production of a beam of a radiation which differs from the ordinary light in several ways. These are nowadays used in laser light shows, compact disk players, surgical incisions, in ophthalmology and gynecology, etc.

HISTORICAL ASPECTS

The great German physicist Max Planck in 1900 presented an explanation of why colors of glowing hot bodies change with temperature. He proposed the quantum theory according to which radiations are discrete quantities or packets of energy. Einstein in 1970 outlined the principles underlying the production of laser radiation as a part of quantum theory. In 1960, Dr Theodore Maiman of Hughes Laboratory of United States of America produced the first burst of ruby lasers. Later, the workers of Bell telephone laboratory produced a helium-neon laser. They also developed carbon dioxide laser which became popular for surgical applications. More recently, the potential clinical use of nonthermal effects of the laser on the tissues came into existence. This therapy got a boost in 1979 by the invention of semiconductor diode laser—gallium-arsenide (GaAs) laser **(Figs. 7.1 and 7.2)**.

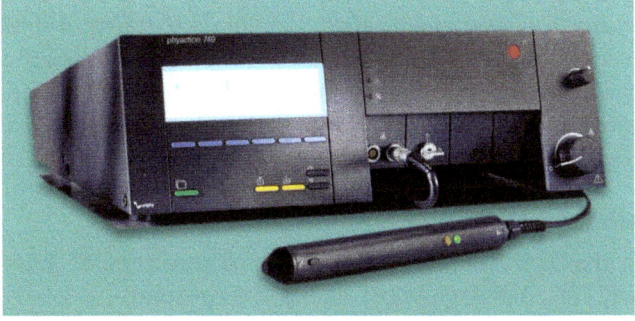

Fig. 7.1: Laser therapy.

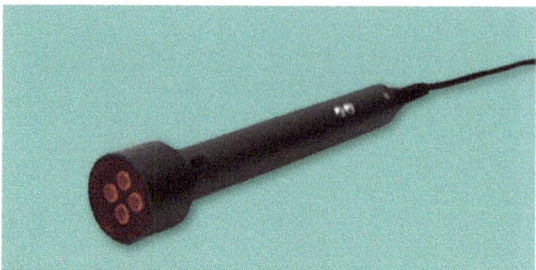

Fig. 7.2: Scanning electrode.

PROPERTIES OF LASER

The laser differs from the ordinary light in the following ways:
- *Monochromaticity:* This means that the laser light has a single color (mono—single, chromaticity—coloration). This is because the lasers are of a single wavelength and thus the definite frequency. Ordinary light however has many wavelengths.
- *Coherence:* Laser radiations are not of the same wavelength but also have same phase. Coherence means similar or synchronous behavior of laser beam, this means two things simultaneously. First, the laser beam is temporarily coherent, means that the photons are in same phase with crests meeting crests and troughs meeting troughs in time. Secondly, the laser beam is spatially coherent, means the photons are unidirectional and stay in same phase over long distances and little spread of beam. Ordinary light on contrary has variable wavelengths.
- *Collimation:* Laser beams remain collimated that means they remain in parallel. They do not diverge much and the energy can be propagated over a larger distance.

PRODUCTION OF LASER

It is recalled that the electrons of an individual atom remain as a "cloud" of negative charge around the positive nucleus. According to the quantum theory, the electrons can only occupy certain energy levels or shells around the nucleus. Under normal circumstances, in the vast majority of the atoms the electrons remain at the lowest energy level, i.e., at the resting or ground state. If enough energy is added to atom, an outer electron may gain sufficient energy to free itself from the nucleus. The atom then becomes a positively charged ion and the electron becomes a free negative charge. When the outer electrons are in one of the higher energy states, they will tend to return to a lower energy state, sometimes to the most stable or ground state. Also, the quantum energy which is expressed in electron volts is inversely proportional to the wavelength. This means the greater the quantum energy; the lesser will be the wavelength. A large number of atoms with the electrons in the excited state can lead to amplification since one photon releases a second and these two can release more and so on.

Components for Laser Production

For the production of a laser radiation, the device must consist of the following components: (1) lasing medium, (2) resonating chamber, and (3) energy source.
- *Lasing medium:* The material which is capable of producing laser is known as lasing medium. It can absorb energy from the external source and then gives off its excess energy as photons

of light. Lasing medium could be solid crystal or semiconductor, liquid or gas. The lasing media in low intensity laser or cold laser are either helium-neon (He-Ne) or semiconductor, i.e., GaAs.

- *Resonating chamber:* The resonating chamber contains the lasing medium which is surrounded by two parallel mirrors at either ends. One of the mirrors has 100% reflectance while the other has slightly less reflectance. The mirror with slightly less reflectance serves as an output device which allows some of the photons to escape through it.
- *Energy source:* A flashgun is used to excite the electrons of the lasing medium. The source of flashgun is usually current electricity.

TYPES OF LASER

The various types of laser are available nowadays. The commonly used lasers are:
- Ruby laser (or crystal laser)
- Helium-neon laser (gas laser)
- Diode laser (or semiconductor laser)

Ruby Laser (Crystal Laser)

Ruby laser is also known as crystal laser because it contains synthetic ruby as a lasing medium. Synthetic medium (aluminum oxide and chromium) is used rather than the natural one to ensure purity of the medium which is necessary to generate physical characteristics of laser. Aluminum oxide with trace of chromium oxide forms a 10 cm long and 1 cm wide synthetic ruby rod. A helical electric discharge tube containing xenon tube is wound around the ruby rod. Both the ends are made reflecting by silvering the surfaces with one end as 100% reflective and other slightly less. The xenon tube is used to give intense flash of white light which excites the ruby molecules and raises the electron to a higher energy level. As the excited state is unstable, the electrons return to ground state by releasing a photon. This is known as *spontaneous emission*. The rate of supply of energy exceeds to a greater extent which leads to a large number of atoms at higher energy levels. This is known as *population inversions*. Atoms in their excited state are encountered by the photons and this leads to further stimulated emissions. The excited electron falls to its resting state and gives off a photon of exactly the same energy as that of photon which collided with it (photon of 694.3 nm wavelength). Hence, a beam of red laser with a wavelength 694.3 nm is emitted.

Helium-Neon Laser (Gas Laser)

Gas laser consists of a mixture of primarily helium and neon in a low pressure tube. This low pressure tube is surrounded by a flashgun which excites the atom to a higher energy level.

Thus, photons released by the spontaneous emission and have a wavelength of 632.8 nm. These photons reflect to and fro to the tube and collide with the atoms of higher energy levels. This leads to stimulated emission with the release of similar photons. Intense beam of light emerges from the narrow partially transmissive which is red in color and has a wavelength of 632.8 nm.

Diode Laser (Semiconductor Laser)

Gallium arsenide is used as a diode or semiconductor to produce an infrared invisible laser with a wavelength of 904 nm. In these with an external electric potential, positively charged "holes" are thrown from the p-type gallium-aluminum-arsenide layer into the active layer of

GaAs. The negatively charged electrons interact with the active layer and thus photon of light is released. The photons are reflected to and fro and emitted as a laser beam from one partially transparent end. By varying the ratio of gallium to aluminum, desired specific wavelengths are obtained. The advantage of semiconductor laser diode is that these can either emit a continuous or a pulsed output.

TECHNIQUES OF APPLICATION

The method of application of laser therapy is quite simple. Generally, the laser energy is emitted by a hand held applicator for therapeutic purposes. The GaAs laser contains the semiconductor or diode element at the tip of the applicator, whereas the helium-neon laser contains their components inside the unit and delivers the laser light to the target area via a fiberoptic tube. This causes divergence of the beam. To administer the laser for therapeutic purposes, two methods are generally used: (1) grid method and (2) scanning method.

1. *Grid method:* The treatment area is divided into a grid each of 1 cm^2. The hand-held applicator should be in light contact with the skin and directly perpendicular to the target tissue. Each cm^2 is stimulated for a specific period of time.
2. *Scanning method:* No contact is made between the tip of the laser and the patient's skin. The tip of the applicator is held at a distance of 5–10 mm. Since the divergence of beam occurs, there is a decrease in the amount of energy applied as the distance increases.

DOSAGE PARAMETERS

- *Wavelength:* It depends on the lasing medium used. For superficial conditions like wounds and ulcers, visible red laser is used. For deep conditions of muscles and bones, infrared laser is used. Cluster probe laser having several diodes are used for the larger area of soft tissues.
- *Power:* The power output is measured in watts. Since the power output of laser beam used therapeutically is quite small, mW is generally used. Moreover, percentage of power output is sometimes used, i.e., 10%, 20% or 30% of the total power output.
- *Energy:* The energy delivered to the treatment tissue is expressed in joules. It is calculated by the following equation:
  Energy (in joules) = Power (in watts) × Time (in seconds)
  Sometimes, when the energy required for the treatment of a particular tissue is known and the power output is available then the total treatment time can also be calculated.
- *Power density:* It decreases as the area between the tip of the applicator and the part to be treated increases. Power density is expressed as:
  Power density = Incident power/Area in cm^2
  Total power used therapeutically is thus calculated by the *inverse square law*.
- *Energy density:* Energy density can be calculated as:
  $$\text{Energy density} = \frac{\text{Power (W)} \times \text{Time (seconds)}}{\text{Area (in cm}^2\text{)}}$$

The dosage in laser therapy is calculated in terms of energy density applied which is expressed in J/cm^2.

INTERACTION OF LASER WITH BODY TISSUES

Low intensity lasers are used therapeutically for their nonthermal effects. Visible radiations are remarkably absorbed in the hemoglobin whereas infrared light is strongly absorbed by water. Absorption results in the transformation of energy in the body tissues. Human body consists of 70% of water and 30% of organic material. Organic material which absorbs visible light contains chromophores. Chromophores are defined as the molecular structures which get excited by the visible spectrum due to its configuration. In human body, hemoglobin and melanin contain chromophores and thus absorb laser energy.

PHYSIOLOGICAL EFFECTS AND THERAPEUTIC USES OF LASERS

- *Wound healing:* Laser therapy is nowadays being effectively used for the treatment of wounds. Healing of wounds is thought to accelerate by the application of laser (Dyson and Young, 1986). It is a complex physiological process which involves chemotactic activity, vascular changes and the release of chemical mediators. Radiations particularly from the red spectrum of light are found effective in the treatment of chronic ulcers. Both untreated chronic ulcers as well as trophic ulcers can be very effectively treated by laser therapy. Laser therapy increases tissue proliferation and thus enhances wound healing caused due to burns, surgical incisions, diabetic ulcers and pressure sores. Both direct contact or grid method as well as scanning method is effectively used for healing of wounds. Wound margins are effectively treated by direct contact technique. For doing this, the laser probe is usually applied at 1-2 cm from the edges. Dosage of 4–10 J/cm^2 is usually sufficient.

   Treatment of wound bed is preferably done by noncontact method. The dosage from 1 to 5 J/cm^2 is usually sufficient for the treatment of wound bed. The low dosages are usually sufficient because the protective layer of dermis is absent in this area.

- *Tensile strength and scar tissue:* The tensile strength of the tissues treated with laser therapy is more than the normally healed ones. This tensile strength is directly related to the increased levels of collagen. Collagen synthesis and thus the tensile strength are fibroblasts mediated functions which are improved significantly by the treatment of laser.

   Also, the wounds exposed to laser therapy have more epithelialization and less exudate formation. Hence, they have less scar tissue formation with a better cosmetic appearance.

- *Musculoskeletal conditions:* The laser therapy is found to be very effective in various overuse tendinitis or bursitis conditions like tennis elbow, golfer's elbow, supraspinatus tendinitis, etc. Also, laser therapy is found effective in some acute conditions like ankle sprain as it enhances the healing process and relieves pain.

   Various arthritic conditions like rheumatoid arthritis, osteoarthritis, ankylosing arthritis, pyogenic arthritis, etc., are benefited by the use of laser therapy. Laser has its effect on prostaglandin synthesis and thus it relieves inflammation. Laser is found to be very effective in the healing of the connective tissues and thus is effective in the treatment of various arthritic conditions.

   Laser therapy has bactericidal effects because of increased phagocytosis by leukocytes. When used in conjunction with antibiotics, laser therapy is found effective in the treatment of various inflammatory conditions.

- *Pain relief:* Laser therapy is found effective in relieving pain, both acute as well as chronic. Acute pain as in ankle sprain is relieved by the laser by reducing swelling and enhancing the healing process. Many musculoskeletal pains as in fibrositis or trigger pain are relieved by the application of laser on trigger points or acupressure points. In postoperative conditions also, the laser is found effective in the enhancing healing process and thus reducing pain. Analgesia is achieved in certain neurogenic conditions also. Pain due to trigeminal neuralgia is found to be relieved by laser therapy. Studies on superficial median or radial nerve conduction velocity have shown a decrease in sensory nerve conduction velocity by a low intensity laser.
- *Bone and articular cartilage:* Studies on the effects of laser on bones and articular cartilage are increasing day-by-day. It has been found that the longer duration of low power laser helps in fracture healing and bone remodulation. It helps in chondral proliferation and remodeling of the articular line. It has also been found useful for the treatment of nonunion of fractures.

DANGERS AND CONTRAINDICATIONS

- *Effects on eyes:* The main danger of low power laser therapy is a risk of eye damage if the beam is applied directly into the eye. So, to avoid the exposure of eye with a beam of laser, protective goggles should be worn by the patient as well as by the physiotherapist.
- *Effects on cancerous growth:* The laser should not be applied over the area of cancerous growth. Laser acts as a photobiostimulatory agent, its exposure to cancerous tissue can lead to acceleration of its growth and metastasis.
- *Effects on pregnant uterus:* Laser should not be applied directly over the pregnant uterus as it may cause abnormal growth.
- *Effects on infected tissues:* When treated in contact with the infected tissue, the laser head needs to be cleaned thoroughly or sterilized. It should be used preferably in conjunction with ultraviolet therapy for the treatment of infected wounds.
- *Hemorrhagic areas or cardiac conditions:* Laser can cause vasodilatation and hence care should be taken while exposing any hemorrhagic area. Patients of certain cardiac conditions are avoided the exposure of laser therapy around the cardiac region.

METHODS OF TREATMENT

TREATMENT OF PATIENT'S CONDITION

- Tennis elbow
- Supraspinatus tendinitis
- Golfer's elbow
- Plantar fasciitis

PROFORMA FOR PATIENT'S ASSESSMENT

- *Receiving the patient:* Good morning, I am a physiotherapist and going to treat you. Please, cooperate with me during the treatment and wait until I go through your case sheet.

- *History taking or going through the case sheet:*
  - Name
  - Father's and Mother's name
  - Age
  - Sex
  - Occupation
  - *Address:* Correspondence and permanent
- *Chief complaints:*
  - History of present illness
  - History of past illness
  - Family history
  - Social and occupational history
  - Treatment history
  - Prognosis of the treatment
  - *Investigations:*
    - Hematological tests
    - Radiological tests: X-rays, magnetic resonance imaging (MRI) scan, etc.
- *Checking for general contraindications:*
  - Hyperpyrexia
  - Hypertension
  - Deep X-ray and cobalt therapy
  - Epileptic patients
  - Noncooperative patients
  - Mentally retarded patients
  - Very poor general condition of the patient
  - Menstruation
  - Pregnant uterus
  - Hemorrhage and infected tissue.
- *Checking for local contraindications:*
  - Skin conditions
  - Tumor
  - Any metal in the treatment area
  - Neoplastic tissue
- *Preparation of trays:*
  - *Two test tubes:*
    - One with hot water
    - One with cold water
  - Cotton
  - Goggles
  - Towels
  - Pillows
  - Sandbags

- *Preparation of apparatus:* The laser apparatus is conveniently positioned. Protective goggles, designed for the particular wavelength being used, are worn to avoid any risk of accidental application of laser beam into the eye.
  - Selection of treatment head
  - Switching on
  - Regulation of power
  - Checking the insulation
  - Checking the plugs
  - Checking the socket
  - Checking the main wire whether it is properly fitted in the main machine
- Gaining the confidence of the patient.
- *Positioning the patient:* Comfortable with good support.
- *Treatment:*
  - Checking of apparatus
  - Placing the applicator
  - Instructions to the patient
    - Warn not to remove goggles
    - Not to move
    - Not to touch the machine
    - Not to sleep
- *Application:* Maintain the laser applicator so that beam is at right angles in order to achieve maximal penetration. Contact may be made. Do not switch on the applicator before application of applicator to the skin.
- *Termination:* Switch off before removing the applicator from the skin contact. Immediate increase or decrease of pain needs to be recorded.
- *Other points:*
  - Knowledge of condition
  - Record of treatment.

Tennis Elbow (Lateral Epicondylitis)

Definition

Tennis elbow is a condition characterized by pain and tenderness on the lateral side of the elbow, usually related to the common extensor tendons of the forearm.

The condition is common in both the sexes almost equally and age of occurrence is between 30 and 45 years.

Etiology

Excessive use of wrist extensors as in:
- Repetitive overuse activity like squeezing clothes
- Wrong technique at sport (e.g., tennis, golf, badminton, fencing)
- Unaccustomed gardening or carpentry.

Pathology

Tear occurs at tenomuscular junction, in the tendon or at tenoperiosteal junction. The resulting inflammation forms to heal the torn tissue. If excessive fibrin is formed, fibrous tissue will result in adhesions the tendon and neighboring tissue. This causes pain and repeated injury to tendon prevent healing and excessive scar tissue form.

Clinical Features

- Pain on exertion.
- Pain over the elbow to the wrist.
- Resisted wrist extension is painful, passive movement is pain-free.
- Tenderness over the tendon.

Treatment

Acute:
- Ice towel for 20 minutes
- Rest
- Splint for wrist extension for 2–8 weeks
- Strapping

Modalities Used

- Laser
- Pulsed electromagnetic energy
- Friction massage for 5–10 minutes for 4 days.

Position of Patient

Sitting on chair with elbow supported and semiflexed.

Position of Therapist

Standing/sitting by the side of patient.

Treatment Dosage

Energy density should be 0.5–1 J/cm^2.

Supraspinatus Tendinitis

History

This may occur as a result of accident (e.g., a fall on the shoulder), over exercise (e.g., aerobics) or a series of minor stresses (e.g., long periods of writing).

Clinical Features

Pain: Toothache type pain is present radiating from the acromion process to the deltoid insertion.

Painful area:
- Abduction to 60° is pain-free.
- 60–120° is painful.
- 120–180° is pain-free.

Movements
Shoulder arm movements are full (but have a painful arc).
- Resisted abduction in outer range is often painful.
- Lowering the arm from elevation is very painful. If this movement is resisted then pain is less.
- Reversed glenohumeral rhythm, the scapula moving more than the humerus.

Functions
Severely limited in patient who has to carry weights (e.g., dresses on coat hangers).

Position of Therapist
Standing by the side of patient.

Position of Patient
Side lying/sitting with the arm supported over a pillow.

Treatment
Energy density should be 4 J/cm^2.

Golfer's Elbow (Medial Epicondylitis)
Definition
This is a condition characterized by pain and acute tenderness on the medial side of the elbow. It affects the common flexor origin.
   Principles of treatment are same as for tennis elbow.

Treatment
Energy density should be 1 J/cm^2.
Pain is produced by extension of elbow, supination and valgus strain.

Position of Patient
Sitting or supine lying with shoulder of the affected arm abducted.

Position of Therapist
Standing or sitting by the side of patient.

Plantar Fasciitis
Definition
This is a common cause of pain in the heel. It occurs as a result of inflammation of the plantar aponeurosis at its attachment on the tuberosity of the calcaneum.
   The pain is worse in the morning and often reduces with the activity.

On Examination
There is marked tenderness over the medial aspect of the calcaneal tuberosity, at the site of attachment of the plantar fascia.

Investigation
X-ray often shows a sharp bone spur projecting forward from the tuberosity of the calcaneum.

Treatment
- Rest
- Analgesics
- Soft heel pad made up of microcellular rubber (MCR)
- Local corticosteroids
- Laser therapy

Energy density of 4 J/cm^2 is usually sufficient.

CHAPTER 8

Superficial Heating Modalities

PARAFFIN WAX BATH THERAPY

Paraffin wax bath therapy is an application of molten paraffin wax over the body parts. The temperature of the paraffin wax is maintained at 40–44°C, whereas its melting point is 51–55°C. If the molten wax at 51–55°C is poured on the body parts, it may cause burn over the body tissues that is why some impurity is added to lower down its melting point such as liquid paraffin or mineral oil. Paraffin wax bath therapy provides about six times the amount of heat available in water because the mineral oil in the paraffin lowers its melting point. The combination of paraffin and mineral oil has low specific heat which enhances the patient's ability to tolerate heat from paraffin better than that from the water of the same temperature. The composition of solid wax:liquid paraffin:petroleum jelly is 7:3:1 or solid wax:liquid paraffin or mineral oil is 7:1. The mode of transmission of heat from paraffin to the patient skin is by means of conduction.

Paraffin Wax Bath Unit

Parts of a typical paraffin wax bath unit are stainless steel container, mains, thermostat, thermostat pilot lamp, power pilot lamp, lid and caster **(Fig. 8.1)**.

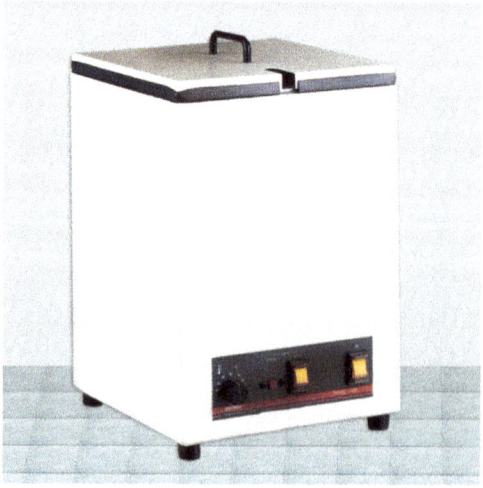

Fig. 8.1: Paraffin wax bath unit.

Initially, heating is quicker with this type because there is no water jacket to be heated. Container contains wax and paraffin oil. Mains function is to switch on or off the heating element, which is located in the casing of paraffin wax bath unit.

Thermostat keeps the temperature fixed or static in the range which is adjusted with knob.

Thermostat pilot lamp indicates whether thermostat is on or off.

Power pilot lamp function is to show whether power is on or off.

Lid covers the container and caster allows the paraffin wax bath container to be moved from one place to another.

Methods

The part to be treated must be cleaned with soap and water. Moisture is to be soaked with towel. Position of the patient should be such that the part to be treated comes closer to the wax bath container. Before application one must ensure that there should be no moisture over the body tissues otherwise burn could occur. The warm wax is placed on body tissues by various techniques and the treatment is given for about 10–20 minutes.

Techniques of Application

Various techniques used for the application of paraffin wax are as follows:
- *Direct pouring method:* The molten wax is directly poured by a mug or utensil on the part to be treated and then wrapped around by a towel. The wax is allowed to solidify for about 10-12 minutes. Several (4-6) layers can be made over the body tissues.
- *Brushing method:* A brush of various sizes (4" or 6") is used for the application of molten wax over the body tissues. Several coats (4-6) are applied over the body tissues and wax is allowed to solidify and wrapped over by a towel.
- *Direct immersion or dipping method*: In this method, the body part to be treated is directly immersed into the container of paraffin wax and taken out. Once the wax solidifies, the part is again immersed to make another layer of paraffin wax and wrapped around by a towel. This method is preferably used for treating distal parts of the body.
- *Toweling or bandaging method*: A towel or a roll of bandage is immersed in molten paraffin wax and then wrapped around the body part. Several layers can be made over the body parts. This method is preferably used for treating proximal parts of the body.

Once the treatment is given by paraffin wax, it can be reused for the next session. Regular cleaning or changing of the wax is necessary to ensure good hygiene.

Effects and Uses

Paraffin wax bath therapy provides superficial heating to the tissues. It increases the local circulation to the area, increases the pliability of the skin, and reduces stiffness and thus reduces pain.

Indications

Paraffin wax therapy is used for the treatment of:
- Rheumatoid arthritis
- Osteoarthritis
- Joint stiffness, adhesions
- Postimmobilization stiffness, scars on the skin, etc.

Contraindications: Paraffin wax bath therapy should not be used in the cases of:
- Open wounds
- Skin rashes
- Allergic conditions
- Impaired skin sensation
- Defective arterial supply, etc.

Maintenance of Paraffin Wax Bath Unit

Sterile the paraffin wax bath by heating it to 212°C Fahrenheit. For reuse, sterilization should be done frequently. Drain the melted paraffin wax, filter it out and replace it back for reuse. Change the wax at least once in 6 months.

PROFORMA FOR PATIENT'S ASSESSMENT

- Receiving the patient
- Knowing details about the condition
- Preparation of trays—two test tubes:
    i. One with cold water
    ii. One with hot water
- Pillows, towels, sandbags
- Preparation of apparatus: The temperature of the wax is checked.

Preparation of patient: The nature of wax treatment is explained and the area to be treated is cleaned and soaked with towel. Any moisture on the area needs to be removed to avoid burning.

Correct positioning of patient: The patient is positioned in such a way that the part to be treated comes in close proximity to the wax bath container.

Checking for Contraindications

- Open wound
- Ischemic disease
- Buerger's disease
- Fungal infection, e.g., paronychia
- Acute dermatitis and eczema.

Testing skin sensation: Two test tubes are used, one with hot and other with cold water. Part to be treated, needs to be checked for its intact sensation before treatment.

Treatment

- *Checking the apparatus:* Check whether thermostat is working properly.
- *Application:* Various methods of applications are used. Each must be followed as explained earlier. Wax is allowed to cool and can be reused for the next treatment session.
  Termination: The patient's skin should be inspected for any burn.

HOT PACKS/HYDROCOLLATOR PACKS

Hot packs are the packs which are immersed in an apparatus called hydrocollator **(Fig. 8.2)**. They provide superficial moist heat to the part where applied. They contain the substance which

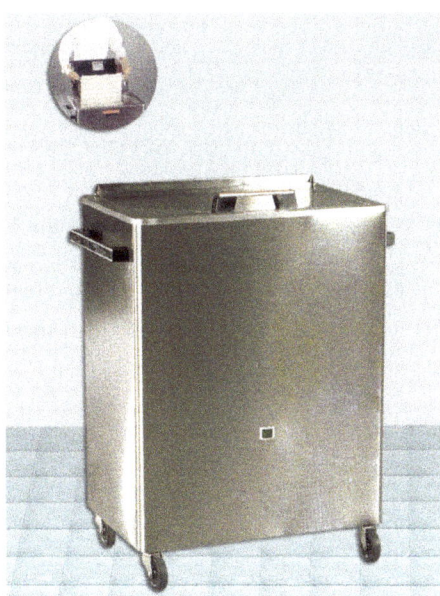

Fig. 8.2: Hydrocollator.

absorbs heat like silica or gel. They are stored in a thermostatically controlled water bath inside the equipment. The temperature inside the hydrocollator ranges between 65° and 80°C. The aim of the hydrocollator pack is to rise the body temperature at 40–45°C.

Hydrocollator packs are available in various sizes and shapes **(Figs. 8.3A to C)**. The size and shape of pack should be chosen on the basis of area being treated. The common sizes are small (for smaller joints like elbow, ankle), large (for large joints like hip and back), contoured (for cervical spine).

When used, hydrocollator packs are taken out of apparatus by means of tongs and wrapped inside a towel. Six to eight layers of towel is made around the pack. The total treatment time is around 8–10 minutes.

Effects and Uses

- *Effect on muscular spasm:* The most important physiological effect of hot pack is that it relieves the muscular spasm very quickly. Moist heat provided by the hydrocollator pack is beneficial for relieving the muscular spasm.
- *Local rise in temperature:* The rise in local body temperature occurs following hot packs application. The heat is transferred by means of conduction from hot packs to skin and superficial tissues. Local rise in temperature has many effects including increasing circulation, relieving spasm and thus relieving pain.
- *Increase of local circulation:* The local circulation around the area is also increased. It provides fresh supply of blood and nutrition. It reduces the waste products of metabolism from the area.
- *Skin and connective tissue:* Skin becomes supple and elasticity of connective tissue is also increased when combined with stretching.
- *Relieve of pain:* Pain is relieved by application of hot packs. Pain relief following hot pack application may occur due to decreased nerve conduction velocity or elevated pain

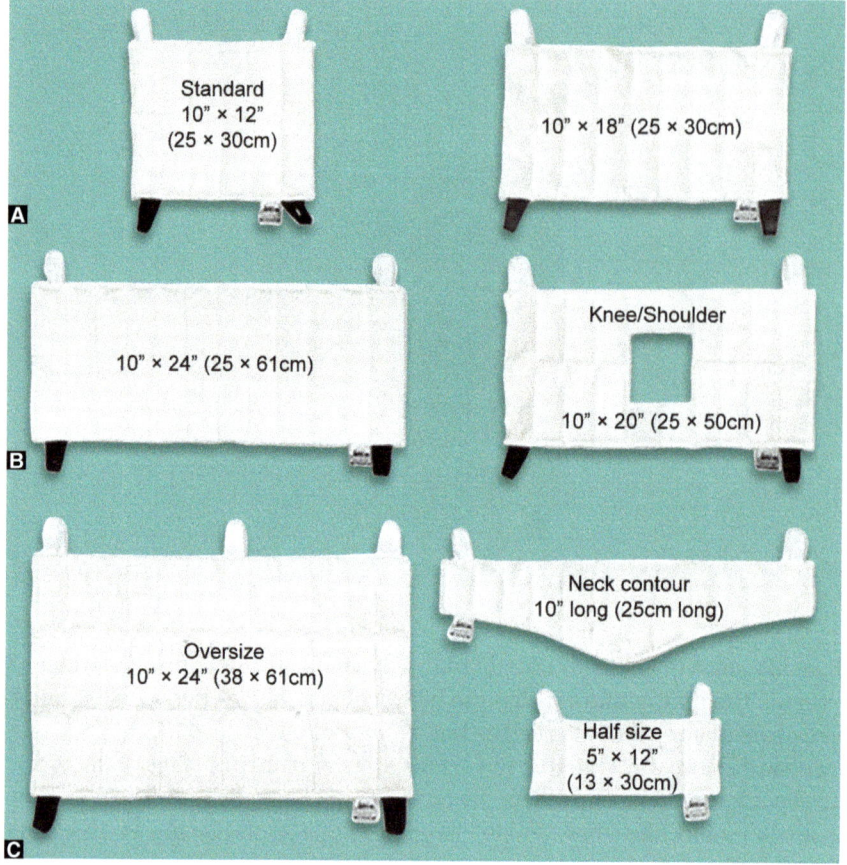

Figs. 8.3A to C: Hydrocollator hot packs.

threshold. It may be due to sedative or counter irritation effect by heat. Pain relieve may be associated with relieve of muscular spasm and increase in joint range of motion.

Contraindications

The hot packs should not be used in the area of:
- Impaired skin sensation
- Open wounds
- Recent hemorrhage
- Skin allergy
- Impaired circulation

ELECTRIC HEATING PADS

Electric heating pads are used to provide raised temperature of 40–45°C to the body parts. It contains an electric heating element inside it and is regulated by a resistor or rheostat. They provide superficial heat to the part where applied. The transmission of heat is by means of conduction.

The main advantage of using electric heating pads is that they can be used at home by the patients themselves and are cheaper and flexible.

Electric heating pads are available in various sizes and shapes. The size and shape of pack should be chosen on the basis of area being treated. The common sizes are small (for smaller joints like elbow, ankle), large (for large joints like hip and back), contoured (for cervical spine).

The common effects produced are increased in local circulation, relief of spasm, relieve of pain and increase in joint range of motion.

Contraindications are impaired skin sensation, open wounds, recent hemorrhage, skin allergy and impaired circulation.

WHIRLPOOL BATH

The use of water for therapeutic purposes is taking place since ancient times. The use of whirlpool bath has becoming an increasingly valuable means of physiotherapeutic treatment. The principle of whirlpool bath therapy is to combine the effects of temperature with the mechanical effects of the water. Warm whirlpool contains water at temperature ranges between 36–45°C and a jet of water or air stream is allowed to produce turbulence in the water. This turbulence can also be produced by electric motor incorporated into the apparatus.

Depending upon the size of the apparatus, whirlpool bath can be used for the treatment of limbs or extremities (upper or lower) or the whole body **(Fig. 8.4)**. Part is immersed into the water and jet of stream is allowed to produce turbulence in the hot water. Treatment is usually given for 15–20 minutes depending upon the area and/or condition of the patient.

Whirlpool baths can be used for various rheumatic disorders, postimmobilization stiffness, joints pain, etc. The warm whirlpool is an excellent postsurgical modality to increase systemic blood flow, removing waste products and thus reduces pain. It is effectively used in sports medicine for relaxation after practice or competition and for the treatment of various injuries.

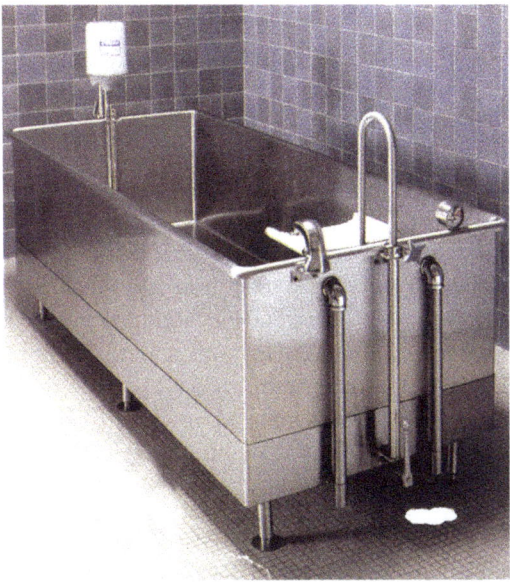

Fig. 8.4: The whirlpool bath.

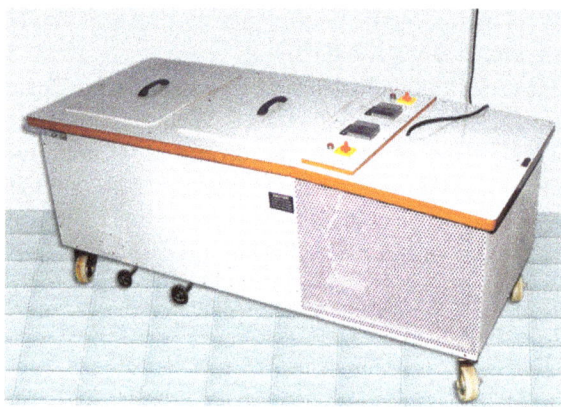

Fig. 8.5: Contrast bath.

To maintain proper hygiene, whirlpool bath needs to be cleaned frequently. Some disinfectant or antimicrobial agent should be used for cleaning the tank, turbine and jet or nozzle.

Contraindications are open wounds, recent hemorrhage, skin allergy, eczema or infection.

CONTRAST BATH

The principle of contrast bath therapy is to combine the effects of both hot as well as cold bath together. The part is immersed alternatively in hot and in cold water tanks **(Fig. 8.5)**. The temperature of hot water ranges from 36° to 45°C and the cold water from 15° to 20°C. The part is immersed first in the hot water and then in the cold water, and the treatment is repeated thereafter. As a general rule, the treatment should begin with the hot water and should end with the cold water.

The total treatment time may vary between 15 minutes and 30 minutes, with immersion in the warm around 3 minutes and in cold around 1 minute. The whole cycle is repeated for about 4–5 times.

Effects

The alteration in warm and cold leads to vasodilatation and vasoconstriction at regular intervals. It leads to reduction in edema and is beneficial in various chronic peripheral circulatory disturbances.

The regular change in temperature also leads to considerable change in the sensory stimulus. This stimulus is relatively vigorous because each time neural stimulation starts to occur, the temperature stimulus is reversed. This strong sensory stimulus acts to suppress pain by means of gate mechanism and accounts for suppression of pain in many patients receiving this treatment.

To maintain proper hygiene, contrast baths are also need to be cleaned frequently. Some disinfectant or antimicrobial agent should be used for cleaning both the tanks.

Contraindications are open wounds, recent hemorrhage, skin allergy, eczema or infection.

HELIOTHERAPY

Helio means sun and *therapy* means treatment. The use of natural sunlight for therapeutic purposes is better known as heliotherapy. The use of sunlight is prevalent since the times of ancient Greeks and Romans. In modern days, persons can be seen taking sunbaths at the beaches in the coastal regions.

Heliotherapy is effective in the treatment of psoriasis and other skin conditions as the sunrays emit ultraviolet radiations.

SAUNA BATH

The use of sauna bath was started from Finland. Its first use came into picture in 1936 in Berlin during the period of Olympic Games. Many players saw Scandinavians using this bath. Its use at a very large scale comes into picture in 1972 during Munich Olympic Games where a large number of sauna bath chambers were made available to the athletes by which it becomes popular worldwide.

Sauna bath is administered in a wooden chamber. One hot oven is used inside the sauna chamber. Stones are placed on the oven and allowed to heat. Water is poured to produce some steam in short bursts. Wooden chamber is used for sauna bath because it absorbs humidity from the inside air and thus restores dryness in the chamber. Regular monitoring of temperature and humidity is done with thermometer and hygrometer.

Sauna is a dry hot air bath. The temperature is kept between 60° and 90°C and relative humidity of the air is maintained between 5 and 10%. One treatment session is about 30–40 minutes and consists of two phases: (1) the sweating phase, and (2) the cooling phase.

Phases of Sauna Bath

Sweating Phase

Intense sweating occurs in the sauna bath chamber. About 500–1,000 gram of water is usually lost in one session. The aim is to open all the pores in the skin. Patient is allowed to sit on the lower benches to start and only gradually move up to the higher ones. Loss of weight is seen due to the loss of water from the body. It can be very quickly regained by a corresponding intake of fluids along with minerals.

Cooling Phase

The sweating phase is followed by a cooling phase, which is an important part of the sauna. To begin cooling with cool air, then take a cold shower and then finally to take a dip into a cool pool of water. The aim is to close all the opened pores after removing waste products along with the sweat. Cooling should always begin from the feet and then moving upwards.

The sauna bath chamber is reentered after a pause of 10–15 minutes. After two or three sessions of sauna, a rest period of at least 30 minutes is absolutely necessary.

Mineral water, herb tea or fruit juice to provide adequate hydration is also necessary after sauna bath. Light food involving lots of salad, fruit, yoghurt, etc., should be given only after half an hour.

Physiological Effects

The physiological effects of sauna bath include increase of general circulation. It provides lots of fresh blood to the tissues. It helps removing waste products of metabolism from the body. It relaxes the body and gives a sense of general wellbeing. Pain is also relieved substantially from the body.

Sauna baths are nowadays used in weight reduction programs. Making weight (reducing or increasing weight) by athletes taking part in competition is not advisable.

CHAPTER 9

Ultrasonic Therapy

INTRODUCTION

In the medical community, ultrasound is the modality that is used for a number of purposes including diagnosis, destruction of tissues and therapy. Diagnostic ultrasound is used for imaging the fetus during pregnancy. Destructive ultrasound is used to produce extreme tissue hyperthermia which has been demonstrated to have tumoricidal effects in cancer patients.

Therapeutic ultrasound is one of the most widely used modalities in physiotherapy department **(Fig. 9.1)**. It has been used as a valuable tool in rehabilitation of many different injuries, to stimulate the repair of soft tissue injuries and to relieve pain. It has been traditionally classified as a deep heating modality and used primarily to elevate tissue temperature.

Ultrasound is not strictly electrotherapy because it is a mechanical vibration, albeit (although) produced electrically. It has sometimes been described as micromassage. The meaning of *ultra* is *beyond* or *extreme*. Sound is defined as the periodic mechanical disturbance of an elastic medium such as air.

Ultrasound refers to mechanical vibrations which are essentially the same as sound waves but of a higher frequency. Such waves are beyond the range of human hearing and therefore, also be called as ultrasonic.

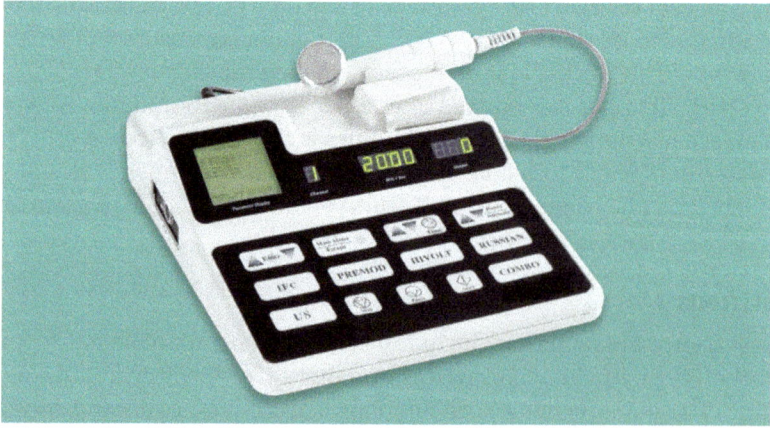

Fig. 9.1: Therapeutic ultrasound.

FREQUENCY OF ULTRASOUND

Ultrasonic energy or ultrasound describes any vibration at a frequency above the audible sound range, i.e., 20–20,000 Hz, but it is frequencies of a few megahertz that are typically used in physiotherapy. Several different therapies are employed in range from 0.5 to 5 MHz. Majority of ultrasound generators are set at a frequency of 1 MHz, although there are ultrasound units that are set at a frequency of 3 MHz **(Fig. 9.2)**. A generator that can be set between 1 and 3 MHz affords the therapist the treatment flexibility.

Ultrasonic energy generated at 1 MHz is transmitted through the more superficial tissue and absorbed primarily in the deeper tissues at depths of 3–5 cm.

A 1 MHz frequency is most useful in individuals with a high percentage of cutaneous body fat and whenever the desired effects are in the deeper structures. At 3 MHz, the energy is absorbed in the more superficial tissues with a depth of penetration between 1 and 2 cm **(Fig. 9.3)**.

PROPERTIES OF WAVES

Sonic waves are a series of mechanical compressions and rarefactions in the direction of travel of the wave; hence, they are called longitudinal waves **(Fig. 9.4)**.

They can occur in solids, liquids and gases and are due to regular compression and separation of molecules. The passage of these waves of compression through matter is, of course, invisible because it is the molecules that vibrate about their average position as a result of the sonic wave **(Fig. 9.5)**.

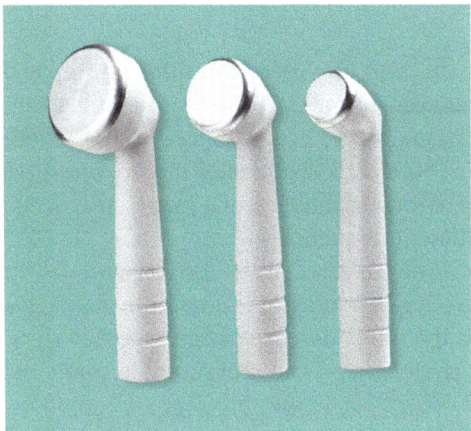

Fig. 9.2: Ultrasound treatment heads.

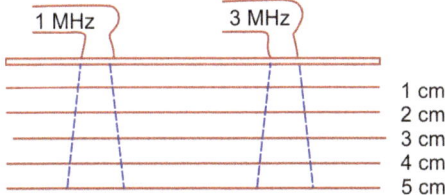

Fig. 9.3: Depth of penetration of ultrasound waves.

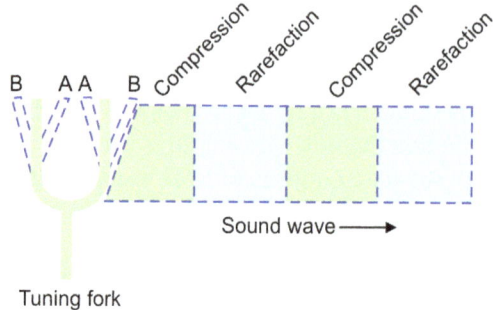

Fig. 9.4: Compression and rarefaction.

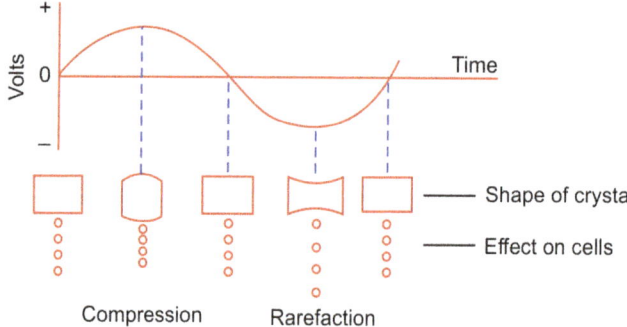

Fig. 9.5: Effect of a change of potential applied to the crystal and the effect of this on adjacent cells.

As sound waves pass through any material, their energy is dissipated or attenuated. Sometimes, all the energy is absorbed at once. Sometimes, the sound wave passes with almost no loss. The molecules of all matter are in constant random motion; the amount of molecular agitation is what is measured as heat. The greater the motion is oscillatory, for instance, the whole molecule may move or rotate to and fro, or it may change shape in an oscillatory way and this may occur at many different frequencies.

The velocity of a wave is the speed at which the wave moves through the medium, and it varies depending upon the physical nature of the medium. Sound waves will pass more rapidly through material in which the molecules are closed together, thus their velocity is higher in solids and liquids than in gases. The velocities of sound in some media are:

- Air   344 m/s
- Water   1,410 m/s
- Muscle   1,540 m/s
- Bone   3,500 m/s.

PRODUCTION OF ULTRASOUND

Ultrasound can be produced by following ways:
- For 1 MHz machine, a vibrating source with a frequency of 1 million cycles per second is needed. This is achieved by using either a *quartz* or a *barium titanate* or a *lead zirconate* or *nickel-cobalt ferrite* crystal. These crystals deform when subjected to a varying potential difference, this is called *piezoelectric effect*.

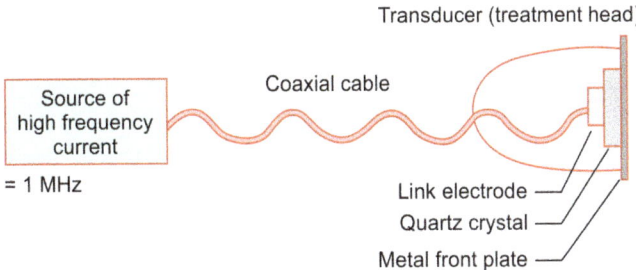

Fig. 9.6: The components of ultrasonic apparatus.

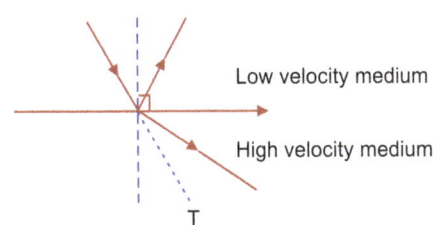

Fig. 9.7: Passing of ultrasonic waves in different medium.

- The basic components of ultrasonic apparatus are shown in **Figure 9.6**. There is a source of high frequency current, which is conveyed by a coaxial cable to a transducer circuit or treatment head or applicator or sound head. Inside the transducer circuit, high frequency current is applied to the crystal being fused to the metal front plate of the treatment head. Any change in the shape of the crystal causes a movement of the metal front plate which, in turn, produces ultrasonic waves.
- Strict frequency control of high frequency current (1 MHz or 3 MHz) ensures a steady and regular rate of deformation (to put out of shape).

Figure 9.5 shows the effects of a change of potential applied to the crystal and the effect this has on adjacent cells. Ultrasonic waves are propagated in a linear fashion up to the end of the near field at which point the beam starts to diverge **(Fig. 9.7)**.

Transmission of Ultrasound

If ultrasonic beam encounters an interface between two media and is transmitted, it may be refracted, i.e., deflected from its original path as light. When traveling from a medium in which its velocity is low into one in which its velocity is high, it is refracted away from the normal.

The significance of refraction is that in **Figure 9.7**, if T was the target, refraction would cause the ultrasonic beam to miss it. As refraction does not occur when the incident waves travel along the normal, treatment should be given with the majority of waves traveling along the normal (i.e., perpendicular to the interface between the media), whenever possible.

Attenuation of Ultrasound

It is the term used to describe the gradual reduction in intensity of the ultrasonic beam once it has left the treatment head. There are two main factors that contribute to attenuation.

Absorption

Ultrasound is absorbed by the tissues and converted to heat at that point. This contributes to the thermal effect of ultrasound.

Scatter (to Spread)

This occurs when the normally cylindrical ultrasonic beam is deflected from its path by reflection at interfaces, bubbles or particles in its path.

The overall effect of these two is such that the ultrasonic beam is reduced in intensity the deeper it passes. This gives rise to the expression "half-value distance" which in depth of soft tissue that reduces the ultrasound beam to half its surface intensity.

The half value distance for soft tissue varies for 1 MHz and 3 MHz output and is 4 cm and 2 cm, respectively. In practical terms, when treating deeper structures, consideration needs to be given to the frequency and intensity of ultrasound chosen.

Ultrasonic Fields

A further consideration relating to depth of penetration and intensity of ultrasonic beam in the division of the beam into a near and far field (**Figs. 9.8A to C**).

The extent of the near field depends upon the radius (r) of the transducer and the wavelength (λ) of the ultrasound in the medium. The depth of the near field can be calculated using the formula r^2/λ. As wavelength and frequency are inversely related, the depth of the near field varies with the frequency of ultrasound.

The near and far fields arise because the wavefronts from different parts of the source have to travel different distances, and consequently there is interference between adjacent fronts. At some points, the interference to constructive and the waves combine their energy and thus, when viewed in both longitudinal and transverse profile, there will be points in the ultrasonic

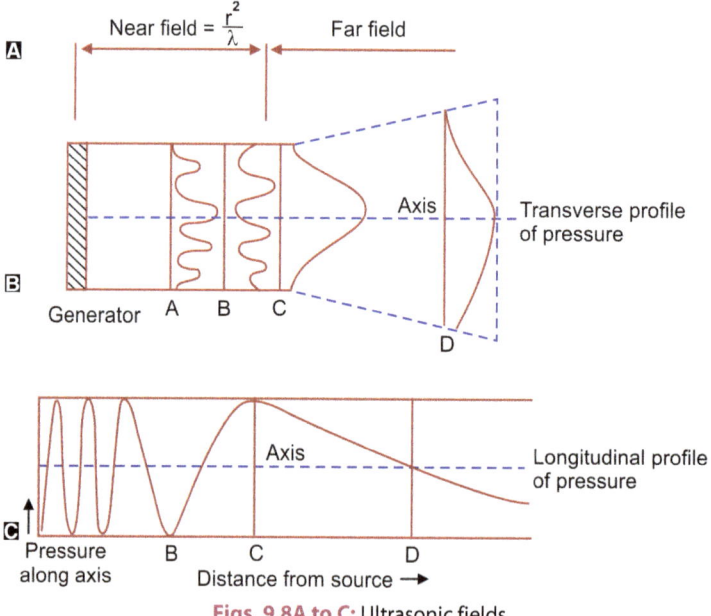

Figs. 9.8A to C: Ultrasonic fields.

beam where intensity is high and points where intensity is low. This is most marked in the near field where there are considerable changes in pressure.

The extent of the near field is of significance in that it is more intense than the far field and may have a more profound effect in the treatment of certain conditions. However, the near field has a much greater variation in intensity than the far field. Consequently, the frequency of the ultrasound and the radius of the transducer may need to be considered when treating tissue at a depth greater than 6.5 cm.

Coupling Media

Ultrasonic waves are not transmitted by air, thus some couplant which does transmit them must be interposed between the treatment head (transducer) and the patient's skin.

Unfortunately, no couplant affords perfect transmission and only a percentage of the original intensity is transmitted to the patient. Even most efficient couplant reduces the applied dose by a quarter.

Air (zero transmission) will in fact, reflect the ultrasound beam back into the treatment head and this could set up standing wave which might damage the crystal. Consequently, the treatment head is never left switched on when not in contact with a transmitting medium.

Some coupling media and their efficiency of transmission are:
- Aquasonic gel   72.6%
- Glycerol   67%
- Distilled water   59%
- Liquid paraffin   19%
- Petroleum jelly   0%
- Air   0%.

Characteristics of a Coupling Media
- An acoustic impedance similar to the tissue
- High transmissivity for ultrasound
- High viscosity
- Low susceptibility to bubble formation
- A chemically inactive nature
- A hypoallergic character
- Relative sterility
- Cheap
- Couplant should also act as a lubricant to allow the treatment head to move smoothly over the skin.

Treatment Parameters

Ultrasound may be used in a continuous mode or in pulsed mode.

In continuous mode, treatment head continuously produces ultrasonic energy. In pulsed mode, the periods of ultrasound are separated by periods of silence.

Intensity

In ultrasound, intensity unit is *watt* but this is a gross measure of the power being emitted by the treatment head, so an averaged intensity is normally used.

- *Space averaged intensity:* Where the average intensity over a specified area is given, e.g., watts per square cm (Wcm^{-2}).
- Time averaged/space averaged intensity can be used when the ultrasound is being applied in a pulsed mode, and gives the average intensity over the whole treatment time (per second) for a specified area (Wcm^{-2}). For example, if 0.5 Wcm^{-2} is applied pulsed 1:4, then in one second, the average intensity (as if the ultrasound was continuous) would be 0.1 Wcm^{-2}. The output meters on some ultrasound generators automatically make this adjustment when using pulsed ultrasound.

Pulsed Mark: Space Ratio

When ultrasound is applied in its pulsed mode, the ratio of the time on to time off should be expressed. This is the mark : space ratio, the mark being the time ultrasound on, space being the silence, both being measured in milliseconds. Some units have a single fixed M:S ratio of 2:8, whereas others have a variable range, e.g., 1:1, 1:4 and 1:7.

Reflection of Ultrasound

Sound obeys the law of reflection and if an ultrasonic beam traveling through one medium encounters another medium which will not transmit (let it pass into the new medium), reflection takes place. Air will not transmit ultrasonic waves, so in ultrasonic treatment, great care is taken to avoid leaving air between the treatment head and the patient to minimize reflection. However, there will always be some reflection at each interface that the ultrasound beam encounters. This gives rise to the term acoustic impedance (Z) which is the ratio between the reflected and transmitted ultrasound at an interface. When the acoustic impedance is low, transmission is high and vice versa.

Testing the Apparatus

Prior to any treatment, it is sensible to check that there is an output from the machine. This can be done by placing the treatment head just below the water surface in a suitable container and observing the disturbance (ripples) which appears **(Fig. 9.9)**.

The apparatus should be on and off with the treatment head below the water. This and other similar methods only indicate the presence of an output but to quantify it, a radiation. Balance should be used regularly.

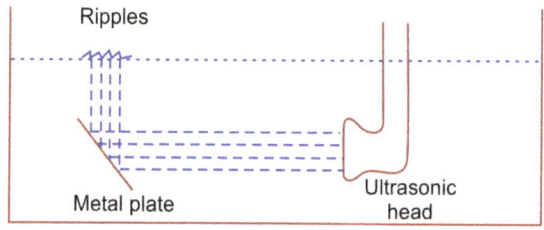

Fig. 9.9: Testing the apparatus.

TECHNIQUES AND METHODS OF APPLICATION

Preparation of Patient
Skin should be washed and hairs should be removed. The nature of the treatment, need for a couplant and stability of the area are all that needs to be explained to the patient. The duration of the treatment as well as any particular cooperation required is indicated.

Examination and Testing
Skin surface to be treated should be inspected; inflammatory skin conditions should be avoided.

Preparation of the Part to be Relaxed
The couplant should be applied to the skin surface.

Setting Up
The patient should be in a comfortable position as skill is needed to apply efficient ultrasound therapy, ensuring close contact, appropriate movement and correct angle of the transducer at all times.

The treatment head is placed on the skin before the output is turned on. This is to avoid damage to the transducer which can occur if the energy is reflected back into the transducer. Some machines have a monitoring system. If the ultrasound energy reaching the tissues becomes much less than the set intensity, the output is greatly reduced, the timer stops and the operation is alerted in some way.

Instructions and Warnings
The patient is asked to keep the part still and relaxed and to report if any increase of pain or other sensations immediately.

Application
The treatment head is moved continuously over the surface while even pressure is maintained in order to iron out irregularities in the sonic field. The emitting surface must be kept parallel to the skin surface to reduce reflection and pressed sufficiently firmly to exclude any air. The rate of movement must be slow enough to allow the tissues to deform and thus remain in complete contact with rigid treatment head but fast enough to prevent *hot spots* developing when using a high intensity treatment. The pattern of movement can be a series of overlapping parallel strokes, circles or figures of eight **(Fig. 9.10)**.

Termination
The intensity is returned to zero, either manually or automatically, before the transducer is removed from the water bath or tissue contact. The skin is cleaned of couplant or dried. The transducer should be cleaned after each use with a noncorrosive, nonabrasive antiseptic lotion.

Recording
The following should be recorded:
* Machine used
* Intensity

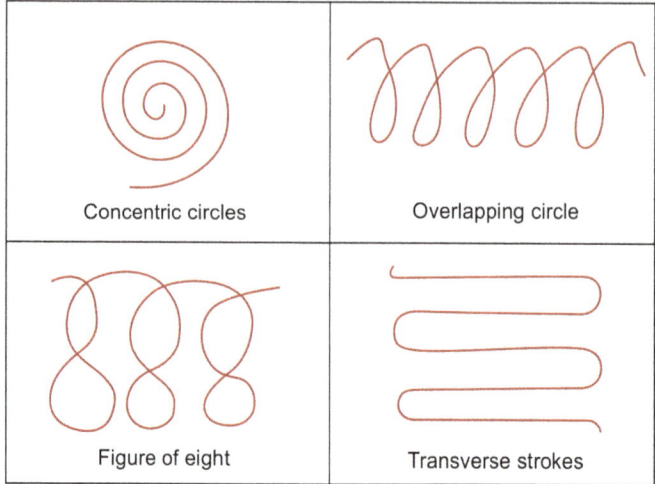

Fig. 9.10: Methods of application.

- Frequency
- Pulse mode
- Insonation time
- Couplant
- Region and area of insonation
- Response of treatment.

Techniques of Application

Direct Contact Method

If the surface to be treated is fairly regular, then a coupling medium is applied to the skin in order to eliminate air between the skin and the treatment head and transmit the ultrasonic beam from the treatment head to the tissues. The treatment head is moved in small concentric circles over the skin in order to avoid concentration at any one point, keeping the whole of the front plate in contact with the patient. This technique is suitable for areas up to three times the size of the treatment head. Large area should be divided and each area treated separately. The size of the area and its exact location should be specified on the treatment head **(Fig. 9.11)**.

Water Bath Method

When direct contact is not possible because of irregular shape of part or because of tenderness, a water bath may be used. As the part to be treated is immersed in water this can only reasonably be applied to the hand, ankle and foot.

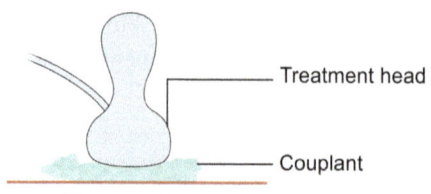

Fig. 9.11: Direct contact method.

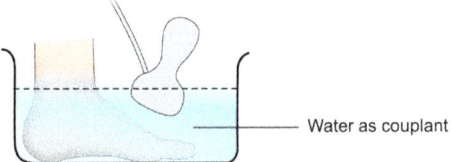

Fig. 9.12: Water bath method.

A water bath filled with degassed water is used, if possible. Ordinary tap water presents the problem that gas bubbles dissociate out from the water, accumulate on the patient skin and the treatment head, and reflect the ultrasound beam. If tap water has to be used, then the gas bubbles must be wiped from these surfaces frequently.

The patient is seated, and part is put in water of a comfortable temperature in such a position that it is suitably supported **(Fig. 9.12)**.

The treatment head is placed in the water and held 1 cm from the skin and moved in small concentric circles, keeping the front parallel to the skin surface to reduce reflection to a minimum.

If the patient's hand is to be immersed in the bath while the application is active, care should be taken to minimize exposure to any reflected or scattered ultrasound. This can be done by wearing a dry knitted glove inside a water-proof rubber or plastic glove.

Water Bag Method

Another method of applying ultrasound therapy to irregular surface which cannot conventionally be placed in a water bath is treated with a plastic or rubber bag filled with water forming a water cushion between the treatment head and the skin.

Rubber bag filled with degassed water can be used. All visible air bubbles should be squeezed out before knotting the neck of the bag to seal it. A coupling medium has to be placed both between the rubber bag and skin and between the rubber bag and the treatment head to eliminate any air **(Fig. 9.13)**.

The bag placed on irregular surface is then held with the help of patient or others. Treatment head is pressed firmly onto the bag so that a layer of water about 1 cm thick separates it from the surface (body). Inevitably, some bubbles will form and it is important to ensure that these are in the sides of the bag and not in the region transmitting the ultrasound. The treatment head is then moved over the surface of the bag. It does, however, present problems in terms of attenuation as many more interfaces have to be crossed by the ultrasound and rubber absorbs

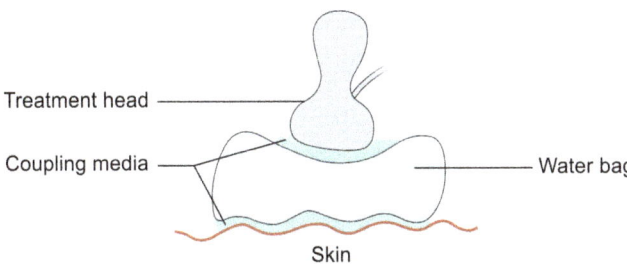

Fig. 9.13: Water bag method.

much of ultrasonic energy. To minimize the problem, condoms or thin balloons are more satisfactory because these are thin, cheap and easy to use.

DOSAGE

Three factors which determine ultrasound dosage are as follows:
1. Size of the treatment area
2. Depth of the lesion from the surface
3. Nature of lesion.

Parameters of Ultrasound
- Mode
- Frequency
- Intensity
- Duration of treatment.

When treating the patients with ultrasound, it is worth remembering that the intensity of ultrasound leaving the treatment head is not the intensity being applied to the deep tissues. Intensity, therefore, has been reduced by:
- Absorption in the coupling medium
- Attenuation of the beam by absorption and scatter
- Refraction of the beam at tissue interfaces which may deflect the beam always from the offending tissue.

Mode

Continuous mode produces more heat so it is used for musculoskeletal conditions such as muscular spasm, joint stiffness, pain, etc.

Pulsed mode produces less heat so it is used for soft tissue repair, e.g., tendinitis.

For example, 0.5 W/cm² pulsed at 1:4 deliver the same energy as 0.1 W/cm² on a continuous mode.

Frequency

Attenuation increases with increase in frequency effectively, lower frequency penetrate further:
- Ultrasonic 3 MHz—superficial tissue
- Ultrasonic 0.75 to 1 MHz—penetrate deeply.

Intensity

Power is the total energy/second supplied by the machine and is measured in Watts:
- Intensity applied is according to the nature of the lesion.
- For acute and immediate post-traumatic: 0.1–0.25 W/cm².
- For chronic and scar tissue: 0.25–1 W/cm².

Duration of Treatment

- Amount of energy depends on intensity and duration of treatment.

- Size of area determines the treatment time.
- 1-2 minutes for every cm².
- Many transducer heads have an area of 5 cm² and the palm of the small hand is about 50 cm².

Minimum	—	1-2 minutes
Maximum	—	8 minutes
Average	—	5 minutes
For chronic	—	Longer treatment time
For acute	—	Lesser treatment time.

Dosage in Acute Lesion or Conditions

In any acute conditions, treatment is applied cautiously to prevent exacerbation of symptoms.
- Initial stage
  Low dose:
   0.25–0.5 Wcm^{-2}
   Time 2–3 minutes
  Progression unnecessary, if condition improves.
- Failure case:
   0.25–0.5 Wcm^{-2}
   Time 4–5 minutes
   or
   0.8 Wcm^{-2}
   Time 2–3 minutes.

Aggravation of symptoms is not always a bad sign as it may indicate repair processes are taking place. During that situation, a reduction in dose in both time and intensity may be indicated (or) treatment with ultrasound may be deferred (to postpone or to put off) until symptoms subside to their original level. It may also be possible to select different M:S pulse ratio and use:
- 1:7 for very acute
- 1:1 for less acute.

Dosage in Chronic Condition

Chronic condition may be treated with pulsed or continuous mode. The maximum intensity of ultrasound which should be used is that which produces mildly perceptible warmth. This usually occurs around 2 W/cm². Initially, low dose is tried—intensity 0.8 W/cm², time 4 minutes.

If improvement occurs, treatment is repeated. If no improvement occurs, dose is gradually increased.
- Maximum dose of ultrasound: 2 W/cm² for 8 minutes.
- If no improvement occurs after 6 sittings, ultrasound treatment has to be discontinued. Progression and timings: Frequency of treatment.
- Recent injuries and acute conditions: once or twice daily.
- Chronic conditions: Every alternate day.

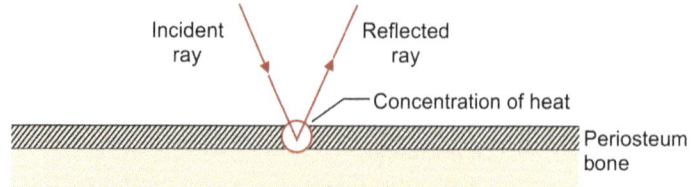

Fig. 9.14: Reflection of ultrasound beam from bone, concentration of heating effect may leads to periosteal pain.

PHYSIOLOGICAL EFFECTS OF ULTRASOUND

Following ultrasonic therapy, the physiological changes that take place are as follows:

Thermal Effects

As the ultrasound waves are absorbed by the tissues, they are converted into heat. The amount of heat developed depends upon:

* Absorption of the tissues, e.g., protein absorbs ultrasound more effectively and therefore produces much heat.
* The number of times the treatment head passes over the part.
* The efficiency of circulation through the insonated tissues.
* When using continuous ultrasound, the amount of heat developed is directly proportional to the intensity and duration of insonation.
* When using pulsed ultrasound, there is less thermal effect than with continuous and a mark:space ratio of 1:4 produces less heat than 1:1.
* Reflection of ultrasound at a tissue interface produces a concentration of heating effect at a specific point **(Fig. 9.14)**. This is particularly likely at the interface between periosteum and bone. As reflection from bone occurs, there is double intensity of ultrasound in the periosteal region, which may cause localized overheating and can manifest itself as periosteal pain. In practical terms, this means that it is best to avoid passing the ultrasound treatment head over the subcutaneous bony points, if possible.

Uses of Thermal Effects

The local rise in temperature could be used to accelerate healing. The extensibility of collagen is increased by rise in temperature and so stretching of scars or adhesions is easier following ultrasound. The thermal effect may also help reducing pain.

In the past, ultrasound was classified as a heat treatment, but recent work has shown that there are many nonthermal effects of ultrasound which may be of use in treatment. These effects are all associated with one another, and arise because of considerable force generated within the tissues by the ultrasound. The nonthermal effects are as follows:

Cavitation

This is the oscillatory activity of highly compressible bodies within the tissues such as gas or vapor filled voids **(Fig. 9.15)**. Cavitation may be stable or unstable cavitation.

Stable Cavitation

Stable cavitation occurs when bubbles oscillate to and fro within the ultrasonic pressure waves but remain intact. It is not dangerous and could be of benefit as it modifies the ultrasonic beam in such a way as to cause microstreaming.

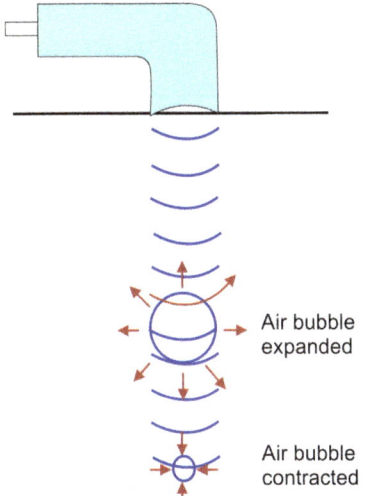
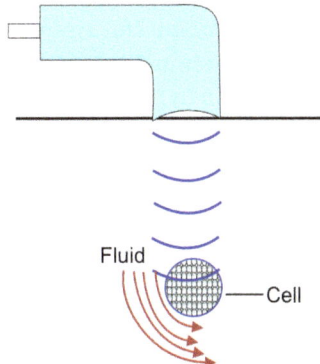

Fig. 9.15: Cavitation—compression and contraction of air bubble due to ultrasonically induced pressure.

Fig. 9.16: Microstreaming.

Microstreaming is the unidirectional movement of fluids along the boundaries of the cell. Due to microstreaming, permeability of cell membrane and direction of movement of molecules into the cells is influenced **(Fig. 9.16)**.

Unstable or Transient Cavitation

This occurs when the volume of the bubbles changes rapidly and then collapse. It is potentially dangerous to the tissues as the collapse of the bubbles cause a great local rise in temperature. It is avoided by moving the treatment head (to prevent standing waves) using a low intensity (below 3 watt/cm^2) and using a high frequency (1-3 MHz).

Mechanical Effect or Micromassage

This occurs where the longitudinal compression waves of the ultrasound beam produces compression and rarefaction of cells, and affect the movement of tissue fluid in interstitial spaces. This can help in reducing edema. Combined with the thermal effect, the extensibility of scars and adhesions could be affected in such a way to make stretching them easier. It is also possible that the mechanical effect could help reduce pain.

Biological Effect

Ultrasound can have some useful effects in all the three stages of repair:
1. *Inflammatory:* Ultrasound probably increases the fragility of lysosome membrane, and thus enhances the release of their contained enzymes. These enzymes will help to clear the area of debris and allow the next stage to occur.
2. *Proliferative:* Fibroblasts and myofibroblasts may have Ca^{++} ions driven into them by the ultrasound. This increases their mobility and encourages their movement toward the area of repair. The fibroblasts are stimulated to produce the collagen fibers to form scar and myofibroblasts contract to pull the edges together.

3. *Remodeling:* Ultrasound has been shown to increase the tensile strength of the scar by affecting the direction, strength and elasticity of fibers which make up the scar easier.

THERAPEUTIC USES OF ULTRASOUND

- *Uses of ultrasound:* Ultrasound is often used after soft tissue injuries as the mechanical effects help to remove the traumatic exudates and reduces the danger of adhesion formation. Heat produced by ultrasound in large diameter nerve fibers may reduce pain through gate mechanism. Accelerated protein synthesis stimulates the rate of repair of damaged tissues.
- *Scar tissue:* Scar tissue is made pliable (capable of bend or twist) by the application of ultrasound, which allows more effective stretching of contracted scars. If the scar is bound down on underlined structures, ultrasound may help in gaining its release.
- *Chronic indurated edema:* The mechanical effects of ultrasound have an effect on chronic edema and helps in its treatment. It also breaks down adhesions formed between adjacent structures.
- *Varicose ulcers:* Ultrasound is found effective to promote the healing of varicose ulcers and pressure sores.
- *Blood flow:* In an investigation of the effect of continuous ultrasound on blood flow, a dose of 1.5 W/cm^2 for 5 minutes applied to the forearm did not alter the skeletal muscle blood flow.
- *Bone injuries:* Ultrasound in the first and second week after bony injury can increase bone union, but given to an unstable fracture during the phase of cartilage proliferation, it may result in proliferation of cartilage and therefore decrease in bone reunion. Ultrasound can also be used in early diagnosis of stress fractures. A moderate dose applied over the site of the fracture leads to intense pain, whereas the same dose applied to the opposite side has no pain. Thus, ultrasound can identify stress fractures.
- *Plantar warts:* Plantar warts are occasionally seen in the athletic population, occurring on the weight-bearing areas of the feet and caused by either a virus or microtrauma. These lesions contain thrombosed capillaries in a whitish colored soft core covered by hyperkeratotic epithelial tissue. Among other more conventional techniques, several studies have recommended as an effective painless method for eliminating plantar warts.
- *Placebo effect:* While the physiological effects of ultrasound have been discussed in detail, it can also have significant therapeutic psychological effects. A number of studies have demonstrated a placebo effect in patients receiving ultrasound.

DANGERS OF ULTRASOUND

- *Burns:* If continuous beam is used and is allowed to remain stationary, excess heat can accumulate in the tissues and eventually leads to burns. However, the danger of burn is effectively eliminated by keeping the treatment head moving, using pulsed beams and avoiding bony prominence, if possible.
- *Cavitation:* Especially unstable cavitation is dangerous and has been described previously.
- *Overdose:* Excessive dose may cause an exacerbation of symptoms.
- *Danger to equipment:* If the treatment head is held in the air while switched on, the reflection of the beam back into the treatment head may set up standing waves which could damage the crystal, consequently the head is never turned on unless it is in contact with the transmitting material.

CONTRAINDICATIONS

* *Vascular conditions:* Conditions such as thrombophlebitis, where insonation may cause emboli to be broken off, are not treated with ultrasound.
* *Acute sepsis:* An area which presents acute sepsis should be treated cautiously with ultrasound because of the danger of spreading the infection, or in some instances, breaking off septic emboli. If the treatment is passed over an infected area (as in the treatment of herpes zoster), it must be sterilized with an appropriate solution before treatment of the next patient.
* *Radiotherapy:* Radiotherapy has a devitalizing effect on the tissue, therefore ultrasound is not applied to a radiated area after 6 months of irradiation.
* *Tumors:* Tumors are not insonated because they may be stimulated or metastasized.
* *Pregnancy:* A pregnant uterus is not treated as the insonation may cause damage to the fetus. Consequently, during pregnancy, the back and abdomen should not be treated.
* *Cardiac disease:* Patients who have had cardiac disease are treated with low intensities in order to avoid sudden pain, and area such as cervical ganglion and the vagus nerve are avoided because of the risk of cardiac stimulation. Patients fitted with cardiac pacemakers are not usually treated with ultrasound in the area of the chest, as the ultrasound generator may have an effect on the pacemakers' rate of stimulation.
* *Hemorrhage:* When bleeding is still occurring or has only recently been controlled, such as an enlarging hemarthrosis or hematoma or uncontrolled hemophilia, ultrasound is contraindicated.
* *Severely ischemic tissue:* Because of the poor heat transfer and possibly greater risk of arterial thrombosis due to statistics and endothelial damage, ultrasound is contraindicated.
* *Nervous system:* Normal doses of ultrasound have been applied for many years to the tissues around the spinal cord without any ill effects. In fact, treatment of the spinal nerve roots and over the apophyseal joints is particularly common. Since the CNS is deeply buried beneath the thick muscles and more importantly bone tissue, it seems reasonable to suppose that only trivial amounts of energy could reach it. Where the nerve tissue is exposed, e.g., over a spina bifida or after laminectomy, ultrasound is avoided.
* *Specialized tissue:* The fluid filled eye offer an exceptionally good ultrasound transmission and retinal damage could occur. Treatment over the gonads, i.e., testes and ovary, are also not recommended.
* *Implants:* Although metal implants in the tissue would reflect the ultrasound at their interfaces and thus leads to more energy absorption in this area, this does not lead to a large temperature rise in the region because the amount of heat generated is easily conducted collar areas. The effect might, however, be different with smaller and more superficial implants like metal bone fixing pins subcutaneously placed, as a precaution low doses are used in these areas. Plastics used in replacement surgery as high intensity polyethylene and acrylic should also be avoided since their effect on ultrasound absorption is unknown.
* *Anesthetic area:* If ultrasonic is given to anesthetic area, there will not be any type of pain or heat experienced by the patient which could lead to burns.

PHONOPHORESIS

Phono means *sound* and phoresis means *migration of the ions through a membrane by the action of an electric current.*

Phonophoresis is defined as the movement of the drugs through skin into the subcutaneous tissues under the influence of ultrasound. It is otherwise called as sonophoresis or ultra sonophoresis.

Principle

Phonophoresis relies on perturbation of the tissue causing more rapid particle movement and thus encouraging absorption of the drug.

Effects of Phonophoresis

The thermal effects of ultrasonic increase tissue permeability and the acoustic pressure created by the ultrasonic beam drives the medication into the tissues. Thus, the medication follows the path of beam. Both pulsed and continuous ultrasonic have been used in phonophoresis. Continuous ultrasonic at an intensity great enough to produce thermal effects may induce a proinflammatory response. If the goal is to decrease inflammation, pulsed ultrasonic with low spatial-averaged temporal peak intensity may be the best choice.

Penetration of Phonophoretically-driven Drugs

The depth to which drugs can be made to penetrate is a matter of particular uncertainty. Once the drug has passed through the epidermis, it is likely to be dispersed in the circulation to an extent which depends on the vascularity of the tissues concerned and the ease with which molecules of the drugs can enter blood vessels. Ultrasonic machine with 0.33–0.25 MHz were found to be more effective. Low frequency leads to greater penetration. It must be realized that deeper penetration does not necessarily infer greater effectiveness. If therapeutic effects occur in the dermis and epidermis, such as cutaneous anesthetic effect of lignocaine, it might be expected that higher frequencies would be more effective, since the ultrasonic energy is largely absorbed in the superficial tissues. This has been shown to occur that 1.5 MHz and 3 MHz ultrasonic appeared to be more effective in achieving absorption of local anesthetic than 0.75 MHz. Interestingly, this same study showed that pulsed was rather more effective than continuous ultrasonic in achieving transfer of this particular analgesic. This provides evidence for a specific effect due to the energy of ultrasonic.

Drug Used in Phonophoresis

The anti-inflammatory drug hydrocortisone has been widely used. High concentration of the drug 10% ointments are more effective when comparing 1% can be driven through the skin with relatively high intensity ultrasonic. Many inflammatory skin conditions have been treated with hydrocortisone.

It is possible that ultrasonic therapy having a proinflammatory and steroid an anti-inflammatory are conflicting therapies.

Other steroid-type drugs can be applied by phonophoresis as well as many nonsteroidal anti-inflammatory drugs, mainly salicylates. An anti-inflammatory analgesic cream (trolamine salicylate) has been recommended. A study to investigate the effectiveness of this agent on delayed onset muscle soreness (DOMS) in normal subjects found that ultrasound alone increases the symptom while ultrasound with trolamine salicylate has no such effect.

It was concluded that the anti-inflammatory activity of this drug was able to offset the increased soreness due to the proinflammatory effect of ultrasound.

Phonophoresis of hydrocortisone has been used in the reactions of many skin conditions including psoriasis, scleroderma and bursitis.

A lotion containing zinc oxide, tannic acid, urea and menthol has been applied by phonophoresis to treat herpes simplex virus type II in both oral and genital infections with good results.

Antibiotics such as penicillin have been given by phonophoresis for the treatment of skin infections.

Applications

The drug to be driven into the tissue is combined in a suitable gel or cream which forms the couplant. It is smeared onto the part using a spatula (an instrument with broad blade for spreading pigments) so that it is not applied by the patient's fingers.

Treatment head is used onto the skin in a usual manner. Relatively high intensities of 1 W/cm^2 and 1.5 W/cm^2 have been used.

The depth of the target tissue determines the frequency used.

The time of treatment depends on the area over which phonophoresis is to be applied.

1 minute treatment for every 10 cm^2 area is reasonable, although some suggest 5 minutes for each 25 cm^2, i.e., about 1 minute for 30 cm^2.

After the completion of treatment, the drug should be removed from both the patient's skin and the transducer head. Because of unnoticeably applied to other patient with same treatment head.

Since the cream or gel containing the drug is being used as the coolant, it is important that it transmits ultrasonic adequately. In general, that gels are more efficient coupling agents than creams, particularly for higher frequency ultrasonic (1.5 and 3 MHz).

Contraindications

The same considerations apply when giving phonophoresis as apply when giving ultrasonic for its intrinsic effects.

The effect of the drug must also be considered; for example, anti-inflammatory drugs may suppress necessary inflammatory reaction, such as local skin infections, allowing them to become more serious.

If local skin anesthetizing drugs are being driven in by ultrasonic waves, it must be remembered that skin sensation under the treatment head will gradually be lost so that the patient may no longer detect excessive heat; high intensities should not, therefore, be used for these drugs.

Keep in mind that allergies and sensitivities to the substance contraindicate its use on the skin as well, for example:
- Patient who cannot eat sea food should not be treated with iodine. If skin irritation and itching occurs, it should be reported. The usual antidote is an antihistamine. An alternative should be selected in future treatment.
- Patient sensitive to metals should not be treated with zinc. These patients usually cannot wear metallic watch bands, jewelry, etc., without having skin reaction and at times, systemic reactions. Dermato3logic consultation should be sought for specific antidotes for offending metals. Nonmetallic substances should be substituted.
- If a patient has a reaction to mecholyl with vasomotor shifting, administer a simple stimulant such as black coffee. Vertigo form orthostatic adjustment is usually momentary.

- Reactions to hydrocortisone are not as common as you think. The culprits are usually the chemicals included in the base of ointment or solution (e.g., novocaine) rather than the steroid itself. Have the patient use an antihistamine skin lotion should any dermal irritation occur.
- Do not treat a patient with salicylates if he or she is sensitive to aspirin. Seek medical consultation for the specific treatment of symptoms. It should be noted that although the above reactions are extremely rare, the efforts taken in the prevention of their occurrence will be well worthwhile.

COMBINATION THERAPY

The application of two therapeutic modalities at the same time and at the same site is described as combination therapy. Ultrasonic therapy is frequently used with other modalities including hot packs, cold packs and electric nerve and muscle stimulating currents.

The most widely used combinations are those of ultrasonic with some form of nerve and muscle stimulating current, for example, ultrasonic and interferential. This can be done because the ultrasonic transducer provides low resistance electrical contact with skin. Electrical stimulating currents are used for analgesia or producing muscle contraction. Ultrasonic and electrical stimulating currents have been recommended to treat myofascial trigger points. Both modalities provide analgesic effects and both are effective in reducing the pain-spasm- pain cycle.

Hot packs and high intensity ultrasonic are used primarily for their thermal effects. Heat is effective in reducing muscle spasm and muscle guarding. It also has an analgesic effect and is useful in pain reduction since hot packs produce an increased blood flow superficially, thus creating a less dense medium for transmission of ultrasonic, attenuation may be increased and depth of penetration of ultrasonic reduced.

Cold packs are most often used for analgesia and to decrease acute blood flow after injury. Because cold is such an effective analgesic, caution must be exercised when using ultrasonic at higher intensities that produce thermal effects, since patient's perception of temperature and pain is diminished. However, in treating acute and postacute injuries, the combination of cold to reduce blood flow (i.e., swelling) and produce analgesia, and low intensity ultrasound, for its nonthermal effects that promote soft tissue healing, may be the treatment of choice. Since cold produces a decrease in blood flow superficially and thus a more dense medium, superficial attenuation of ultrasonic may be decreased, facilitating transmission to deeper tissues.

The production, application and therapeutic effects are those of the individual therapies as described in this text. The justification for the use of combination therapy is principally the beneficial effect of both modalities that may be achieved at the same time, thus making the therapy efficient, at least in terms of time committed by both therapist and patient.

A second justification is that there may be an enhancing effect of one therapy upon the other, making the combination more effective than each therapy alone.

SHOCK WAVE THERAPY

Shock wave therapy (SWT) **(Fig. 9.17)** is a technique in which high pressure sound waves are used for the treatment of various musculoskeletal conditions. In earlier days, shock waves were used in breaking up of kidney stones. Presently, it is being used for the treatment of plantar

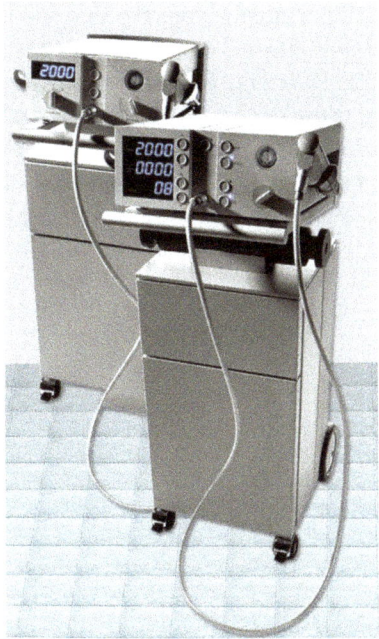

Fig. 9.17: Shock wave therapy apparatus.

fasciitis and tennis elbow tendinitis. It has also been found to be effective in the treatment of patellar tendinitis, supraspinatus tendinitis, bicipital tendinitis, rotator cuff injuries, Achilles tendinitis, pseudoarthrosis, stress fractures, delayed union, early stages of avascular bone necrosis and shoulder calcification. There is also a Food and Drug Administration (FDA) study to treat recalcitrant diabetic wounds.

Basically two forms of shock waves are currently used:
1. Extracorporeal shock wave therapy (ESWT)
2. Radial shock wave therapy (RSWT).

Extracorporeal shock wave therapy devices contain converging focused shock waves. Maximum energy is reached at a specific point in the body. These devices produce a medium to high energy level.

Radial Shock wave therapy devices contain radial diverging shock waves. The energy is spread over a large surface area. These devices produce a low-to-medium energy level.

Physical Principles

A shock wave is defined as a sonic pulse characterized by:
- High peak pressure (500 bar)
- A short lifecycle (10 ms)
- Fast pressure rise (<10 ns)
- A broad frequency spectrum (16 Hz–20 MHz).

There are a couple of theories as to how ESWT helps promote better healing. The most accepted one is that the microtrauma of the repeated shock wave to the affected area creates neo-vascularization (new blood flow) into the area. It is this new blood flow that promotes tissue healing. The second theory is that in chronic pain, the brain has "forgotten" about the pain and is doing nothing to heal the area. By having SWT, a new inflammatory process is created and the brain can react to it by sending the necessary body nutrients to the area to promote healing.

Contraindications for this procedure include: neurological and vascular disease of the foot, history of rupture of the plantar fascia ligament, open bone growth plates, pregnancy, implanted metal in the area (bone screws and pins) and people on medication that interferes with blood clotting such as coumadin and prophylactic aspirin.

Dosage Parameters
- Energy: 5–20 J/cm^2
- Pressure: 2–5 bar
- Number of shocks: 500–2000
- Treatment sessions: 3–5.

METHODS OF TREATMENT

TREATMENT OF PATIENT'S CONDITION
- Tennis elbow
- Golfer's elbow
- Supraspinatus tendinitis
- de Quervain's disease
- Bicipital tendinitis
- Subdeltoid bursitis
- Subacromial bursitis
- Metatarsalgia.

ULTRASOUND THERAPY

PROFORMA FOR PATIENT'S ASSESSMENT
- Receiving the patient:
  Good morning, I am a physiotherapist and going to treat you. Please, cooperate with me during the treatment and wait until I go through your case sheet.
- History taking or going through the case sheet:
  - Name
  - Father's and mother's name
  - Age
  - Sex
  - Occupation
  - Address: Correspondence and permanent
  - Chief complaints
  - History of present illness
  - History of past illness

- Family history
- Social and occupational history
- Treatment history
- Prognosis of the treatment
- Investigations:
    - Hematological tests
    - Radiological tests—X-rays, MRI scan, etc.
- Checking for general contraindications:
    - Hyperpyrexia
    - Hypertension
    - Deep X-ray and cobalt therapy
    - Epileptic patients
    - Noncooperative patients
    - Mentally retarded patients
    - Very poor general condition of the patient.
- Checking for local contraindications:
    - Skin condition
    - Wound
    - Tumor
    - Any metal in the treatment area
    - Pregnant uterus.
- Preparation of trays:
  Two test tubes
    - One with hot water
    - One with cold water

  Cotton
  Gel (Coupling media)
  Towels
  Pillows
  Sand bags.

❖ Preparation of the apparatus:
  - Selection of treatment head
  - Switching on
  - Regulation of amplitude
  - Checking the insulation
  - Checking the plugs
  - Checking the socket
  - Checking the main wire whether it is properly fitted in the main machine.

❖ Gaining the confidence of the patient.

❖ Positioning the patient:
  - Comfortable with good support

❖ Treatment:
  - Checking the apparatus
  - Placing the treatment head
  - Instructions to the patient
  - Knowledge of the details of technique of application

- Other special points:
  - Comfort and consideration of patient
  - Knowledge of condition
  - Position and posture of physiotherapist
  - Care of apparatus and patient
  - Maintaining the record of treatment.

TENNIS ELBOW (LATERAL EPICONDYLITIS)

Definition

Tennis elbow is a condition characterized by pain and acute tenderness on the lateral side of the elbow usually related to the common extensor tendon.

Age: 30–45 years
Sex: Equally common in both the sexes
Cause: Excessive use of wrist extensors
For example: a. Carrying a heavy weight
 b. Wrong technique at sports (e.g., tennis, golf, badminton, fencing)
 c. Unaccustomed gardening or carpentry.

Pathology

Tear occurs at the tenomuscular junction, in the tendon, or at the tenoperiosteal junction. The resulting inflammation produces exudates in which fibrin forms to heal the torn tissue. If excessive fibrin is formed, fibrous tissue will result in adhesions of the tendon and neighboring tissues. This causes pain, and repeated use and minor injury to tendon prevent healing and excessive scar tissue form.

Clinical Features

- Pain on exertion
- Pain over the elbow toward the wrist
- Elbow and wrist, restricted range of motion due to pain
- Resisted wrist extension is painful, passive movement is pain-free
- Tenderness over the tendon.

Treatment

- Acute
  - Ice towel for 20 minutes
  - Rest
  - Splint for wrist extension for 2–8 weeks
  - Strapping.

Modalities Used

- Friction (Circular or transverse) massage for 5–10 minutes for 4 days
- Ultrasound 1 W/cm² in continuous mode for up to 8 minutes
- Pulsed electromagnetic energy
- Laser.

Positioning of the Patient

Sitting with arm on the pillow placed over the couch.

Mode : Continuous/Pulsed
Duration : 5–8 minutes
Intensity : 0.75–1.5 W/cm²

GOLFER'S ELBOW (MEDIAL EPICONDYLITIS)

Definition

This is a condition characterized by pain and acute tenderness on the medial side of the elbow. It affects the common flexor origin.

Principles of treatments are the same as for tennis elbow.

Position of the Patient

Sitting with arm on the pillow placed over the couch.

Mode : Continuous/pulsed
Duration : 5–8 minutes
Intensity : 0.75–1.5 W/cm².

SUPRASPINATUS TENDINITIS

Etiology

This may occur as a result of one accident (e.g., a fall on the shoulder), over exercise (e.g., aerobics) or a series of minor stresses (e.g., long periods of writing).

Clinical Features

Pain: Toothache type pain is present radiating from the acromion process to the deltoid insertion.

Painful area:
- Abduction to 60° is pain-free.
- 60–120° is painful.
- 120–180° is pain-free.

Movements:
- Shoulder, arm movements are full (but have a painful arc).
- Resisted abduction in outer range is often painful.
- Lowering the arm from elevation is very painful. If this movement is resisted, the pain is less. This is a test used to determine whether it is bursitis or tendinitis. Bursitis remains painful on resisted lowering of the arm.
- Reversed glenohumeral rhythm—the scapula moving more than the humerus.

Function: Severely limited in patient who has to carry (e.g., dresses on coat hangers).

Management

- Hydrocortisone injection
- Nonsteroidal anti-inflammatory drug.

Physiotherapy
- Rest in an arm sling
- Ultrasound—remove inflammatory exudates. It must be applied to the tendon that is with the shoulder in extension El medial rotation.
- Ice towel to the superior aspect of shoulder (10–20 minutes).

Exercise
- Auto-assisted elevation through flexion adduction should be produced once every hour to prevent adhesion formation, re-education of glenohumeral rhythm.
- Frictions.

DE QUERVAIN'S DISEASE (TENOSYNOVITIS)

Tenosynovitis is inflammation of the synovial sheath of the tendon (Tendinitis is inflammation of the tendon which does not have a sheath).
 De Quervain's disease is a chronic constructive tenosynovitis affecting the abductor pollicis longus and extensor pollicis brevis tendons of the thumb at the wrist.

Clinical Features
- Pain along the lateral aspects of the distal end of the radius
- Swelling along the tendons
- Tender on palpation
- Active extension against resistance and passive flexion of the thumb are painful.

Cause
Overuse (Using scissors excessively).

Treatment
- Rest
- Splinting the wrist and thumb in full extension
- Administration of the anti-inflammatory drugs
- Ultrasound
- Low dosage (0.25 W/cm²)
- Pulsed mode
- Apply along the length of the tendon
- Later stages, administration of hydrocortisone.

BICIPITAL TENDINITIS

This tends to occur when the tendon of the long head lies in the bicipital groove. Pain is provoked by resisted supination of the forearm and flexion of the elbow. Frictions and ultrasound are the treatment of choice.

SUBDELTOID BURSITIS

Bursitis is inflammation of a bursa. A bursa is a membranous sac lined with endothelial cells. It may or may not communicate with the synovial membrane of the joint. The function of the bursa is to prevent friction between two structures (e.g. tendon and bone or tendon and muscle) or to project bony points.

Common Sites
- Prepatellar bursitis (Housemaid's knee)
- Suprapatellar bursitis
- Subdeltoid bursitis
- Miner's or student's elbow (olecranon bursitis)
- Achillodynia (Inflammation of the one of the bursa around the Achilles tendon).

Causes
- Trauma
- Associated diseases— rheumatoid arthritis, gout.

Clinical Features
Pain and swelling.

SUBACROMIAL BURSITIS

This condition is characterized by a painful arc on shoulder abduction. It is present between 60° on both active and passive movements when the bursa is passing underneath the acromion process together with supraspinatus tendon, the long head of biceps and the capsule of the glenohumeral joint, e.g., pulsed electromagnetic energy (PEME) and ultrasound.

METATARSALGIA

This is the condition in which there is pain in the metatarsal region. It is usually felt under the metatarsal heads and is commonly found in the middle-aged or elderly and more often in women than men.

Causes
Metatarsalgia may be due to weak intrinsic muscle allowing the anterior arch to collapse. It also occurs secondary to hallux valgus, flat feet, talipes equinus or pes cavus. Patients suffering from rheumatoid arthritis also develop metatarsalgia. Unsuitable footwear predisposes this.

Clinical Features
- Pain
- Walking pattern is affected.
- Metatarsal heads are usually prominent on the sole of the foot with callosities forming over the heads.

Treatment
- Re-education of muscles
- Ultrasound.

10
CHAPTER
Cryotherapy

INTRODUCTION

The application of cold for various therapeutic purposes is called *cryotherapy*. Cryotherapy is commonly used in the treatment of acute trauma and subacute injuries. The temperature of the body tissue is reduced and the heat is transferred from the body tissue to the cold medium. The magnitude of cooling depends upon the area of the body tissue exposed, temperature of the cooling agent and the duration of exposure. The depth of penetration is also related to intensity and duration of cold application and the circulatory response to the body segment exposed. Thus, for a constant source of cooling, the temperature drop in the tissues will depend upon:

- *Temperature difference between the coolant and the tissues:* The colder the application, the greater the heat loss from the tissues.
- *Thermal conductivity of the tissues:* This differs from one area to another. In general, water-filled tissues, such as muscles, have a high thermal conductivity as compared to fat or skin. The normal layer of subcutaneous fat serves as a thermal insulation for the inner tissues so that the heat loss through the tissues and the cold penetration is largely dependent upon the blood flow.
- *Length of time for which the cold is applied:* The amount of energy loss is fully dependent upon the length of exposure.
- *Size of area that is being cooled:* The smaller the area, more will be cooling.

TECHNIQUES OF APPLICATION

The various techniques that are used for administering cold are:
- Ice massage
- Ice towels
- Immersion in cold or cold whirlpool
- Ice packs or cold packs
- Evaporative cooling or vapocoolant sprays
- Excitatory cold.

- *Ice massage:* In this technique, ice is placed in a polyethylene bag and applied over the body tissue. Ice cubes, crushed ice or flaked ice, etc., can be used. The ice bag is placed over the patient's tissue and the patient is not allowed to lie over the pack. The pressure of application should be minimal and the movement of the bag should be to and fro and circular. The ice can be placed over the body tissue for a period of 10–20 minutes.

- *Ice towels:* This is a popular method of application because there is little danger of producing an ice burn. Prepare the ice solution by filling a bucket or bowl with two parts of flaked or crushed ice to one part water in which two terry towels are immersed. The surplus water is wrung from towel, leaving as much ice clinging to it as possible. It is then applied to the part being treated. The towels are changed after every 30 seconds to 2 minutes. Up to ten towels can be applied consecutively with total treatment time of 15–20 minutes.
- *Immersion in cold or cold whirlpool:* The part of the body is immersed in cold water or a whirlpool in which temperature of water is lowered up to 0–10°C. Flaked ice or crushed ice is used in a solution with water to form slush. Extremities of the body can be effectively treated with immersion in the cold. The total duration of the treatment is around 10 minutes in which the patient can immerse in either for a single 10 minutes session or for a series of shorter immersions until accumulative total of 10 minutes have been reached.
- *Cold packs:* Commercially used cold packs are used for administering cold. These cold packs contain special material which retains the cold like the silicate gel. These are available in various sizes and shapes. Different body parts are treated with different sizes and shapes of cold packs **(Fig. 10.1)**. These packs are stored in a special refrigeration or freezer for at least 20 minutes to 1 hour before use **(Fig. 10.2)**. The main advantages of these cold packs are that they are reusable and can contour or mold themselves according to the body part treated.
- *Evaporative cooling or vapocoolant sprays:* The use of vapocoolant sprays is increasing nowadays. These are being used very commonly in sporting activities or athletic injuries. The commonly used sprays are fluoromethane or ethyl chloride. The jet of spray is usually applied from a distance of about 1 feet or 12 inches. Gentle stretch is applied to the tissues after application of vapocoolant sprays.
- *Excitatory cold:* The marked sensory stimulus of ice on the skin can be used to facilitate contraction of inhibited muscle. Ascertain the spinal root level supply (myotome) of inhibited

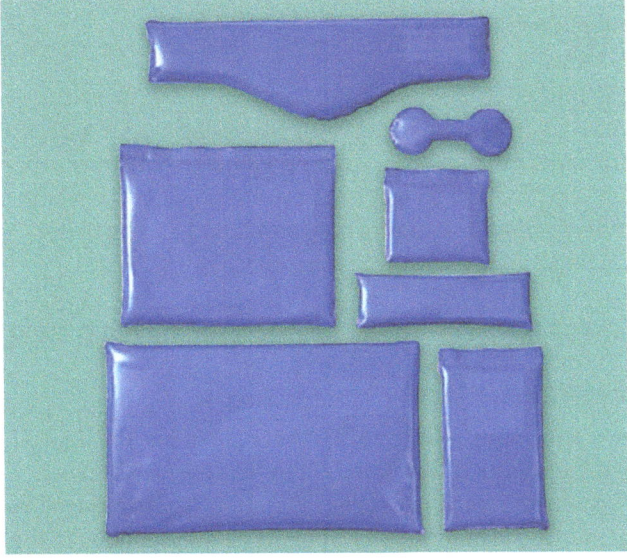

Fig. 10.1: Cold packs.

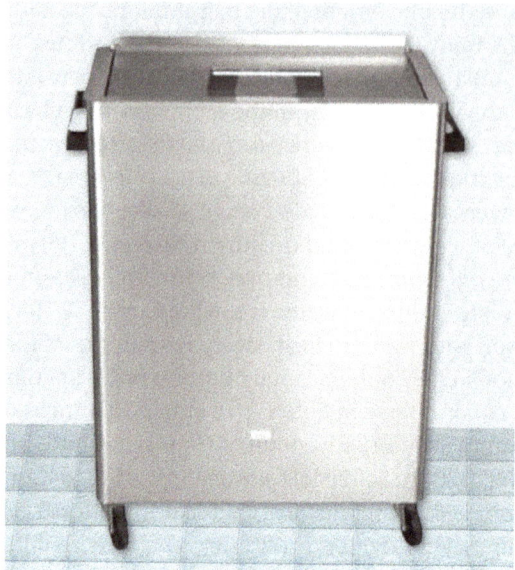

Fig. 10.2: Cold packs unit.

muscle and find the area of skin which has same root supply (dermatome). The ice is stroked quickly three times over the dermatome and skin is then dried. This sensory stimulus passes via the peripheral nerve and enters the cord through posterior horn. It raises the level of excitation around the anterior horn cell [as acetylcholine (ACh) has connection with these sensory fibers]. The increased excitation may supplement the patient's willing effort to make the muscle contract. This technique of "quick ice" is often a useful stimulus in aiding voluntary contraction of muscle.

BASIC PRINCIPLES

When cold therapy is applied to the tissues, the heat is absorbed from the tissues by the cooling agent. Ice changes its state from solid to liquid by absorbing heat. *A specific amount of energy is required to change the solid form of ice into water which is called latent heat of fusion.* One gram of ice at 0°C requires 336 joules of energy to convert it into 1 g of water at 0°C, whereas 1 g of water at 0°C requires 155 joules of energy to convert it into 1 g of water at 37°C. Thus, for cooling the body tissues, it is better to use ice for treatment rather than water.

PHYSIOLOGICAL EFFECTS AND THERAPEUTIC USES OF COLD THERAPY

Effects on Circulatory System and Uses

The initial response of the body tissue to cold is that to preserve the heat. This is accomplished by an initial phase of local vasoconstriction. When homeostasis is reached and the body part has become cooled, there follows phase of vasodilatation. Then there follows alternate periods of vasoconstriction and vasodilatation. This appears as hunting toward the mean point and is known as Lewis's hunting reaction **(Fig. 10.3)**.

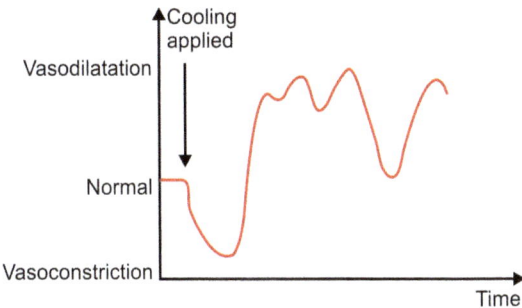

Fig. 10.3: Lewis's hunting reaction.

The initial phase of vasoconstriction helps to reduce the flow of blood into the tissues following recent injury. This helps to limit swelling and the extent of tissue damage.

The alternate phase of vasoconstriction and vasodilatation helps removing the waste products of metabolism like the lactic acid and thus delays fatigue.

Effects on Nervous System and Neural Tissues

The rate of conduction of the nerve fibers is reduced by cold. The A fibers are affected first followed by B and C fibers.

The major effects of ice application are to relieve pain. The probable mechanism involved is the stimulation of cold receptors which send back the impulses, which have to pass into the spinal cord via the posterior root. These impulses which arrive through the relatively large diameter nerves effectively block the pain impulses attempting to gain access to the cord and thus the pain gate is closed.

The cold stimulus is itself, is a noxious one and can stimulate the midbrain which may release beta-endorphin or enkephalin (the body's opiate like substances) into the posterior horn and thus reduces pain.

It is also possible that the increased circulation by the cold could carry away chemical substances which are stimulating nociceptors and thus the pain is reduced.

One of the major effects of cold therapy is on the muscle tone. The short, brisk application of cold is thought to enhance the muscle tone (i.e., excitatory cold), while the prolonged use of cold (as in immersion of cold) reduces the muscle tone to a greater extent.

DANGERS AND CONTRAINDICATIONS

- *Cardiac conditions:* The administration of cold therapy in cardiac patients needs special attention. In patient with a recent myocardial infarction, the application of cold may cause further drop in blood pressure and further reduces the blood supply of the heart. The weak heart may collapse immediately.
- *Peripheral nerve injuries:* In cases with peripheral nerve injuries, the blood supply of the peripheral nerves reduces further and may cause its further damage. Also, the nerve supply of the blood vessels is further delayed causing loss of the normal response of its cooling. Thus, in the patients with peripheral nerve injuries, the application of cold should be avoided.

- *Peripheral vascular disease or vasospastic disease:* The application of cold should be avoided in cases of peripheral vascular disease, as the cold may further reduce an already inadequate blood supply. In cases of vasospastic disease, such as the Raynaud's disease, the condition may worsen by the application of cold.
- *Psychological or cold sensitive:* The patients having fear of the cold may react adversely. Following the application of cold, they start producing histamine, such as substance causing urticaria with skin rash and itching. The application of cold in psychologically apprehensive persons and the cold sensitive patients is avoided.

METHODS OF TREATMENT

PROFORMA FOR PATIENT'S ASSESSMENT

- *Receiving the patient:* Good morning, I am a physiotherapist and going to treat you. Please, cooperate with me during the treatment and wait until I go through your case sheet.
- *History taking or going through the case sheet:*
  - Name
  - Father's and mother's name
  - Age
  - Sex
  - Occupation
  - Address: Correspondence and permanent

  Chief Complaints:
  - History of present illness
  - History of past illness
  - Family history
  - Social and occupational history
  - Treatment history
  - Prognosis of the treatment
  - Investigations:
    - Hematological tests
    - Radiological tests—X-rays, magnetic resonance imaging (MRI) scan, etc.
- *Checking for general contraindications:*
  - Hypertension
  - Deep X-ray and cobalt therapy
  - Epileptic patients
  - Noncooperative patients
  - Mentally-retarded patients
  - Anemia
  - Very poor general condition of the patient
  - Menstruation
- *Checking for local contraindications:*
  - Skin condition
  - Wound
  - Tumor

- *Preparation of trays:*
    - Two test tubes:
        - One with hot water
        - One with cold water
    - Towels
    - Pillows
    - Sandbags
- Preparation of the cold pack or cryotherapy unit
- Gaining the confidence of the patient
- *Positioning the patient:* Comfortable with good support
- *Preparation of the patient:*
    - Explain (Remove the clothing where the area is to be treated)
    - Testing the skin sensation
    - Inspection of the part to be treated.
    - Palpation of the part to be treated.
- *Application to the patient:*
    - Development of appropriate cold level
    - Duration
    - Safety
- *Termination:*
    - Inspection of the part (erythema) or cold burn
    - Palpating the part (pain).
- *Record about the patient condition:*
    - Duration of the treatment
    - Name
    - Address
- *Knowledge of dangers:* If cold burn occurs, gently rub the part.
- Knowledge of contraindications.
- Home instructions.
- General information.

ANKLE SPRAIN

It is one of the most frequent injured structures in sports, particularly in basketball and football. Ankle sprain is the most common of all the sprains. Lateral ligament sprain accounts for 85% of all ankle sprains.

Mechanism of Injury

The sudden forceful inversion, plantar flexion and adduction cause lateral ligament sprain. Lateral ligaments comprise of the following, e.g., the anterior talofibular ligament, posterior talofibular ligament and the calcaneofibular ligament. The sudden forceful inversion, plantar flexion and adduction of these ligaments cause sprain.

Grades of Sprain

Grade 1: Minimal pain and disability—weight-bearing not impaired
Grade 2: Moderate pain and disability—weight-bearing difficult
Grade 3: Severe swelling, no pain, discoloration, no weight-bearing possible, significant functional loss.

Investigation

X-ray: Anteroposterior (AP), lateral (to see any associated fracture).

Treatment

Sports injuries can be treated safely using the PRICES. The acronym stands for:
- **P** : Prevention from the injury
- **R** : Rest (relative rest) to the part
- **I** : Icing (to prevent swelling and pain)
- **C** : Compression (by crepe bandage) of the part
- **E** : Elevation of the part
- **S** : Support

Cryotherapy is used to prevent swelling and to minimize pain.

Ice bag or cold pack is used for at least 20 minutes. Swelling is minimized and further injury of the ligament fibers by swelling is also reduced. Compression is followed by crepe bandage. Ice bag can be used along with compression also. Initially ice can be used for a period of 24 hours, but can be extended up to 72 hours (depending upon the severity) following injury.

Gradual exercises are started after 72 hours of the injury. Once swelling and pain subsides, partial weight-bearing can be started.

When partial weight-bearing is pain-free, full weight-bearing is allowed and early return to activities is suggested.

MUSCLE CONTUSION/HEMATOMA

Very common in contact sports, cause of injury is direct blow or hit by a blunt object or by a ball.

Quadriceps contusion is common in football and is also called "Charley horse".

Hematoma occurs when a large sized vessel is damaged and blood starts accumulating in the area.

Clinical Features

Contusion: Pain, swelling, decreased ROM and ecchymosis.

Hematoma: Mass of firm, jelly-like consistency, ecchymosis, decreased range of motion (ROM) and pain.

Investigations

X-rays are usually normal, but beneficial to exclude any fracture.

Treatment

Initial application of ice is very beneficial.

Cold pack is used for subsidizing swelling and to reduce pain. Ice is applied for a period of at least 20 minutes, and response is seen. If there is reduction in swelling and hematoma, it can be continued for another 20 minutes after an interval of 10 minutes.

Aspiration of hematoma under strict sterile conditions is indicated in recurrent and nonsubsidizing hematomas.

CHAPTER 11

Biofeedback

INTRODUCTION

Biofeedback is an instrumentation and technique which is used to accurately measure, process and feedback some reinforcing information via auditory or visual signals by electronic or electromechanical device especially for therapeutic purposes.

It can also be simply defined as *the process of furnishing an individual information of his body function, so as to get some control over it.*

Biofeedback can be used to assess the physiological functions and then to improve it by having proper control over it. The information regarding various physiological functions, such as heart rate, blood pressure, skin temperature, force generated by muscular contraction or relaxation, range of motion of joints, etc., are recorded and displayed in front of the patient. Various forms of information can be reinforced back to the patient, such as kinesthetic, visual, auditory, cutaneous, vestibular, etc. The patient is made to visualize the functions. The target is set at the higher or lower sides of the patients normal capacities. The aim is to achieve the desired targets.

This is not different in principle from the re-education given by the physiotherapist in providing feedback for the correction of posture or for the initiation of muscle contraction. Information from the muscle spindles, joint position, joint range of motion, etc., all gives a source of feedback. Motor functions are thus improved and well controlled by the patient. It is also considered that feedback should be proportional to the response. A strong contraction of muscle produces a strong signal. Also, a visual signal by a digital display is thought to be more effective than an auditory feedback as comparisons are to be made during further contractions.

BIOFEEDBACK INSTRUMENTATION

Biofeedback instruments are designed to monitor some physiologic event, objectively quantify these monitorings and then interpret the measurements as meaningful information.

Sometimes, these units cannot measure a physiologic event directly. Instead they record some aspects that are highly correlated with the physiologic event.

The most commonly used instruments include these that record *peripheral skin temperatures* indicating the extent of vasoconstriction or vasodilation; *finger photo transmission units* (photoplethysmograph) that also measure vasoconstriction and vasodilatation; units that record *skin conductance activity* indicating sweat gland activity; and units that measure electromyographs (EMG) indicating amount of electrical activity during muscle contraction.

Additionally, there are other types of biofeedback units available including electroencephalographs (EEG), pressure transducers and electrogoniometers.

Peripheral skin temperature: Peripheral skin temperature is an indirect measure of the diameter of peripheral blood vessels. As vessels dilate, more warm blood is delivered to a particular area, thus increasing the temperature in that area. This effect is easily seen in the fingers and toes where the surrounding tissue warms and cools rapidly. Variations in skin temperature seem to be correlated with affective states with a decrease occurring in response to stress or fear. Temperature changes are usually measured in degrees Fahrenheit.

Finger photo transmission: The degree of peripheral vasoconstriction can also be measured indirectly using a photoplethysmograph. This instrument monitors the amount of light that can pass through a finger or toe, reflex off a bone, and pass back through the soft tissue to a light sensor. As the volume of blood in a given area increases, the amount of light detected by the sensor decreases thus giving some indication of blood volume. Only changes in blood volume can be detected since there are no standardized units of measures. These instruments are used most often to monitor pulse.

Skin conductance activity: Sweat gland activity can be indirectly measured by determining electrodermal activity most commonly referred to as the galvanic skin response (GSR). Sweat contains salt, which increases electrical conductivity. Thus, sweaty skin is more conductive than dry skin. This instrument applies a very small electrical voltage to the skin, usually on the palmar surface of the hand or the volar surface of the fingers. Measuring skin conductance is a technique useful in objectively assessing psychophysiologic arousal and is most often used in lie detector testing.

Electromyogram biofeedback: EMG biofeedback is certainly the most typically used of all the biofeedback modalities in a therapeutic setting. Muscle contraction results from the more or less synchronous contraction of individual muscle fibers that compose a muscle. Individual muscle fibers are innervated by nerves that collectively comprise a motor unit. The axon of that motor unit conducts an action potential to the neuromuscular junction where a neurotransmitter substance (acetylcholine) is released. As this neurotransmitter binds to receptor sites on the sarcolemma, depolarization of that muscle fiber occurs in both directions along the muscle fiber, creating movement of ions and thus an electrochemical gradient around the muscle fiber. Changes in potential difference or voltage associated with depolarization can be detected by an electrode placed in closed proximity to the muscle fiber.

The raw EMG activity is usually displayed visually on an oscilloscope. On most biofeedback units, integrated EMG activity is visually presented as a line traveling across a monitor, as a light or series of lights that go on and off, or as a bar graph that changes dimensions, all of which change in response to the incoming integrated signal. If the biofeedback unit uses some forms of a meter, it may either be calibrated in objective units, such as microvolts or given some relative scale to measure. Meters may either be analog or digital. Analog meters have a continuous scale and a needle that indicates the level of electrical activity within a particular range. Digital meters display only a number. They are very simple and easy to read. However, the disadvantage of a digital meter is that it is more difficult to tell where in a given range the signal falls.

On some biofeedback units, raw EMG activity is presented in an audio format. The majority of biofeedback units have audio feedback along with which produces some tone, buzzing, beeping or clicking. An increase in the pitch of a tone, buzz or beep or an increase in the frequency of clicking indicates an increase in the level of EMG activity. This would be most useful for individuals who need to strengthen muscle contractions. Conversely, decreases in pitch or frequency indicating a decrease in EMG activity would be most useful in teaching athletes to relax.

Specific treatment protocols are required for reproducible results, such as skin preparation, application of electrodes, selection of feedback or output modes, and sensitivity settings.

GENERAL PRINCIPLES

A behavioral positive reinforcement or "reward" model is usually employed with biofeedback techniques. Simply stated, when patients generate appropriate motor behaviors, they are positively reinforced. The audio and visual feedback stimuli, and other nonverbal information, are usually much faster and more accurate than the therapist's comments. Unlike other interventions, the benefits of accomplishing small changes in motor behavior in the desired direction can be reinforced, which should speed the rehabilitation process. In behavioral learning terminology, the therapist uses the biofeedback signal to shape the motor behavior by reinforcing the patient's successive approximations to the goal behavior or functional outcome.

When the patient succeeds in controlling the signal, the therapist must relate it to the underlying motor behavior and then re-establish the expected outcomes. Reinforcing already-learned behaviors is of course, futile, so the machine's threshold should be monitored frequently, increasing the task's difficulty as motor skills progress.

Feedback can be intrinsic or extrinsic. Intrinsic feedback is the body's internal feedback mechanism, which uses visual, auditory, vestibular and proprioceptive mechanisms. Extrinsic feedback is any feedback derived from an external source (e.g., a biofeedback signal or physical therapists comments) that augments intrinsic feedback.

BIOFEEDBACK IN REHABILITATION

When using biofeedback, the patient must:
- Understand the relationship of the electronic signal with the desired functional task
- Practice controlling the biofeedback signals
- Perform the functional task until it is mastered and the patient no longer needs the biofeedback.

Conventional neuromuscular re-education is based heavily on providing patients with helpful comments (feedback) to assist their recovery of previously acquired skills. The therapist's job is to focus the patient's attention on the underlying motor programs and biomechanical schema required to recoup those skills.

Recent applications of biofeedback have been directed at muscle imbalances and the fine tuning of motor control. The focus, for example, with the quadriceps, might be a balanced vastus medialis oblique:vastus lateralis (VMO:VL) ratio and not merely gross strength.

Biofeedback is simply one technique that therapists may employ to help convey their message about motor programs and biomechanical schemata to the patient. Biofeedback can assist the rehabilitation process by:
- Providing a clear treatment outcome or goal for the patient to achieve.
- Permitting the therapist and patient to experiment with various strategies (processes) that generate motor patterns to achieve the desired outcome or goal.

- Reinforcement for getting the appropriate motor behavior.
- Providing a process which gives orientation, time and accurate knowledge of results for the patient's efforts.

The machine should be set to give auditory or visual feedback that corresponds to the desired motor behavior. For example, if spastic antagonists are to be monitored, the patient should be instructed to decrease the EMG activity; the biofeedback device is set to flash a light in order to provide signal of this outcome. Alternatively, an electrogoniometer can be used which changes the pitch of a buzzer as the joint is moved in the appropriate direction. In brief, biofeedback techniques are used to augment the patient's sensory feedback mechanism through specific and precise information about the body physiologic processes that might otherwise be inaccessible.

USE OF ELECTROMYOGRAM BIOFEEDBACK FOR NEUROMUSCULAR RE-EDUCATION

Electromyogram (EMG) biofeedback is useful for neuromuscular re-education. The basic EMG device comprises of one ground and two surface electrodes, an amplifier, an audio speaker and a video display. A surface EMG for skeletal muscle activity can be compared with electrocardiography (ECG) being done for heart. The EMG signal is transmitted from the muscle through the skin, through the electrode paste, through the electrodes, through the wires and then to the amplifier. The equipment is quite complex and for skilled use a good understanding of the EMG signal's characteristics is required. The EMG display bears an approximate relationship to the magnitude of the muscle contraction which causes it. The relationship is quite complicated because the motor unit action potential that occurs cannot all be equally detected and recorded. However, for biofeedback purposes the overall effect of stronger contractions leads to louder clicks and a large display on the screen are adequate.

LIMITATIONS OF BIOFEEDBACK

The biofeedback must be relevant, accurate and rapid to enhance motor learning. If any of these three elements is missing, the traditional form of feedback, i.e., verbal feedback can be used which is more convenient.

- *Relevancy:* Useful relevant information is important for the desired motor response. It should neither be too short or too long. EMG biofeedback can provide relevant information about the motor unit activity which cannot be available otherwise.
- *Accuracy:* The biofeedback device and the way, it is used, should provide an accurate information. Many believe that the EMG signals are not sufficient to constitute true process of feedback. They use specific devices that directly measure force or joint range of motion. For obtaining accurate results, appropriate biofeedback device and proper technique of application should be used.
- *Rapid information:* All EMG processes delay electrical events during signal amplification and conversion to audio speaker and visual meter because of inherent delays from the electrical circuits. Most commercial EMG biofeedback instruments give 50–100 ms delay before the signal reaches to the ears and eyes of the patients. Biofeedback to be useful must provide immediate rapid information. While biofeedback is employed, the movements are necessarily closed loop.

In brief, the information used to be feedback to patients must be accurate, relevant and rapid for effective therapeutic use. Therapists must choose the appropriate instrument or device that provides the most meaningful information to the patients.

USES OF BIOFEEDBACK

- *Peripheral nerve injuries:* Biofeedback can be used in the treatment of recovering peripheral injuries. Once a motor unit activity has been detected on EMG, voluntary repetition can be encouraged. EMG biofeedback provides a means of extending the recognition of least possible motor activity and then quantifying it to some extent. In cases of nerve transplant or tendon transplant, biofeedback can be useful to provide assistance to the patient to learn the new muscle action.
- *Spinal cord injury:* Biofeedback techniques have been recommended and applied in the rehabilitation of spinal cord injury patients. Feedback is provided to the patient to perform voluntary action in paralyzed muscle. After several repetitions, gradual positive response can be seen.
- *Hemiplegia:* Several studies have found biofeedback to be useful method of treatment in hemiplegia. Biofeedback is commonly used into re-educate controlled dorsiflexion of foot and thus to improve gait. It can also be used for deltoid in order to improve shoulder control.
- *Dystonic conditions:* Dystonic conditions in which the patient suffers uncontrollable movements and postures can also be treated with EMG biofeedback. Spasmodic torticollis is one such condition in which voluntary muscle contractions are used to inhibit inappropriate neck movements.
- *Treating spasticity:* Several spastic conditions, such as cerebral palsy, multiple sclerosis, head injury, etc., can be treated with biofeedback in order to reduce and control spasticity. It should be noted that in all neurological disorders treated by biofeedback, it is assumed that there are some intact neuronal pathways available to suppress spasticity.
- *Postural control:* Biofeedback devices are used to have appropriate postural control. A trunk inclination monitor which signal tilt can be used for the treatment of low backache. A tilt away from normal can provide an audio feedback and thus helps correcting posture.
- *Muscle strengthening:* Muscle strength training devices have an electronic display which indicates the strength in a muscle and acts as a biofeedback to the exercising muscles. It provides a feedback by display of force produced by the contracting muscle and thus helps to strength the muscle further.
- *Functional re-education:* Biofeedback can be effectively used in improving functional re-education. The biofeedback devices can be used in various ways to encourage repeated practice of a particular movement to improve function.
- *Providing relaxation:* The electrical resistance of hand or fingers is measured and displayed. Increase or decrease in stress is reflected in the amount of sweating that occurs which in turn determines the skin resistance. Biofeedback devices are used effectively for providing general relaxation to the body. Pulse rate or respiratory rate is recorded by some apparatus and findings are displayed to the patient. The patient tries to control and regulate the pulse and respiratory rate and thus inducing relaxation.

12
CHAPTER
Electromyography

INTRODUCTION

Electromyography (EMG) is basically the study of motor unit activity. In EMG, the study of the electrical activity of contracting muscle provides information concerning the structure and function of the motor units. Motor units are composed of one anterior horn cell, one axon, its neuromuscular junctions and all the muscle fibers innervated by the axon (**Fig. 12.1**). The nerve cell and the muscle fiber that it supplies are defined as *motor unit*.

Whenever a muscle fiber contracts, the surface membrane undergoes depolarization so that an action potential is recorded from the fiber. When the fibers of a motor unit are activated, they contract nearly but not quite synchronously and their action potential is added up and hence relatively large complex potential known as motor unit action potential (MUAP) is recorded. EMG makes it possible to localize the site of pathology affecting either muscle or its innervation and also provides evidence regarding the nature of pathological process.

Electromyography is a technique by which the action potentials of contracting muscle fibers and motor units are recorded and displayed. Recording the EMG requires a three phase system:
i. An input phase

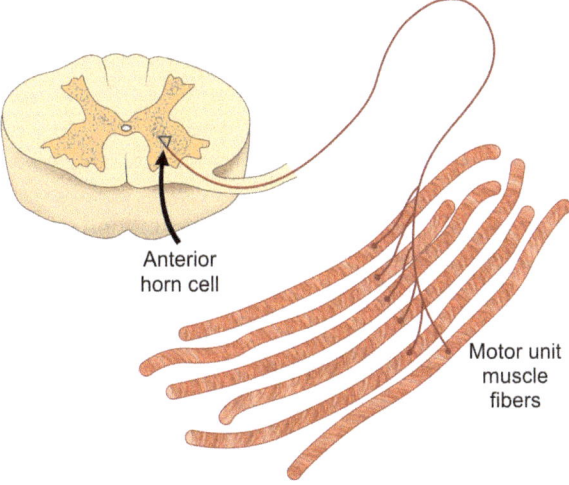

Fig. 12.1: The motor unit.

ii. A processor phase
iii. An output phase

An input phase includes electrodes to pick up electrical potential from contracting muscle, a processor phase amplifies the very small electrical potentials and an output phase includes the display and analysis of electrical potential by visual and auditory means.

TYPES OF ELECTROMYOGRAPHY

- Diagnostic or clinical EMG
- Kinesiological EMG

Diagnostic or Clinical Electromyography

It is used for the study of diseases of muscles, neuromuscular junctions and nerves. It is used for the purpose of electrodiagnosis. The electric potentials from the skeletal muscle fibers are recorded and analyzed for the study of some disease processes. Diseases in which the structure and function of the motor unit is affected, the MUAP may have an abnormal configuration and the pattern of motor unit activity during voluntary contraction may be altered. Healthy muscle fibers contract only when they are activated by neurons and hence under normal conditions, only the MUAPs are seen. In neuromuscular disease, single muscle fiber may contract apparently spontaneously and this may be recognized by the action potential derived from small group of fibers.

Kinesiological Electromyography

It is used in the study of muscle activity and to establish the role of various muscles in specific activities. Kinesiological EMG is beneficial for producing the objective means for documenting the effects of treatment on muscle impairments. It is used to examine the muscle function during the specific, purposeful tasks or therapeutic regimen.

MOTOR UNIT ACTION POTENTIAL

The motor unit action potential (MUAP) means when the depolarization of muscle fibers, which results in the electrical activity and graphically recorded by electromyogram, it represents potential derived from group of muscle fibers that are contracting nearly synchronously and are situated fairly close together and frequently activated by a single neuron. The MUAP therefore represents a sample of activity of the fibers of motor unit and its characteristics are influenced by position of electrodes in relation to fibers of unit. The muscle action potential can be recorded as a monophasic wave in a nonconducting medium. Recording in a conducting medium, the current flow generated by the potential is same as a relative positive wave when recorded from a distance. Electromyography refers to recording of action potentials of muscle fibers firing singly or in groups near the needle electrode in a muscle. The distance of recording electrodes from the muscle fiber determines the rise time and fall time of the muscle fibers.

COMPONENTS OF ELECTROMYOGRAPHY

The components of EMG apparatus are:
- Electrodes
- Amplifier system
- Display system

Electrodes

They are used in the input phase for picking up of electrical potentials from the contracting muscle fibers. The electrodes are of following types:
- Surface electrodes
- Needle electrodes
- Fine wire indwelling electrodes
- Single fiber needle electrodes
- Macroelectrode
- Intracellular electrode
- Multi-lead electrode

Surface Electrodes

Surface electrodes are basically used for kinesiological investigations. These are made up of small disc of electrodes most commonly of silver or silver chloride. The diameter of electrode is generally 3–5 mm **(Fig. 12.2)**. Skin preparations are important in order to reduce skin resistance. Skin preparation includes washing of skin, rubbing to remove dry and dead cells and cleaning with alcohol to remove dust. They are generally considered adequate for monitoring large superficial muscles or muscle groups. They are not considered selective enough to record activity accurately from an individual motor unit or from specific small or deep muscles unless special recording procedures with adequate amplifiers and filtering procedures are used.

Needle Electrodes

Needle electrodes are used for clinical EMG for recording single motor unit potential from different parts of a muscle. The different types of needle electrodes used are:

1. *Concentric (coaxial) needle electrode:* This type of electrode consists of a stainless steel cannula through which a single wire of platinum or silver comes out. The cannula shaft and wire are insulated from each other and only their tips are exposed. They act as electrodes and potential difference between them is thus recorded **(Fig. 12.3A)**.
2. *Monopolar needle electrode:* These are composed of single fine needle which is insulated except at its tip. A second surface electrode is placed on the skin near the site of insertion which serves as a reference electrode. These electrodes are less painful than concentric electrodes because they are much smaller in diameter **(Fig. 12.3B)**.
3. *Bipolar needle electrode:* These consist of a cannula containing two insulated wires with their bare tips. The bared tips of both wires act as the two electrodes and the needle serves as the ground **(Fig. 12.3C)**.

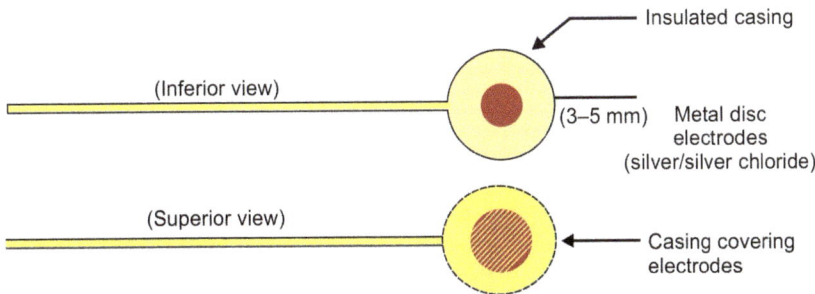

Fig. 12.2: Surface electrodes.

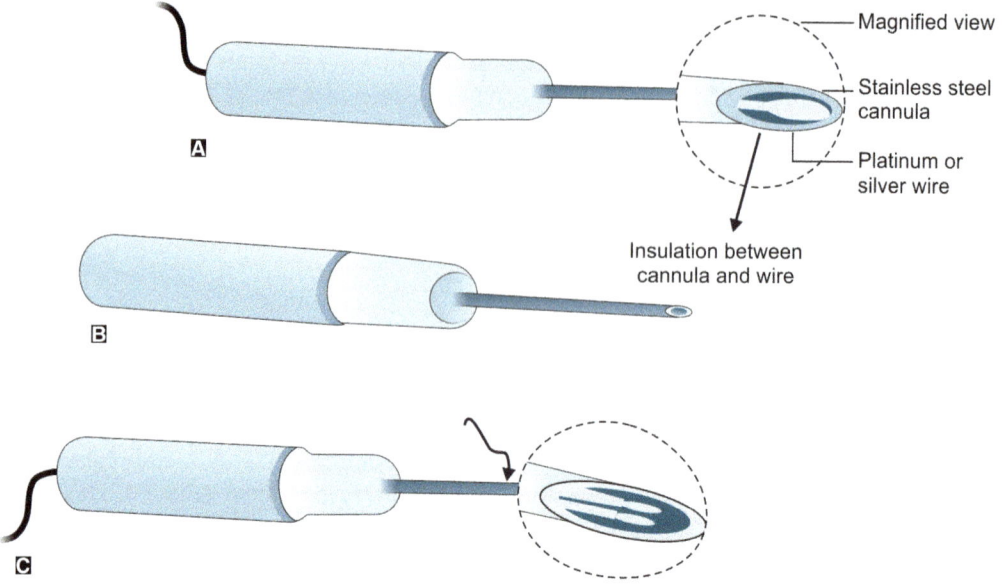

Figs. 12.3A to C: Different types of needles electrodes; (A) Concentric (coaxial) needle electrode; (B) Monopolar needle electrode; (C) Bipolar needle electrode.

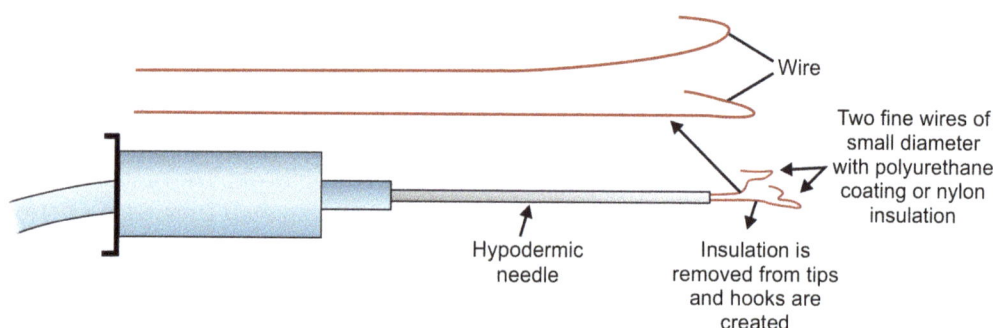

Fig. 12.4: Fine-wire indwelling electrodes.

Fine Wire Indwelling Electrodes

These are used for kinesiological study of small and deep muscle. It is made by using two fine wires of small diameter with polyurethane coating or nylon insulation. Insulation is removed from the tip of the wires and hooks are created to keep the wires imbedded while the needle is removed from the muscle **(Fig. 12.4)**.

Single Fiber Needle Electrodes

These are concentric wires of 25 µm diameter and contain stainless steel cannula of 0.5 mm diameter. This gives information about propagation velocity along the muscle fibers. Single fiber needle records from a small area and hence it cannot be used for motor estimation of motor unit size. Single fiber EMG is employed to study neuromuscular transmission abnormality and fiber density.

Electrodes

They are used in the input phase for picking up of electrical potentials from the contracting muscle fibers. The electrodes are of following types:
- Surface electrodes
- Needle electrodes
- Fine wire indwelling electrodes
- Single fiber needle electrodes
- Macroelectrode
- Intracellular electrode
- Multi-lead electrode

Surface Electrodes

Surface electrodes are basically used for kinesiological investigations. These are made up of small disc of electrodes most commonly of silver or silver chloride. The diameter of electrode is generally 3–5 mm **(Fig. 12.2)**. Skin preparations are important in order to reduce skin resistance. Skin preparation includes washing of skin, rubbing to remove dry and dead cells and cleaning with alcohol to remove dust. They are generally considered adequate for monitoring large superficial muscles or muscle groups. They are not considered selective enough to record activity accurately from an individual motor unit or from specific small or deep muscles unless special recording procedures with adequate amplifiers and filtering procedures are used.

Needle Electrodes

Needle electrodes are used for clinical EMG for recording single motor unit potential from different parts of a muscle. The different types of needle electrodes used are:
1. *Concentric (coaxial) needle electrode:* This type of electrode consists of a stainless steel cannula through which a single wire of platinum or silver comes out. The cannula shaft and wire are insulated from each other and only their tips are exposed. They act as electrodes and potential difference between them is thus recorded **(Fig. 12.3A)**.
2. *Monopolar needle electrode:* These are composed of single fine needle which is insulated except at its tip. A second surface electrode is placed on the skin near the site of insertion which serves as a reference electrode. These electrodes are less painful than concentric electrodes because they are much smaller in diameter **(Fig. 12.3B)**.
3. *Bipolar needle electrode:* These consist of a cannula containing two insulated wires with their bare tips. The bared tips of both wires act as the two electrodes and the needle serves as the ground **(Fig. 12.3C)**.

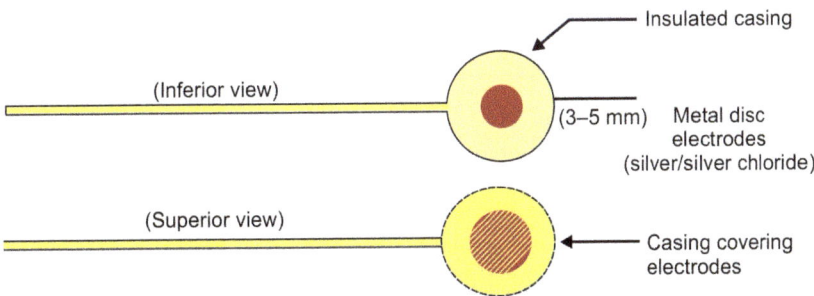

Fig. 12.2: Surface electrodes.

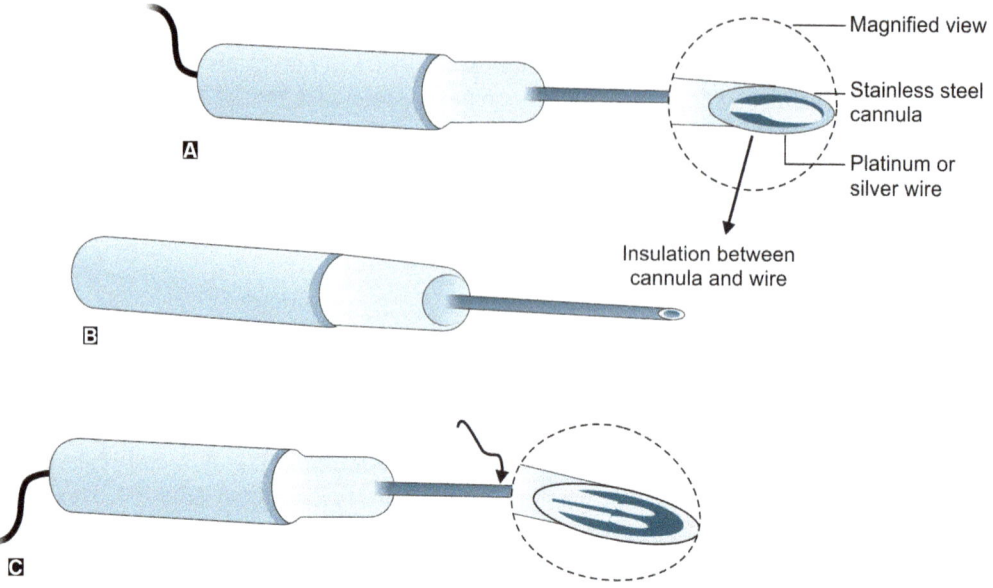

Figs. 12.3A to C: Different types of needles electrodes; (A) Concentric (coaxial) needle electrode; (B) Monopolar needle electrode; (C) Bipolar needle electrode.

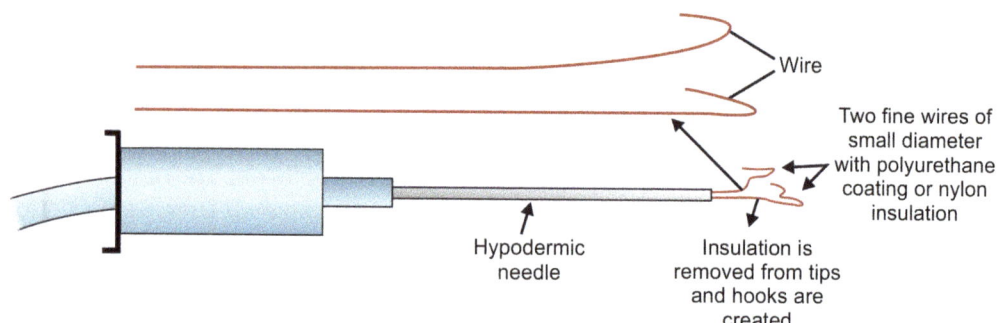

Fig. 12.4: Fine-wire indwelling electrodes.

Fine Wire Indwelling Electrodes

These are used for kinesiological study of small and deep muscle. It is made by using two fine wires of small diameter with polyurethane coating or nylon insulation. Insulation is removed from the tip of the wires and hooks are created to keep the wires imbedded while the needle is removed from the muscle **(Fig. 12.4)**.

Single Fiber Needle Electrodes

These are concentric wires of 25 μm diameter and contain stainless steel cannula of 0.5 mm diameter. This gives information about propagation velocity along the muscle fibers. Single fiber needle records from a small area and hence it cannot be used for motor estimation of motor unit size. Single fiber EMG is employed to study neuromuscular transmission abnormality and fiber density.

Macroelectrode

Macroelectrode is a concentric needle electrode of 15 mm shaft. It records from a large number of motor units along the shaft of the needle. The recording from one motor unit is separated by using a single fiber needle attached to macroelectrode in the midshaft. This method gives information concerning the whole motor unit but has not at present widely applied to the study of pathological motor units.

Intracellular Electrode

This is an extremely fine electrode of diameter 0.5 μm and is used to record the potential changes inside the membrane across a cell. It is made so fine so as to penetrate deep inside a cell or intracellular matrix.

Multi-lead Electrode

This electrode consists of a common steel cannula which comprises of at least three insulated electrodes at regular intervals inside it.

In addition to recording electrodes (surface or needle), a ground electrode must be applied in order to cancel the interference effect of the external electrical noise and vibrations, such as caused by mobile phones, fluorescent lights, broadcasting facilities, elevators and other electrical appliances. The ground electrode is a surface electrode which is attached to the skin near the recording electrode but usually not over the muscle.

The Myoelectric Signal

The EMG electrodes convert bioelectric signal resulting from muscle or nerve depolarization into an electrical potential capable of being processed by an amplifier. The difference of electric potential between the two recording electrodes is processed. The potential difference is measured in volts. The amplitude or height of potential is measured in microvolts. The potential difference and the amplitude are directly proportional to each other, the greater the potential difference between the electrodes the greater the amplitude. The amplitude of motor unit potential is measured from the highest to the lowest point (i.e., from peak to peak).

The Amplifier System

Before the motor unit potential can be visualized, it is necessary to amplify the small myoelectric signals. An amplifier converts the electric signal large enough to be displayed.

Differential Amplifier

The electric potential is composed of the EMG signal from the muscle contraction and unwanted noise from the static electricity in the air and power lines. To control for the unwanted part of the signal, the differential amplifier is used, as noise is transmitted to the amplifier as a common mode signal when the difference of potential is reduced at both the ends, the noise being cancelled out both the ends of amplifier.

Common Mode Rejection Ratio

Actually, noise is not eliminated completely in the differential amplifier. Some of the recorded voltage includes noise. The common mode rejection ratio (CMRR) is a measure of how much the desired signal voltage is amplified relative to the unwanted signal. A CMRR of 1000:1 indicates that the wanted signal is amplified 1000 times more than the noise. It can also be expressed in decibels (dB). A good differential amplifier should have a CMRR exceeding 100000:1. The higher is this value, the better it is.

Signal to Noise Ratio

Noise can be generated internally by the components of the amplifier system, such as resistors, transistors, or the circuit. This noise can be observed by the hissing sound on an oscilloscope. The factor that reflects the ability of the amplifier to limit this noise relative to the amplified signal is the signal to noise ratio. This ratio can also be described as the wanted signal to the unwanted signal.

Gain

The gain refers to the ratio of the output level of signal to the input level of signal. This characteristic refers to the amplifier's ability to amplify the signals. A higher gain will make a smaller signal to appear larger on the display system.

Input Impedance

Impedance is a resistive property present in the alternating current circuits. Impedance is present at the input of the amplifier and as well as at the output of the electrodes and they are directly related to the voltage. As per law, if the impedance at the amplifier is more than the impedance at the electrodes, the voltage will drop more and more accurately it represents the signal. On contrary, if the impedance at the electrodes is more than the impedance at the amplifier, the voltage drop will be less. Also, the impedance depends on many factors, such as skin resistance, material of the electrodes, size of the electrodes, length of the leads and electrolyte, etc. Blood, skin and adipose tissue also offer resistance to the electrical field.

Frequency Band Width

The EMG waveforms as processed by an amplifier are actually the summation of signals of varying frequencies. The frequency is measured in Hertz (Hz). The frequency of an EMG signal is inversely proportional to the interelectrode separation. Consequently, the frequency spectrum extends from 10 Hz to 500 Hz for most surface electrodes and from 10 Hz to 1,000 Hz for fine wire electrodes.

The Display System

The amplified or processed signal is displayed in a useful manner. The form of output used depends upon the desired information and the instrumentation available. The electrical signal can be displayed visually on a cathode ray oscilloscope or computer monitor for analysis.

A cathode ray oscilloscope consists of the electron gun, screen, horizontal and vertical plates. The working of the cathode ray oscilloscope is the electron gun which projects the electron beam toward the screen interiorly is phosphorescent in nature. There are two set of plates that is vertical and horizontal arranged, as the electron beam passes there is deflection in the vertical plate and sweep at the horizontal plate this is shown at vertical plate signal voltage in microvolts and sweep at the horizontal plate shows the duration of signal in millisecond but by conversion there is positive as well as negative deflection and below base line. These signals are displayed by the loudspeaker which records both the cathode ray oscilloscope image sound

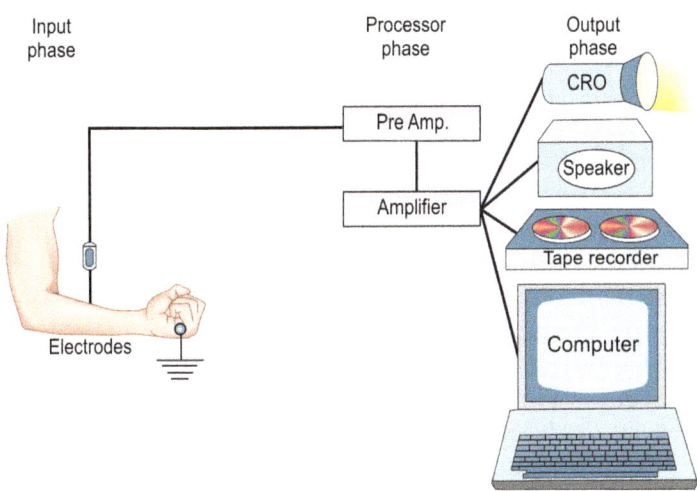

Fig. 12.5: The electromyography recording system.

and ink pen writers are also sometimes used, but they are limited to frequencies. Alternatively, camera can be connected to the cathode ray oscilloscope and then photographs can be made for permanent record. Computers can also be used so that it performs the complex analysis of motor unit potentials and send results to printer.

The data received can also be stored and monitored on a computer-based system (**Fig. 12.5**). It can be stored in an analog or digital form. The conversion process is referred to as analog to digital conversion and the device that is used to perform this task is called A to D converters. The motor unit potential can also be converted into the sound in the same way as the radio signal is processed. For the same reason that every motor unit potential will look different it will also sound different. Normal and abnormal potentials have distinctive sounds that are helpful in distinguishing them.

THE ELECTROMYOGRAPHIC EXAMINATION

An EMG is used to assess the integrity of neuromuscular system including the upper and lower motor neuron, the neuromuscular junction and muscle fibers. The test is done for detecting the muscle action potential in a group or individual in the different stage of contraction. Peripheral nerve lesions are also detected by electromyography.

The Technique of Electromyography Recording

The patient is asked to relax and the needle is inserted inside the muscle, simultaneously spontaneous burst of potential is observed. The insertion activity is observed when the needle breaks the fiber membrane. The equipment of EMG recording is set up at sweep speed 5–10 ms/div; amplification 50 mV/div for studying spontaneous activity and 200 mV/div for motor unit potentials and filter setting 20–10000 Hz, the duration of motor unit potentials should be measured at a gain of 100 mV/div and sweep speed of 5 ms/div and low filter at 2–3 Hz.

In needle EMG, following types of activities are recorded:
- Insertional activity
- Spontaneous activity

* Motor unit potential
* Recruitment pattern

Insertional Activity

Introduction of the needle into the muscle normally produces a brief burst of electrical activity due to mechanical damage by needle movement and it lasts slightly exceeding the needle movement (0.5–0.10 sec). It appears as positive or negative high frequency spike in a cluster. Insertional activity may be increased in denervated muscles and myotonia whereas it is reduced in periodic paralysis during the attack and myopathies when muscle is replaced by connective tissue or fat. Prolonged insertional activity is sometimes found in normal individual which is diagnosed by its widespread distribution. Trains of regularly firing positive waves sometimes are familial and may be due to a subclinical myotonia. On the other hand in muscular individuals, the insertional activity is reduced especially in the calf muscles.

Spontaneous Activity

When the cessation or decay of insertional activity occurs after a second or so, there is no spontaneous activity in a normal muscle, which is called electrical silence. Observation of silence in the relaxed state is an important part of the EMG examination. In the end plate zone however miniature end plate potentials are spontaneously recorded instead of silence. On needle recording, end plate potentials appear as monophasic negative waves of less than 100 mV and duration of 1-3 ms. The end plate potentials are usually seen with an irregular baseline and are called as end plate noise. In the end plate region, action potentials which are brief, spiky, rapid and irregular with an initial negative deflection are known as end plate spikes. These are compared with the sound of sputtering fat in a frying pan. End plate spikes are due to mechanical activation of nerve terminals by the needle. To avoid the normally occurring spontaneous end plate activities, the needle should be introduced slightly away from the motor point.

Normal Motor Unit Action Potential

The normal MUAP is the sum of electrical potential of the muscle fibers present in the single motor unit, having the capability of being recorded by the electrodes. The normal MUAP depends on the given five factors that are amplitude, duration, shape, sound and frequency.

In normal muscle, the *amplitude* of a single MUAP may range from 300 mV to 5 mV from peak to peak. The total *duration* measured from initial baseline will normally range from 3 to 16 m/sec.

The *shape* of a MUAP is diphasic or triphasic with a phase representing a section of potential. There are sometimes polyphasic potentials in two or more phase.

The *sound* is a clear distinct thump and there is capability of the motor unit that it will fire up to 15 times per second with strong contraction, usually when muscle is at rest it represents electrical silence but if there is an activity it is considered as abnormal and denoted by spontaneous activity which is not represented by normal voluntary muscle contraction.

Duration of motor unit action potential: The duration of MUAP is measured from the initial take off to the point of return to the baseline. The duration of MUAP normally varies from 5 ms to 15 ms depending upon the age of the patients, muscle examined and temperature. The facial muscles have a very short duration 4.3–7.5 cm compared to limb muscles. Duration of biceps brachii is 7.3–12.8 ms and that of interossei is 7.9–14.2 ms. The duration of the MUAP is greatly

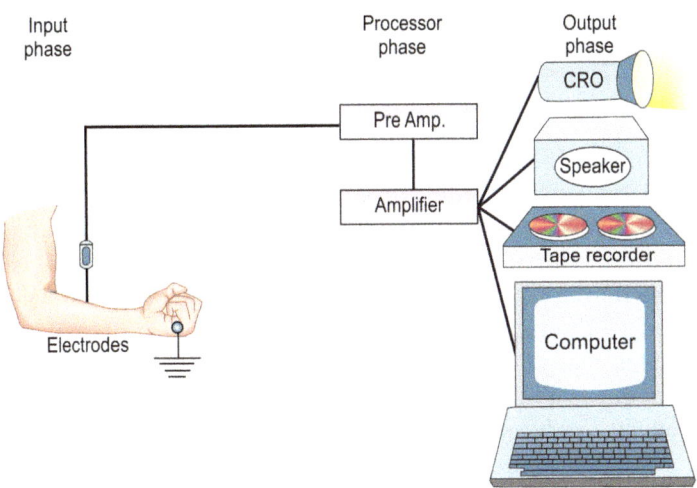

Fig. 12.5: The electromyography recording system.

and ink pen writers are also sometimes used, but they are limited to frequencies. Alternatively, camera can be connected to the cathode ray oscilloscope and then photographs can be made for permanent record. Computers can also be used so that it performs the complex analysis of motor unit potentials and send results to printer.

The data received can also be stored and monitored on a computer-based system **(Fig. 12.5)**. It can be stored in an analog or digital form. The conversion process is referred to as analog to digital conversion and the device that is used to perform this task is called A to D converters. The motor unit potential can also be converted into the sound in the same way as the radio signal is processed. For the same reason that every motor unit potential will look different it will also sound different. Normal and abnormal potentials have distinctive sounds that are helpful in distinguishing them.

THE ELECTROMYOGRAPHIC EXAMINATION

An EMG is used to assess the integrity of neuromuscular system including the upper and lower motor neuron, the neuromuscular junction and muscle fibers. The test is done for detecting the muscle action potential in a group or individual in the different stage of contraction. Peripheral nerve lesions are also detected by electromyography.

The Technique of Electromyography Recording

The patient is asked to relax and the needle is inserted inside the muscle, simultaneously spontaneous burst of potential is observed. The insertion activity is observed when the needle breaks the fiber membrane. The equipment of EMG recording is set up at sweep speed 5-10 ms/div; amplification 50 mV/div for studying spontaneous activity and 200 mV/div for motor unit potentials and filter setting 20-10000 Hz, the duration of motor unit potentials should be measured at a gain of 100 mV/div and sweep speed of 5 ms/div and low filter at 2-3 Hz.

In needle EMG, following types of activities are recorded:
- Insertional activity
- Spontaneous activity

- Motor unit potential
- Recruitment pattern

Insertional Activity

Introduction of the needle into the muscle normally produces a brief burst of electrical activity due to mechanical damage by needle movement and it lasts slightly exceeding the needle movement (0.5–0.10 sec). It appears as positive or negative high frequency spike in a cluster. Insertional activity may be increased in denervated muscles and myotonia whereas it is reduced in periodic paralysis during the attack and myopathies when muscle is replaced by connective tissue or fat. Prolonged insertional activity is sometimes found in normal individual which is diagnosed by its widespread distribution. Trains of regularly firing positive waves sometimes are familial and may be due to a subclinical myotonia. On the other hand in muscular individuals, the insertional activity is reduced especially in the calf muscles.

Spontaneous Activity

When the cessation or decay of insertional activity occurs after a second or so, there is no spontaneous activity in a normal muscle, which is called electrical silence. Observation of silence in the relaxed state is an important part of the EMG examination. In the end plate zone however miniature end plate potentials are spontaneously recorded instead of silence. On needle recording, end plate potentials appear as monophasic negative waves of less than 100 mV and duration of 1–3 ms. The end plate potentials are usually seen with an irregular baseline and are called as end plate noise. In the end plate region, action potentials which are brief, spiky, rapid and irregular with an initial negative deflection are known as end plate spikes. These are compared with the sound of sputtering fat in a frying pan. End plate spikes are due to mechanical activation of nerve terminals by the needle. To avoid the normally occurring spontaneous end plate activities, the needle should be introduced slightly away from the motor point.

Normal Motor Unit Action Potential

The normal MUAP is the sum of electrical potential of the muscle fibers present in the single motor unit, having the capability of being recorded by the electrodes. The normal MUAP depends on the given five factors that are amplitude, duration, shape, sound and frequency.

In normal muscle, the *amplitude* of a single MUAP may range from 300 mV to 5 mV from peak to peak. The total *duration* measured from initial baseline will normally range from 3 to 16 m/sec.

The *shape* of a MUAP is diphasic or triphasic with a phase representing a section of potential. There are sometimes polyphasic potentials in two or more phase.

The *sound* is a clear distinct thump and there is capability of the motor unit that it will fire up to 15 times per second with strong contraction, usually when muscle is at rest it represents electrical silence but if there is an activity it is considered as abnormal and denoted by spontaneous activity which is not represented by normal voluntary muscle contraction.

Duration of motor unit action potential: The duration of MUAP is measured from the initial take off to the point of return to the baseline. The duration of MUAP normally varies from 5 ms to 15 ms depending upon the age of the patients, muscle examined and temperature. The facial muscles have a very short duration 4.3–7.5 cm compared to limb muscles. Duration of biceps brachii is 7.3–12.8 ms and that of interossei is 7.9–14.2 ms. The duration of the MUAP is greatly influenced by age of the subject; MUAP is short in children, longer in adults and still longer in elderly persons. Temperature also influences the duration significantly; 7°C cooling increases the duration of MUAP by 10–30%. The duration of MUAP is a measure of conduction velocity, length of muscle fiber, membrane excitability and synchrony of different muscle fibers of a motor unit. The initial and the terminal low amplitude portions of motor unit potential are also contributed by the fibers more than 1 mm away from the recording electrode. The duration of MUAP, therefore, is much less influenced by the distance of recording electrode compared to the amplitude.

Rise time of motor unit action potential: The rise time of MUAP is the duration from initial positive to subsequent negative peak. It is an indicator of the distance of needle electrode from the muscle fiber. A greater rise time is attributed to resistance and capacitance of the intervening tissue.

Amplitude of motor unit potential: The amplitude of MUAP is measured peak to peak. It depends upon size and density of muscle fiber, synchrony of firing, proximity of needle to the muscle fiber, age of the subject, and muscle examined and muscle temperature. Decreasing muscle temperature results in higher amplitude and longer duration of MUPs.

Phase of motor unit action potential: Motor unit potential recorded by a concentric or monopolar needle reveals as inverted triphasic potential (positive-negative-positive). The phase is defined as the portion of MUP between departure and return to the baseline. A MUAP with more than four phases is called as polyphasic potential. Some potentials show directional changes without crossing the baseline and these are known as turns.

Recruitment Pattern

The firing rate of MUAP for a muscle is constant. When voluntary contractions are initiated, the motor units are recruited in an orderly fashion, the smallest appearing first, larger later and largest still later. This pattern of recruitment is based on Hanneman's size principle. If there is loss of MUAP, the rate of firing of individual potentials during muscle contraction will be out of proportion to the number of firing and it is termed as a reduced recruitment. During strong voluntary contraction, normally there is dense pattern of multiple superimposed potentials which are called as interference pattern. Less dense pattern may occur with a loss of motor units, poor effort or in upper motor neuron lesions.

Abnormal Spontaneous Potentials

As a normal muscle at rest exhibits electrical silence, any activity seen during the relaxed state is considered as abnormal. These activities are termed as spontaneous because these are not produced by the voluntary contraction of the muscles. The common abnormal spontaneous activities are:
- Fibrillation potential
- Positive sharp waves
- Fasciculation potential
- Repetitive discharges

Fibrillation Potential

Fibrillations are spontaneously occurring action potentials from a single muscle fiber. Fibrillation potential is seen in the denervated muscle as they give spontaneous discharges due to circulating acetylcholine. Fibrillation potential is classically indicative of lower motor neuron disorders, such as peripheral nerve lesions, anterior horn cell disease, radiculopathies, and polyneuropathies with axonal degeneration. Fibrillation potentials are found to a lesser extent in myopathic diseases, such as muscular dystrophy, dermatomyositis, polymyositis and myasthenia gravis.

Positive Sharp Waves

Positive sharp waves are found in denervated muscles at rest and are usually accompanied by fibrillation potentials. These are recorded as a biphasic with a sharp initial positive deflection followed by slow negative phase. Positive sharp waves are seen in primary muscle disease, such as muscular dystrophy, polymyositis but sometimes, it is also seen in upper motor neuron lesions.

Fasciculation Potential

Fasciculation potentials are random twitching of muscle fiber or a group and may be visible through skin. These are spontaneous potentials seen with irritation or degeneration of anterior horn cell, nerve root compression and muscle spasm or cramps. They may be biphasic, triphasic or polyphasic.

Repetitive Discharges

These are also called as bizarre high-frequency discharges. These are characterized by an extended train of potentials of various forms. These are seen with lesions of the anterior horn cells, peripheral nerves and with the myopathies.

Normalization of Electromyography

It is not reasonable or justified to compare the EMG activity of one muscle to another or from one person to another. This is because of the variability inherent in the EMG signal and interindividual differences in anatomy and movement. Therefore, some form of normalization is required to validate these studies, as for many studies the quantified EMG signal is used to compare activity between different muscles or subjects.

KINESIOLOGICAL ELECTROMYOGRAPHY

Kinesiological EMG is used to study the muscle activity and to establish the role of various muscles in specific activities. Surface EMG can be used as a kinesiological tool to examine muscle function during specific and purpose tasks. Kinesiological EMG presents an objective means for documenting the effect of treatment on muscle impairments. Surface as well as fine wire indwelling electrodes is used for kinesiological study. Smaller muscles obviously require the use of smaller electrodes, with a small interelectrode distance. The ground electrode should be located reasonably close to the recording electrodes. The EMG signal can be stored, averaged and sampled in a variety of ways to permit detailed and complete analysis. For kinesiological EMG the therapist should be interested at looking the overall muscle activity and quantification of the signal is often desired to describe and compare changes in the magnitude and pattern of the muscle response.

NERVE CONDUCTION VELOCITY

Nerve conduction velocity (NCV) tests are used to determine the speed with which a peripheral motor or sensory nerve conducts an impulse. EMG and NCV are two important diagnostic procedures that can provide complete information about the extent of nerve injury or muscle disease. These data can be valuable for diagnosis of disease and determination of rehabilitation goals for patients with musculoskeletal and neuromuscular disorders.

Nerve conduction velocity can be tested for any superficial nerve that is superficial enough to be stimulated through the skin at two different points. Most commonly NCV test is performed on ulnar, median, peroneal and posterior tibial nerves and less commonly on radial, femoral and sciatic nerves.

Principles of Motor Nerve Conduction

Motor nerve conduction velocity is calculated measuring the distance between two points of stimulation in mm which is divided by the latency difference in ms. The nerve conduction velocity is expressed as m/sec. Measurement of latency difference between the two points of stimulations eliminates the effect of residual latency.

$$\text{Conduction velocity} = \frac{D}{PL - DL}$$

Where,
D = distance between proximal and distal stimulation in mm
DL = distal latency in m/sec
PL = proximal latency in m/sec

The motor nerve is stimulated at least at two points along its course **(Fig. 12.6)**.

The stimulating electrode is typically a two pronged bipolar electrode with the cathode and anode. Small surface electrodes are usually used to record the evoked potential from the test muscle, although needle electrodes may be used when responses are very weak. A ground electrode is placed between the stimulating and recording electrodes. The pulse is adjusted to record a compound muscle action potential. A biphasic action potential with the initial negativity is thus recorded. For accurate motor nerve conduction velocity measurement, the distance between two points of stimulation should be at least 10 cm. This reduces the error due to faulty distance measurement. Stimulation at shorter segments of the nerve, however, is necessary in the evaluation of focal compressive neuropathies, e.g., carpal tunnel syndrome. In a diseased nerve, the excitability is reduced and the current requirement may be much higher than normal.

The measurement for motor nerve conduction study includes the onset latency, duration and amplitude of compound muscle action potential (CMAP) and nerve conduction velocity. The onset latency is the time in ms from the stimulus artifact to the first negative deflection of

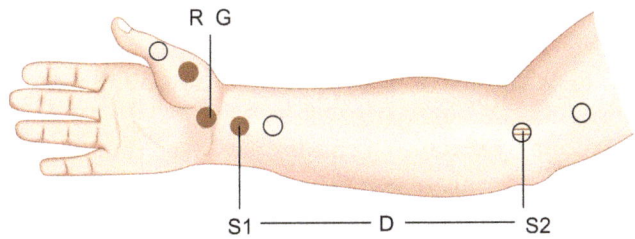

Fig. 12.6: Principles of motor nerve conduction.

R = Recording electrode
G = Ground electrode between stimulating and recording electrode
S1 = Stimulation at wrist
S2 = Stimulation at elbow

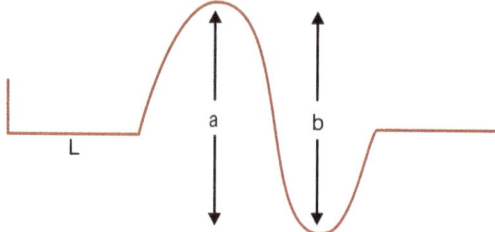

Fig. 12.7: Measurement of compound muscle action potential latency and amplitude.
L = Onset latency
a = Base to peak amplitude
b = Peak to peak amplitude

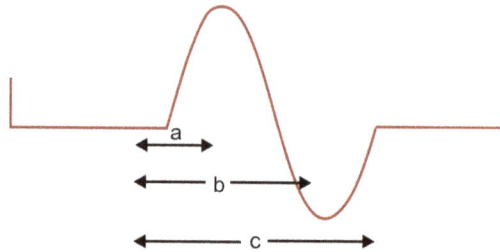

Fig. 12.8: Measurement of duration of compound muscle action potential.
a = Onset to negative peak
b = Onset to positive peak
c = Onset to final return to base line

CMAP. The amplitude of CMAP is measured from baseline to the negative peak (base to peak) or between negative and positive peaks (peak to peak) **(Fig. 12.7)**.

The duration of CMAP is measured from the onset to the negative or positive peak or the final return of waveform to the baseline **(Fig. 12.8)**.

Principles of Sensory Nerve Conduction

The sensory conduction can be measured orthodromically or antidromically. In orthodromic conduction, a distal portion of the nerve, e.g., digital nerve is stimulated and sensory nerve action potential (SNAP) is recorded at a proximal point along the nerve **(Fig. 12.9)**. In antidromic sensory nerve conduction, the nerve is stimulated at a proximal point and nerve action potential is recorded distally. In antidromic sensory nerve conduction measurement, the action potential may be obscured by superimposed muscle action potential, which is elicited due to simultaneous stimulation of motor axon in the mixed nerve. For orthodromic conduction, ring electrodes are preferred to stimulate the digital nerve; whereas surface stimulating electrodes are commonly used for antidromic stimulation.

Recording is also done by surface electrodes; however, in difficult situations needle electrode may be tried. Similar to motor nerve conduction study, the sensory nerve conduction measurement includes onset latency, amplitude, duration of SNAP and nerve conduction velocity **(Fig. 12.10)**.

The latency of orthodromic potential is measured from the stimulus artifact to the initial positive or subsequent negative peak. The latency following orthodromic stimulation is shorter compared to antidromic. In practice, however, both orthodromic and antidromic methods

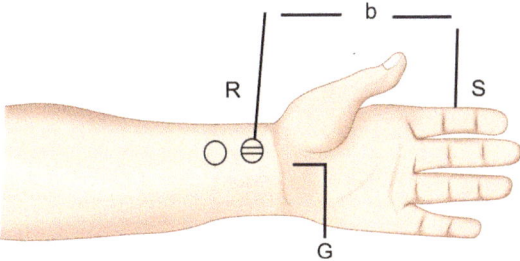

Fig. 12.9: Principles of orthodromic sensory conduction.
R = Recording electrode
G = Ground electrode between stimulating and recording electrode
S = Stimulating site

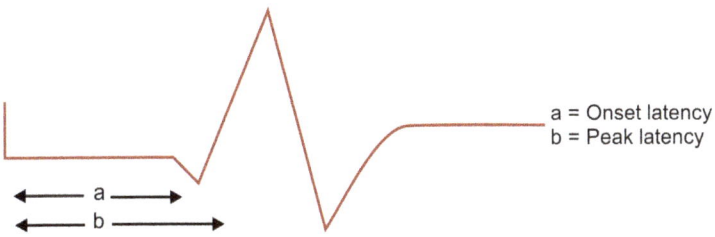

Fig. 12.10: Measurement of latency of sensory nerve action potential.

provide the desired information. The initial positive peak in SNAP giving it a triphasic appearance is a feature of orthodromic potential. In antidromic potential, the initial positivity in SNAP is lacking.

The SNAP amplitude is measured from baseline to negative peak or from positive to negative peak **(Fig. 12.11)**. The SNAP recorded with a surface electrode is of higher amplitude in antidromic recording compared to orthodromic; because nerves are closer to the recording electrode especially in digital nerves.

The duration of SNAP is measured from the initial positive peak to the intersection between the descending phase and the baseline or to the negative or subsequent positive peak or return to the baseline **(Fig. 12.12)**. The amplitude of SNAP is variable not only in different normal subjects but also in the same individual on two sides. SNAP unlike motor conduction velocity may be measured by stimulating at a single stimulation site; because the residual latency which comprises of neuromuscular transmission time and muscle propagation time is not applicable in sensory nerve conduction. Thus, the sensory conduction velocity is calculated by dividing the distance (mm) between stimulating and recording site by the latency (ms). The SNAP amplitude shows a pronounced reduction on proximal recording in orthodromic nerve conduction studies. The SNAP amplitude is also reduced in antidromic studies on proximal stimulation of nerve compared to distal. In contrast to this, the SNAP amplitudes remain stable or there is minimal change on proximal stimulation in motor nerve conduction studies.

H-reflex

The H-reflex was described by Hoffman in 1918 and hence named as H-reflex. It is a useful diagnostic measure for radiculopathy and peripheral neuropathy. The H-reflex is a monosynaptic

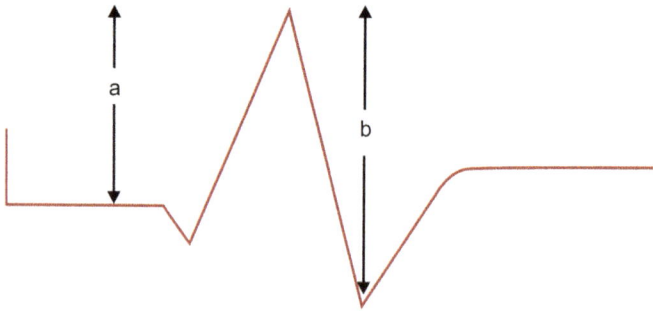

Fig. 12.11: Measurement of sensory nerve action potential amplitude.
a = base to peak
b = peak to peak

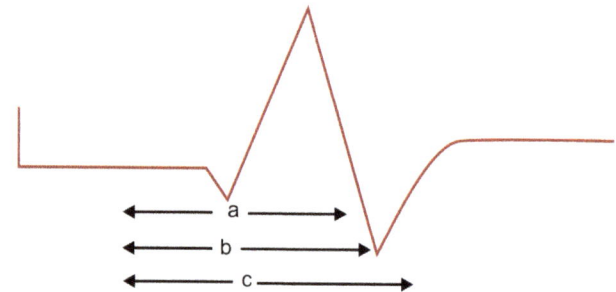

Fig. 12.12: Measurement of duration of sensory nerve action potential.
a = Onset to negative peak
b = Onset to positive peak
c = Onset to return to baseline

reflex elicited by submaximal stimulation of the tibial nerve and recorded from the calf muscle. In normal adults, it can also be recorded in other muscles of the limbs but not from the small muscles of hands and feet except in children below 2 years. H-reflex can be enhanced by the maneuvers which increases motor neuron pool excitability, such as muscle contraction. H-reflex has the advantage of evaluating the proximal sensory and motor pathways. It is therefore especially helpful in the evaluation of plexopathies and radiculopathies. In Guillain Barre syndrome, H-reflex may be absent, delayed or dispersed. In S1 radiculopathy, the soleus H-reflex may be absent. Similarly, flexor carpi radialis H-reflex may be abnormal in C6–C7 radiculopathy. H-reflex is influenced by a number of spinal or supraspinal variables. The H-reflex studies, therefore, provides useful information which are helpful in understanding the pathophysiology of various central nervous system abnormalities.

F-wave

The F-wave was first described by Magladary and McDougal in 1950 in small muscles of the foot. The F-wave is a useful supplement to nerve conduction studies and electromyographic measures and is most helpful in the diagnosis of conditions where the most proximal portion of the axon is involved. It is elicited by the supramaximal stimulus of a peripheral nerve at a distal site, leading to both orthodromic and antidromic impulses. While the orthodromic impulse travels to the distal muscle, the antidromic response travels to the anterior horn cell. The F-wave studies are valuable in the conditions, such as Guillain Barre syndrome, thoracic outlet syndrome, brachial plexus injuries and radiculopathies.

Variables Affecting the Nerve Conduction Study

A number of physiological and technical variables can influence the results of nerve conduction velocity. It is important to be aware of these factors and eliminate these as far as possible for reliable and reproducible results.

Physiological Variables

Age: The nerve conduction velocity in a full term infant is nearly half of the adult value. As the myelination progresses, the nerve conduction velocity attains the adult value by 3–5 years of age. The conduction velocity begins to decline after 30–40 years of age but the values normally change by less than 10 m/s at the sixth or even in the eight decades.

Upper versus lower limb: The median and ulnar nerve conduction velocity is higher compared to tibial and peroneal. An inverse relationship between height and nerve conduction velocity suggests that the longer nerves conduct slower than the shorter nerves. These variables may also account for the faster conduction in the proximal nerves compared to distal.

Temperature: Temperature significantly influences the conduction velocity and the amplitude compound muscle action potential. Low temperature results in slowing of nerve conduction velocity and increase the amplitude. For each degree Celsius fall in temperature, the latency increases by 0.3 ms. This is attributed to the effect of cooling on sodium channel. On increasing the temperature, the velocity increase by 5% degree from 29–38°C. The laboratory temperature, therefore, should be maintained between 21°C–23°C. If skin temperature is below 34°C, the limb should be warmed by infrared lamp, by warm water immersion or making appropriate correction of the results.

Technical Variables

Stimulating system: Failure of the stimulating system may result in unexpectedly small responses. The nerve may be stimulated submaximally or the applied current may not reach the intended target. An important source of failure of stimulating system is shunting of current between anode and cathode either by sweating or by the formation of a bridge by conducting jelly.

Recording system: Faulty connection in the recording system may results in errors in spite of optimal stimulation. The integrity of the recording system can be tested by asking the patient to contract the muscle with the electrode in position. The motor unit potentials are displayed on the oscilloscope if the recording circuit is operational.

Inadvertent stimulation of unintended nerves: Spread of stimulating current to an adjacent nerve or root not under study is frequent and failure to recognize, it results in errors in latency measurement. Needle electrodes are helpful in recording from restricted area of a muscle and are especially helpful in studying the innervation of individual motor branches or pattern of anomalies.

CLINICAL IMPLICATIONS OF ELECTROMYOGRAPHY

The EMG is invaluable in diagnosing the characteristic changes in primary muscle disorders and those following neurogenic disease. The EMG findings, however, such as any other investigation needs to be interpreted with the clinical picture presented by the patient. The study of the disease can be classified under two major categories:
1. Neurogenic disorders
2. Myogenic disorders

Neurogenic disorders may include:
- Disorders of the peripheral nerves
- Polyneuropathies
- Motor neuron disorders

Myogenic disorders may include:
- Myopathies
- Inflammatory muscle disease

Neurogenic Disorders

Disorders of the Peripheral Nerves

The electromyography findings are valuable in the disorders of the peripheral nerves especially in cases of axonal degeneration. In the disorders of the peripheral nerves, the lesions are of three types:
1. Neuropraxia
2. Axonotmesis
3. Neurotmesis

They may be due to traumatic injury or due to entrapment. These disorders typically cause weakness and atrophy of the muscles innervated distal to the lesion.

Neuropraxia: Neuropraxia involves some form of local block which slows or stops nerve conduction. Conduction above or below the block is usually normal. Bell's palsy, Saturday night palsy, carpal tunnel syndrome, etc., are the common causes of conduction block. Nerve conduction measurement shows increased latency across the blockage but normal above and below the blockage.

Axonotmesis: In axonotmesis, the neural tube is intact with axonal damage. On EMG testing there will be fibrillation potential and positive sharp waves in two to three weeks following degeneration depending on the axon from the cell body.

Neurotmesis: In neurotmesis, there is disruption of neural tube along with axonal damage. A nerve conduction velocity test cannot be performed because no evoked response can be obtained. In EMG spontaneous potential will appear with the muscle at rest and no activity is produced with the attempted voluntary contraction.

Polyneuropathies

In polyneuropathy, there is axonal damage or demyelination of axons. Polyneuropathies typically results in sensory changes with distal weakness and diminished reflexes. The common neuropathic conditions are:

- Diabetic neuropathy
- Alcoholic neuropathy
- Neuropathy related with renal disease or carcinoma
- Uremic neuropathy
- Nutritional neuropathies, such as vitamin B_{12} deficiency neuropathy or vitamin E deficiency neuropathy
- Neuropathy due to infections, such as leprosy or Guillain-Barré syndrome
- Toxic neuropathies

With axonal damage, recruitment will be severely affected. Partial interference pattern may be observed with maximal effort. The motor unit duration and amplitude may be decreased. There are typical fibrillation potentials, positive sharp waves and fasciculation.

Motor Neuron Disorders

Motor neuron disorders most commonly involve degenerative diseases of the anterior horn cells. These include:
- Poliomyelitis
- Syringomyelia

Diseases that are characterized by degeneration of both upper and lower motor neuron, such as:
- Amyotrophic lateral sclerosis
- Progressive muscular atrophy
- Progressive bulbar palsy
- Spinal muscular atrophy

Diseases of the anterior horn cell are classically indicated by fibrillation potentials and positive sharp waves at rest. They also present by reduced recruitment with voluntary contraction due to the loss of motor neurons. Polyphasic motor unit potentials of increased amplitude and duration are often seen later in the course of motor neuron disease due to re-innervation and collateral sprouting. This is a typical finding in post-polio paralysis and amyotrophic lateral sclerosis where enlarged motor units are found in partially denervated muscles.

Myogenic Disorders

The electromyographic findings provide information regarding the electrical activity of muscle that supplements the clinical, biochemical and histological investigations in the diagnosis of the muscle disease. The EMG not only supplements the other laboratory investigations of muscle disease but also provides information which cannot be obtained by other means, such as neuromuscular transmission abnormalities, myotonic disorders and periodic paralysis. The common myogenic disorders are:

Inflammatory Muscle Diseases

Inflammatory muscle diseases include polymyositis, dermatomyositis, inclusion body myositis, viral myositis and parasitic myositis.

The classical triad of EMG findings in inflammatory muscle diseases includes:
- Increased insertional activity with complex repetitive discharges
- Fibrillations and positive sharp waves

- Small polyphasic short duration motor unit potential recruited rapidly in relation to the strength of contraction.

Muscular Dystrophy

The common types of muscular dystrophies include Duchenne muscular dystrophy, Becker muscular dystrophy, facioscapulohumeral muscular dystrophy, limb-girdle muscular dystrophy, oculopharyngeal muscular dystrophy and myotonic dystrophy.

Myopathies

- Congenital myopathies
- Metabolic myopathies
- Endocrine myopathies, etc.

In primary muscle disease, such as the dystrophies or polymyositis, the motor unit remains intact but degeneration of muscle fibers is evident. The typical findings are a decrease in duration and amplitude of motor unit potential, full recruitment pattern during full effort in spite of weakness and wasting. These changes may occur with/without spontaneous electrical activity.

Glossary

Absolute refractory period: Brief time period (0.5 μsec) after membrane depolarization during which the membrane is incapable of depolarizing again.

Accommodation: When a constant current flows, the nerve adapts itself. This phenomenon is known as accommodation.

Actinotherapy: Actinotherapy is the application of various radiations over the skin for therapeutic purposes.

Active electrode: The smaller of the two electrodes under which greatest current density occurs or the electrode that is used to drive ions into the tissues.

All-or-none response: The depolarization of nerve or muscle membrane is the same once a depolarizing intensity threshold is reached; further increases in intensity do not increase the response. Stimuli at intensities less than threshold do not create a depolarizing effect.

Alternating current: Current that periodically changes its polarity or direction of flow.

Ammeter: An ammeter is a low resistance galvanometer. It is used to measure the current in a circuit in amperes.

Ampere: Unit of measure that indicates the rate at which electrical current is flowing.

Ampere circuital law: Ampere's circuital law states that the line integral of magnetic field induction around any closed path in vacuum is equal to μ_0 times the total current threading the closed path.

Amplifier: A device using electrical components to increase electrical power.

Amplitude: Describes the magnitude of the vibration in a wave. It is the maximum distance from equilibrium that any particle reaches. It is also referred to as the intensity of current flow as indicated by the height of the waveform from baseline.

Analgesia: Absence of pain or loss of sensibility of pain.

Anions: The ions which carry negative charge and moves toward the anode during electrolysis are called anions. The ions formed when chemical reaction involves addition of electrons (i.e., reduction) are called anions.

Anode: Positively charged electrode in a direct current system.

Arndt-Schultz principle: It states that no reaction or changes can occur in the body tissues if the amount of energy absorbed is insufficient to stimulate the absorbing tissues. Addition of threshold energy and above quantity of energy will stimulate the absorbing tissue to normal function and if too great a quantity of energy is absorbed then added energy will prevent normal function or will destroy tissue.

Atom: An atom is the smallest particle of an element. The diameter of the atom is of the order of 10^{-10} m.

Attenuation: Attenuation is the term used to describe the gradual reduction in intensity of the ultrasonic beam once it has left the treatment head.

Average current: The amount of current flowing per unit of time.

Axonotmesis: More severe compression injury may cause sufficient damage to the nerve axon. Degeneration of the axon takes place including the myelin sheath. Once the nerve fiber has degenerated, alteration in electrical reaction occurs.

Bandwidth: A specific frequency range in which the amplifier will pick-up signals produced by electrical activity in the muscle.

Beat frequency: Beat frequency is produced as a result of interference of two currents.

Biofeedback: Biofeedback is the technique which is used to accurately measure, process and feedback some reinforcing information via auditory or visual signals by electronic or electromechanical device especially for therapeutic purposes.

Biot-Savart's law: Biot-Savart's law deals with the magnetic field induction at a point due to a small current element. It states that the magnetic field induction at a point due to small current carrying element depends upon the length of the conductor and current flowing through it and is inversely proportional to the square of distance between the conductor and that point.

Bursitis: Inflammation of the bursa between bone and muscle tendon.

Capacitance: The capacitance of an object is the ability of the body to hold an electrical charge. Its unit is Farad.

Capacitor electrodes: Air space plates or pad electrodes that create a stronger electrical field than a magnetic field.

Cathode: Negatively charged electrode in a direct current system.

Cations: The ions which carry positive charge and move toward the cathode during electrolysis are called cations. The ions formed when chemical reaction involves removal of electrons (i.e., oxidation) are called cations.

Cavitation: This is the oscillatory activity of highly compressible bodies within the tissues such as gas or vapor-filled voids. Cavitation may be stable or unstable cavitation.

Cell: Cell is a device by which chemical energy is converted into electrical energy. It is of two types—primary cell and secondary cell.

Chronaxie: The chronaxie is the duration of shortest impulse that will produce a response with a current of double the rheobase.

Circuit: The path of current from a generating source through the various components back to the generating source.

Clinical electromyography: Clinical electromyography is used for the study of diseases of muscles, neuromuscular junctions and nerves. It is used for the purpose of electrodiagnosis.

Coaxial cable: Heavy well-insulated thick wire where centrally thick wire is surrounded by a cylindrical mesh of thin wire.

Combination therapy: The application of two therapeutic modalities at the same time is described as combination therapy. The most widely used combinations are those of ultrasonic with some form of nerve and muscle stimulating currents.

Compound: A compound is a substance formed by the union of two or more elements via the electrons of the atoms involved to form a molecule of the compound. Compounds may be either electrovalent or covalent.

Conductance: The ease with which a current flows along a conducting medium.

Conduction: Heat loss or gain through direct contact.

Conductors: Materials that permit the free movement of electrons.

Continuous wave ultrasound: The sound intensity remains constant throughout the treatment and the ultrasound energy is being produced 100% of the time.

Continuous wave: An uninterrupted beam of laser light as opposed to pulsed wave.

Contraindication: The circumstance or the symptom which renders the use of a procedure inadvisable.

Contraplanar method: Contraplanar method is used in short wave diathermy for the deeper structures of the body where through and through heating is required, e.g., hip, shoulder joint. The electrodes are placed over the opposite aspects of the limb or joint, i.e., medial and lateral aspect or anterior or posterior aspect.

Contrast bath: The principle of contrast bath therapy is to combine the effects of both hot as well as cold baths together. It is most useful for treating various vascular disorders.

Convection: Heat loss or gain through the movement of water molecules across the skin.

Coplanar method: Coplanar method is used in short wave diathermy in which the two electrodes are used in the same plane. This method is particularly suitable for the superficial structures and spine.

Cosine law: Cosine law states that the proportion of rays absorbed varies as per the cosine of the angle between the incident and the normal. Thus, larger the angle at which the rays strike at the body surface, lesser will be the absorption and vice versa.

Coulomb: Measurement indicating the number of electrons flowing in a current.

Coulomb's law: According to Coulomb's law, the force of interaction between any two point charges is directly proportional to the product of charges and inversely proportional to the square of distance between them.

Coupling media: As the ultrasonic waves cannot transmit through the air, some form of coupling media is applied for the proper transmission of the waves. It should have the properties of high transmissivity, high viscosity and hypoallergic nature, etc.

Crossfire method: Crossfire method is used in short wave diathermy. In this technique, half of the treatment is given with the placement of electrodes in one direction, i.e., medial or lateral aspect and another half is used with the placement of electrodes in other direction, i.e., anterior or posterior aspect. This method is commonly used for the treatment of the knee joint, sinuses (frontal, maxillary and ethmoidal) and for pelvic organs.

Current density: Amount of current flow per cubic area.

Current electricity: When charges flow through a conductor it is known as current electricity.

Current modulation: Current modulation refers to any alteration in the magnitude or any variation in duration of the pulses. Modulation may be continuous, interrupted, burst, or ramped.

Current: The flow of charge in a conductor is known as electric current. Its unit is Ampere.

Decay time: The time required for a waveform to go from peak amplitude to 0 V.

Depolarization: Process or act of neutralizing the cell membrane's resting potential.

Diathermy: The application of high-frequency electrical energy that is used to generate heat in body tissues resulting from tissue resistance to the passage of energy.

Didynamic current: These are sinusoidal, direct currents being rectified mains type currents with frequency of 50–100 Hz.

Dielectric constant: The dielectric constants of the various tissues differ considerably. The tissues of low impedance such as blood and muscles have higher dielectric constants. The tissues of high impedance such as fibrous tissues and fat have low dielectric constant.

Differential amplifier: Monitors separate signals from the active electrodes and amplifies the difference, thus eliminating extraneous noise.

Diode laser: A solid-state semiconductor used as a lasing medium.

Dipoles: Molecules whose ends carry opposite charges.

Eddy currents: Small circular electrical fields induced when a magnetic field is created that result in intramolecular oscillation of tissue contents, causing heat generation.

Efferent: Conduction of a nerve impulse away from an organ.

Electric heating pads: Electric heating pads are used to provide raised temperature of 40–45°C to the body parts. The main advantage of using electric heating pads is that they can be used at home by the patients themselves and are cheaper and flexible, and are available in various sizes and shapes.

Electric shock: Electric shock is a painful stimulation of sensory nerves caused by sudden flow of current, cessation or pause of flow of current or variation of the current passing through the body.

Electrical current: The net movement of electrons along a conducting medium.

Electrical field: The lines of force exerted on charged ions in the tissues by the electrodes that cause charged particles to move from one pole to the other.

Electrical impedance: The opposition to electron flow in a conducting material.

Electrical potential: The difference between charged particles at a higher and lower potential.

Electricity: It is a form of energy which is produced due to electric charge. It is of two types—static and current electricity.

Electrodes: These are the two conducting plates or pads which are used for the transmission of current.

Electrolysis: The process of decomposition of electrolyte solution into ions on passing the current through it is called electrolysis.

Electrolyte: The substance which decomposes into positive and negative ions on passing current through it is called electrolyte. For example: acids, bases, salts, dissolved in water, alcohol, etc., are common electrolytes. Pure salt like NaCl, KCl are electrolytes, in their molten state.

Electromagnetic spectrum: The range of frequencies and wavelengths associated with radiant energy.

Electromyography: Electromyography is the study of the electrical activity of contracting muscle which provides information concerning the structure and function of the motor units. It is a technique by which the action potentials of contracting muscle fibers and motor units are recorded and displayed.

Energy: Energy is the ability to do work. Its unit is Joule.

Excited state: State of an atom that occurs when outside energy causes it to contain more energy than normal.

Faradic current: Faradic type current is short duration interrupted direct current with pulse duration of 0.1–1 ms and frequencies between 50–100 Hz, used for the stimulation of innervated muscles.

Fibrosis: Formation of fibrous tissue following injury.

Filter: Changes pulsating DC current to smooth DC.

Fleming's right hand rule: According to this rule, if we stretch the first finger, central finger and thumb of our right hand in mutually perpendicular directions such that first finger points along the direction of the field and thumb is along the direction of motion of the conductor, then the central finger would give us the direction of induced current.

Frequency: The number of cycles or pulses per second.

Galvanic current: Galvanic currents are direct current which has a unidirectional flow of electrons toward the positive pole.

Ground state: The normal unexcited state of an atom.

Ground: A wire that makes an electrical connection with the earth.

Hemarthrosis: Accumulation of blood in the joint cavity.

Heliotherapy: The use of sunlight for therapeutic purposes is known as Heliotherapy.

Hot packs: Hot packs provide superficial moist heat to the body parts. They contain the substance which absorbs heat-like silica or gel. Applications of hot packs are most useful for relieving muscular spasm and thus pain.

Hydrotherapy: Cryotherapy and thermotherapy techniques that use water as the medium for heat transfer.

Impedance: The resistance of the tissue to the passage of electrical current.

Indication: The reason to prescribe a remedy or procedure.

Indifferent or dispensive electrode: Large electrode used to spread out electrical charge and decrease current density at that electrode site.

Induction electrodes: Cable or drum electrodes that create a stronger magnetic field than electrical field.

Infrared radiations: The infrared radiations are electromagnetic radiations with the wavelengths of 750 to 400000 nm and frequency 4×10^{14} Hz to 7.5×10^{11} Hz. It lies beyond the red boundary of visible spectrum.

Insertional activity: Insertional activity is seen in Electromyography which is due to mechanical damage by the needle. Normally it produces a brief burst of electrical activity.

Insulators: Materials that resist current flow.

Intensity: A measure of the rate at which energy is being delivered per unit area.

Interferential therapy: Interferential therapy is the application of two medium frequency currents to produce a low frequency effect. It is based on the principle of Interference, as a result of which a beat frequency is produced.

Interpulse interval: The interruptions between individual pulses or group of pulses.

Interrupted direct current: Interruption is the most usual modification of direct current, the flow of current commencing and ceasing at regular intervals.

Intrapulse interval: The period of time between individual pulses.

Inverse square law: The intensity of radiation striking a particular surface varies inversely with a square of the distance from the radiating source.

Iontophoresis: Iontophoresis is a therapeutic technique, which involves the introduction of ions into the body tissue through the patient's skin. The basic principle is to place the ion under an electrode with the same charge, i.e., negative ion placed under cathode and positive ion placed under anode.

Ions: The charged constituents of the electrolyte which are liberated on passing current are called ions.

Kinesiological electromyography: Kinesiological electromyography is used in the study of muscle activity and to establish the role of various muscles in specific activities. It is used to examine the muscle function during the specific, purposeful tasks or therapeutic regimen.

Laser: The word LASER is an acronym for Light Amplification of Stimulated Emission of Radiation.

Law of Grothus-Drapper: It states that the rays must be absorbed to produce the effect and the effects will be produced at that point at which the rays are absorbed.

Law of inverse square: Law of inverse square explains the effect of distance on the intensity of infrared rays. It states that the intensity of a beam of rays from a point source is inversely proportional to the square of the distance from the source.

Lenz law: This law gives us the direction of current in a circuit. According to this law, the induced current will appear in such a direction that it opposes the change (in magnetic flux) responsible for its production.

Lewis Hunting reaction/response: The alternate phases of vasoconstriction and vasodilatation leads to hunting toward the mean point and is known as Lewis-Hunting reaction.

Longitudinal wave: The primary waveform in which ultrasound energy travels in soft tissue, with the molecular displacement along the direction in which the wave travels.

Macroshock: An electrical shock that can be felt and has a leakage of electrical current of greater than 1 mA.

Magnetic field: When current is passed through a coiled cable that affects surrounding tissues by inducing localized eddy currents within the tissues, then field created is called magnetic field.

Maxwell corkscrew rule: According to this rule, if we imagine a right handed screw placed along the current carrying linear conductor, be rotated such that the screw moves in a direction of flow of current, then the direction of rotation of the thumb gives the direction of magnetic lines of force.

Medical galvanism: Creation of either an acidic or alkaline environment that may be of therapeutic value.

Medium frequency currents: Medium frequency currents are the currents whose frequency falls between the range of 1000 to 10000 Hz. They are being used therapeutically due to their advantage of greater penetration and with a higher tolerance and comfort over the low frequency current.

Microshock: An electrical shock that is imperceptible because of a leakage of current of less than 1 mA.

Microwave diathermy: Microwave diathermy is the use of microwaves for therapeutic purposes. The frequency and wavelength ranges from 300 MHz to 300 GHz and 1 cm to 1 m. The commonly used frequencies are 2456 MHz, 915 MHz and 433.92 MHz with wavelengths of 12.24, 32.79 and 69 cm respectively.

Modified faradic current: For better result in the treatment faradic current is always surged to produce a near-normal tetanic-like contraction and relaxation of muscle. This is called modified faradic current. Various forms of surge are available, such as trapezoidal, triangular and saw-tooth.

Monochromaticity: When a light source produces a single color or wavelength.

Monophasic current: It is another name for direct current, in which the direction of current flow remains the same.

Monopolar method: It is used in short wave diathermy in which only one electrode is placed over the treatment area and other electrode is placed at a distance site or is not used at all. The electrode used produces a radial electric field.

Motor nerve conduction velocity: The conduction velocity of a motor nerve is called motor nerve conduction velocity.

Motor point: Motor point is that point where the nerve enters the muscle or impulses have maximum contraction at that point. It is usually located at a point of upper one-third and lower two-thirds of the length of muscle.

Motor unit action potential: The motor unit action potential is the sum of electrical potential of the muscle fibers present in the single motor unit.

Mutual induction: Mutual induction is the property of two coils by virtue of which each opposes any change in the strength of current flowing through the other by developing an induced emf.

Myofascial pain: A type of referred pain associated with trigger points.

Nerve conduction velocity: Nerve conduction velocity is the speed with which a peripheral motor or sensory conducts an impulse.

Neuropraxia: Temporary mild compression of the nerve which leads to the conduction block is called neuropraxia.

Neurotmesis: Instead of minor compression if the injury is such as to disrupt all tissues of the nerve fiber such as a cut through the nerve, then the distal segment degenerates completely. Such lesion often requires surgery to ensure that the two cut ends are sufficiently approximated to allow successful growth.

Ohm's law: Ohm's law states that the current flowing through a metallic conductor is directly proportional to the potential difference across its ends and inversely proportional to the resistance, provided that all physical conditions remain constant.

Pain gate theory: Pain gate theory states that the afferent inputs mainly passes through posterior root of the spinal cord and all afferent information must pass through synapses in the substantia gelatinosa and nucleus proprius of the posterior horn. It is at this level that the pain gate operates.

Paraffin wax bath therapy: Paraffin wax bath therapy is an application of molten paraffin wax on the body parts. It provides more amount of heat than water because the mineral oil in the paraffin lowers its melting point.

Phonophoresis: Phonophoresis is the movement of the drugs through skin into the subcutaneous tissues under the influence of ultrasound waves.

Piezoelectric effect: The deformation of quartz or barium titanate or lead zirconate crystal occurs due to the application of a varying potential difference. This is called piezoelectric effect.

Polarized state of nerve: In resting nerve, the nerve is positive outside and negative inside. At this time, the nerve is not permeable to Na$^+$ ions, so it is called as Polarized state of nerve. The change in polarized stage causes the impulse to travel.

Potential: The electric potential of a body is the condition of that body when compared to the neutral potential of the Earth. Its unit is Volt. It is directed from an area of low potential to an area of high potential.

Power: It is the rate of doing work. The rate at which work is done by the source of EMF in maintaining the current in electric circuit is called the electric power of the circuit. Its unit is Watt.

Pulse: The individual waveform as shown by an oscilloscope is referred to as a pulse.

Pulsed short wave diathermy: Pulsed short wave diathermy is referred to as pulsed electromagnetic energy which is created by interrupting the output of continuous short wave diathermy at regular intervals.

Pure faradic current: Pure faradic current was the type of current produced by the first faradic coil and was unevenly alternating current with each cycle consisting of two unequal phases, low intensity long duration and high intensity short duration current phase.

Radiation therapy: Radiation therapy is the application of various radiations over the skin for therapeutic purposes. The various radiations used are infrared radiations and ultraviolet radiations, etc.

Rebox-type currents: Rebox-type currents are medium frequency currents derived from a device called rebox. The current produced consists of unipolar rectangular pulses of between 50 and 250 μs at 3000 Hz.

Recruitment pattern: In electromyography examination when voluntary contractions are initiated, the motor units are recruited in an orderly fashion.

Resistance: It is the obstruction to the flow of electrons in a conductor. The unit of electrical resistance is the Ohm.

Rheobase: The rheobase is the smallest current that produces a muscle contraction if the stimulus is of infinite duration.

Rheostat: Rheostat is a device used to regulate current by altering either the resistance of the current or potential in the part of the circuit. It consists of a coil of high resistance wire wound onto an insulating block with each turn insulated from adjacent turns.

Russian currents: Russian currents are evenly alternating currents with a frequency of 2500 Hz (between 2000–10,000 Hz). These are applied with a series of separate bursts, i.e., polyphasic AC waveforms. There are thus 50 periods of 20 ms duration consisting of 10 ms burst and 10 ms interval. Each 10 ms burst contains 25 cycles of alternating current, i.e., 50 phases of 0.2

ms duration. These bursts reduces the total amount of current given to the patient thus increases patients tolerance.

Sauna bath: Sauna bath is the application of dry hot air in a wooden sauna chamber. The temperature is kept between 60–90°C and relative humidity of the air is maintained between 5–10%.

Self-induction: Self-induction is the property of a coil by virtue of which, the coil opposes any change in the strength of current flowing through it by inducing an emf in itself. Self-induction is also called the inertia of electricity.

Sensory nerve conduction velocity: The conduction velocity of a sensory nerve is called sensory nerve conduction velocity.

Shock: Shock is a stage of unconsciousness which could be due to so many causes.

Short wave diathermy: Short wave diathermy is the use of high frequency electromagnetic waves of the frequency ranging between 10^7 to 10^8 Hz and a wavelength between 30 and 3 m to generate heat in the body tissues. The therapeutically used frequencies and wavelengths are 27.12 MHz, 40.68 MHz, 13.56 MHz and 11 m, 7.5 m, 22 m respectively. It is the deepest form of heat available to the Physiotherapist.

Sinusoidal currents: Sinusoidal currents are evenly alternating sine wave currents of 50 Hz. This gives 100 pulses or phases in each second of 10 ms each, 50 in one direction and 50 in another.

Spontaneous activity: No spontaneous activity occurs in normal electromyography after a brief burst of insertional activity.

Sprain: An injury of a ligament, partial or complete is known as sprain.

Static electricity: When the charges on the body do not flow, it is called static electricity. The simplest way of producing a static electric charge is to rub two materials together.

Strain: An injury of a muscle or tendon, partial or complete is known as strain.

Strength-duration curve: Strength-duration curve shows the relationship between the magnitude of the change of stimulus and the duration of the stimulus. The curve provides valuable information regarding the state of excitability of a nerve.

Surging: For better result in the treatment, faradic current is always surged to produce a near-normal tetanic-like contraction and relaxation of the muscle. The circuit is modified to give surges of various durations, frequencies and waveforms. Surging is done to avoid accommodation of the current to the nerve fibers.

Tendinitis: Inflammation of a tendon is called tendinitis.

TENS: Transcutaneous electrical nerve stimulation (TENS) is the application of low frequency current in the form of pulsed rectangular currents through surface electrodes on the patient's skin to reduce pain.

Transducer: A device that changes energy from one form to another is known as transducer.

Transformer: A transformer is an electric device which is used for changing the AC voltages. A transformer which increases the AC voltages is called a step-up transformer. A transformer which decreases the AC voltages is called a step-down transformer.

Trigger point: Any localized area of body when subjected to pressure causes pain in a specific area.

Tuning of the circuit: Tuning of the circuit is done in the application of short wave diathermy so as to have maximum transfer of energy to the patient's tissues.

Ultrasonic waves: Ultrasonic waves are the sound waves with a frequency well above the audible sound waves of 20–20,000 Hz.

Ultraviolet radiations: Ultraviolet radiations are the electromagnetic energy which falls between visible rays and X-rays and have wavelength between 10 and 400 nm.

van't Hoff's law: van't Hoff's law states that 'any chemical change which is capable of being accelerated is accelerated by the rise in temperature'. Therefore, all the chemical changes of the body that can be accelerated are accelerated by heat.

Voltameter: The vessel in which the electrolysis is carried, is called a voltameter. It contains two electrodes and a solution electrolyte. It is also known as electrolytic cell.

Voltmeter: A voltmeter is a high resistance galvanometer. It is used to measure the potential difference between two points of a circuit in volts.

Vasoconstriction: Decrease in the lumen (diameter) of the vessel.

Vasodilatation: Increase in the lumen (diameter) of the vessel.

Wallerian degeneration: Wallerian degeneration is a process by which the nerve degenerates proximally to nearest node of Ranvier and distally throughout its whole length. Debris is cleared by macrophagic activity. Process takes up to 21 days to complete and is a preparation for regeneration.

Water bag method: For the transmission of the ultrasound to the irregular patient's tissue, water bag method is applied.

Water bath method: When direct contact is not possible because of irregular shape of part or because of tenderness, a water bath method may be used. As the part to be treated is immersed in water this can only reasonably be applied to the hand, forearm, ankle and foot.

Whirlpool bath: Whirlpool bath is used therapeutically so as to combine the effects of temperature with the mechanical effects of the water. These are used for various rheumatic disorders, postimmobilization stiffness, joints pain, etc.

Suggested Reading

1. Barbara BJ, Susan ML. Physical Agents: Theory and Practice for the Physical Therapist Assistant. FA Davis Company, Philadelphia; 1996.
2. Baxter D. Therapeutic Lasers: Theory and Practice. Churchill Livingstone, Edinburgh; 1994.
3. Bellew J, Michlovitz S, Nolan T. Michlovitz's Modalities for Therapeutic Intervention. FA Davis; 2016.
4. Bonica JJ. The Management of Pain. Lea Febiger: Malvern PA; 1990.
5. Braddom RL. Physical Medicine and Rehabilitation. Elsevier: India; 2008.
6. Chartered Society of Physiotherapy. Guidance for the clinical use of electrotherapy agent; 2006.
7. Dolphin S, Walker M. Healing Accelerated by Ionozone Therapy, Physiotherapy, 1979;65: 81-82.
8. Foster A, Palastanga N. Clayton's Electrotherapy: Theory and Practice (9th edn). AITBS Publishers, New Delhi; 2000.
9. Gersh MR. Electrotherapy in Rehabilitation. FA Davis, Philadelphia; 1992.
10. Johnson EW. Practical Electromyography (4th edn). Lippincott Williams & Wilkins; 2006.
11. Kahn J. Principles and Practice of Electrotherapy (3rd edn). Churchill Livingstone: New York; 1994.
12. Khandpur RS. Handbook of Biomedical Instrumentation. Tata McGraw Hill Publishing Company Ltd: New Delhi; 1987.
13. Kitchen S, Bazin S. Clayton's Electrotherapy (10th edn). PRISM, Indian edition.
14. Kitchen S. Electrotherapy: Evidence based Practice. Churchill Livingstone, Edinburgh; 2002.
15. Kottke F. Handbook of Physical Medicine and Rehabilitation (3rd edn). WB Saunders: Philadelphia; 1982.
16. Kovacs R. Electrotherapy and Light Therapy. Lea and Febiger: Philadelphia; 1949.
17. Krusen FH, Kotke FJ, Euwood PM. Handbook of Physical Medicine and Rehabilitation. WB Saunders Company: Philadelphia; 1971.
18. Kuprian W. Physical Therapy for Sports (2nd edn). WB Saunders Company: Philadelphia; 1995.
19. Lehman GF, De Lateur BJ. Therapeutic Heat and Cold (3rd edn). Williams and Wilkins: Baltimore; 1982.
20. Licht S. Electrodiagnosis and Electromyography (3rd edn). Elizabeth Licht: New Haven, Waverly; 1971.
21. Low J, Reed Ann. Electrotherapy Explained: Principles and Practice, Butterworth Heinemann, London; 1990.
22. Mannheimer J, Lampe G. Clinical Transcutaneous Electrical Nerve Stimulation. FA Davis: Philadelphia; 1984.
23. Michloeitz SL. Thermal Agents in Rehabilitation. FA Davis: Philadelphia; 1990.
24. Mishra UK, Kalita J. Clinical Neurophysiology: Nerve Conduction, Electromyography and Evoked Potentials. BI Churchill: Livingstone; 1999.
25. Nanda BK. Electrotherapy Simplified (3rd edn). Jaypee Brothers Medical Publishers, New Delhi; 2020.
26. Nelson R, Currier D. Clinical Electrotherapy. Appleton and Lange: Norwalk, Conn; 1991.
27. Newton RA. Electrotherapeutic Treatment. Preston Clinton, NJ; 1984.
28. Nikolova L. Treatment with Interferential Therapy. Churchill Livingstone: New York; 1987.

29. Ottawa Panel. Ottawa panel evidence-based clinical practice guidance for electrotherapy and thermotherapy interventions in the management of rheumatoid arthritis in adults. Physical Therapy. 2004;84(11):1016-43.
30. Prentice WE. Therapeutic Modalities in Sports Medicine. Times Mirror Mosby College Publishing: St. Louis; 1990.
31. Rennie S. Diadynamic Current Therapy. In: Peat M (Ed). Current Physical Therapy. Toronto: BC Decker; 1988.
32. Robertson V, Ward A, Low J. Electrotherapy Explained: Principle and Practice (4th edn). Elsevier, Oxford; 2006.
33. Robinson AJ, Madder LS. Clinical Electrophysiology (2nd edn). Williams and Wilkins: Baltimore; 1994.
34. Savage B. Interferential Therapy. Faber and Faber: Boston; 1984.
35. Scott P. Clayton's Electrotherapy and Actinotherapy (5th and 7th edns). Baltimore: Williams and Wilkins; 1965 and 1975.
36. Shriber WA. Manual of Electrotherapy (4th edn). Lea and Febiger: Philadelphia; 1975.
37. Stillwell GK. Therapeutic Electricity and Ultraviolet Radiations. Sidney Licht (Ed) (3rd edn). Williams and Wilkins: Baltimore; 1983.
38. Sullivan SB, Schmitz TJ, Fulk G. Physical Rehabilitation: Assessment and Treatment (5th edn). FA Davis; 2006.
39. Sullivan SB, Schmitz TJ. Physical Rehabilitation: Assessment and Treatment (4th edn). FA Davis; 2001.
40. Sunderland S. Nerves and Nerve Injuries. Williams and Wilkins: Baltimore; 1968.
41. Wadsworth H, Chanmugan AP. Electrophysical Agents in Physiotherapy. Marrickville, NSW, Australia, Science Press; 1983.
42. Walsh DM, McAdams ET. TENS: Clinical Applications and Related Theory. Churchill Livingstone, New York; 1997.
43. Watkins AL. A Manual of Electrotherapy (3rd edn). Lea and Febiger: Philadelphia; 1968.
44. Watson T. Electrotherapy Evidenced Based Practice. Churchill Livingstone; 2008.
45. Watson T. The Role of Electrotherapy in Contemporary Physiotherapy Practice. Manual Therapy. 2000;5(3):132-41.
46. Wolf SL. Electrotherapy. Churchill Livingstone, New York; 1981.

Index

Page numbers followed by *f* refer to figure and *t* refer to table.

A

Abductor pollicis brevis, paralysis of 100
Absorption 240
Acetylcholine 264, 271
Achillodynia 261
Achromycin 215
Acne vulgaris 205, 211
    clinical features 211
    management 211
    pathology 211
Acoustic impedance 242
Actinotherapy 1, 293
A-delta fibers 127
Adhesion
    loosening of 92
    prevention of 92
Adjacent cells 238*f*
Air 241
Air bubble
    compression of 249*f*
    contraction of 249*f*
Air-cooled lamp 203
Aldoril 215
Alkali accumulator 27, 27*f*
Alopecia 206, 215
    areata 215
    classification 215
    etiology 215
    general health 215
    totalis 215
    treatment 215
    universalis 215
Alternating current 76, 293
    generator 52
Aluminum oxide 219
Amalgamated zinc rod 24
Ammeter 36, 36*f*, 293
Ammonium chloride solution, concentration of 25
Ampere circuital law 33, 293
Amplifier system 276, 279, 293
Amyotrophic lateral sclerosis 291
Analgesia 222, 293
Anions 21, 293
Ankle 184, 185
    ligaments of 184
    sprain 267
        investigation 268
        mechanism of injury 267
        treatment 268
Ankylosing spondylitis 196
Annular tears 196
Anode 21, 26, 294
Anterior horn cell 291
    diseases of 291
Antibiotic effect 205
Antifungal agents 215
Anti-inflammatory activity 252
Anti-inflammatory analgesic cream 252
Aortic aneurysm, abdominal 196
Ape thumb deformity 100
Aperture 64
Apparatus
    checking of 98, 106, 113
    choice of 190
    preparation of 97, 100, 142, 144
Argon ionization, process of 201
Arndt-Schultz principle 192, 294
Arterial disease 164
Articular cartilage 177, 222
Aspirin 216
Atom 3, 294
    structure of 3
Attraction, force of 4
Audio speaker 273
Autoimmune disease 71
Autotransformer 55
Axilla 105
Axonotmesis 85, 103, 106, 290, 294

B

Back, motor points of 121*f*
Bacterial infections, effects in 160
Balanced vastus medialis oblique 272
Bandaging method 229
Bandwidth 294
Barbiturates 215
Beat frequency 294
    production of 134*f*
Becker muscular dystrophy 292
Bell's palsy 108
Benzodiazepines 215
Benzoyl peroxide gel 211
Bicipital tendinitis 260
Biofeedback 270, 294
    devices 274
    instrumentation 270
    limitations of 273
Biot-Savart's law 30, 31*f*, 294
Bipolar needle electrode 277
Blood flow 250
Body tissues
    effect on 93
    temperature of 262

Body, effects on metabolism of 159
Bone
    aseptic necrosis of 196
    cartilage 222
    injuries 250
Bound electrons 4
Brachial plexus injuries 289
Breaking off septic emboli 251
Broad frequency spectrum 255
Brushing method 229
Bulbar palsy, progressive 291
Burns 71, 162, 166, 193, 250
    danger of 202
Bursitis 294
Burst
    modulation 90, 91f
    transcutaneous electrical nerve stimulation 130

C

Cable method 157
Calcium
    absorption of 205
    chloride 126
Calf muscle 288
Capacitance 9, 294
Capacitor
    electrodes 294
    field method 151
    grouping of 10
Carcinogenesis 204
Cardiac disease 251
Cardiac pacemakers 163, 166
Cathode 21, 26, 294
Cations 21, 294
Cavitation 248, 249f, 250, 294
Celiac rickets 214
Cell 23, 294
    primary 23
    secondary 23, 25, 26f
Cellular changes 72
Central nervous system abnormalities 288
Cervical spondylosis 170, 178
    clinical features 170
    contraindications 171
    etiology 170
    incidence 170
    investigations 170
    pathogenesis 170
    placement of electrodes 171
    positioning of 171
Chemical agents 94, 71
Chemotaxis 73
Chlorine 126
Chromium 219
Chromophores 221
Chronaxie 125, 295
Chronic inflammatory disease 211
Chronic pain 74
    relief of 137
Circuit 295
    tuning of 303

Circular coil carrying current 31f
    center of 31
Circulatory defects 167
Circulatory disorders 196
Circumflex nerve 111
Clinical electromyography 276, 295
Coal tar 216
Coaxial cable 295
Cobalt therapy 164, 167, 207
Cold packs 263, 263f, 264f
Cold sensitive 266
Cold therapy
    physiological effects of 264
    therapeutic uses of 264
Collimation 218
Combination therapy 254, 295
Comedones 211
Common motor points 119
Complete denervated muscle 124f
Compound muscle action potential, measurement of
    duration of 286f
Compression 238f
Concave spherical mirror 63
Concentric needle electrode 277
Conductance 295
Conduction 5, 295
Conductor 295
    area of 9
    capacitance of 9
    factors affecting capacity of 9
Constant current 124f
Constant voltage 123f, 124f
Continuous modulation 90, 91f
Continuous wave 295
    ultrasound 295
Contraction
    strength of 84
    type of 137
Contraplanar method 182f, 295
Contraplanar technique 181, 184
Contrast bath 234, 234f, 295
    effects 234
Convection 5, 295
Convex electrodes 153f
Cooling phase 235
Coplanar method 175, 175f, 295
Copper loss 55
Cosine law 208, 295
Cotton 97, 139
Coulomb's law 6, 38, 296
Counter-balanced height adjustment 190f
Counter-irritation effect 206
Coupling media 241, 296
    characteristics of 241
Covalent compounds 4
Crossfire technique 157f, 181, 296
Cryotherapy 75, 262
    methods of treatment 266
    techniques of application 262
Crystal laser 219

Current 296
　carriers 11, 12
　carrying coil 45f
　chemical effects of 18
　density 13, 296
　electricity 5, 11, 296
　feel of 106
　flow
　　direction of 86
　　phases of 86
　heating effects of 19
　intensity 126
　modulation 90, 296
　selection of 99, 106, 108, 111, 113
　sudden flow of 59
　thermal of 18
Curvature, center of 64
Curve, shape of 123
Curved mirrors, applications of 64
Cylindrical wavefront 65
Cysts, subchondral 180

D

Dangers equipment 164
Daniel cell 24, 24f
de Quervain's disease 260
　cause 260
　clinical features 260
　treatment 260
Deep X-ray 164, 167, 207
Deformity 100, 180
Degenerative diseases 196
Deltoid inhibition 95, 111
Denervated muscle, stimulation of 93, 94
Denervation, process of 85
Density 68
Depolarization 296
Derivatives 216
Dermatomyositis 291
Desquamation 205
Dexamethasone 126
Diabetic neuropathy 291
Diathermy 50, 296
Didynamic current 296
Dielectric constant 296
Digital nerve 286
Diode laser 219, 296
Dipole 296
　field 9
　moment 8
　rotation of 152f
Dipping method 229
Direct contact method 244
Direct current 76
Direct monophasic current 79f
Direct pouring method 229
Discontinuous curves 8
Disk lesion 196
Dispersion 64
Display system 276, 280
Dithranol 216

Doburil 215
Dopants 16
Dosage parameters 220, 256
Dry cell 25, 26f
Duchenne muscular dystrophy 292
Duodenal ulcer 175
Dynamo 52, 54
Dystrophies 292

E

Earth
　circuit 60
　magnetic field of 42
　shock 60
　　causes of 60
Eddy currents 48, 49f, 50, 296
　applications of 50
Edema
　absorption of 199
　chronic indurated 250
Edison cell 27, 27f
Efferent 296
Effusion 180
Elbow 105
　joint, dislocation of 100
　level of 100
Electric charge, quantization of 6
Electric conductivity 15
Electric current 11, 12, 28
　chemical effects of 21
　magnetic effects of 28, 28f
　thermal effects of 18
　direction of 13, 13f
Electric device, efficiency of 20
Electric dipole 8, 9f
Electric field intensity 6
　direction of 7
Electric field
　concentration of 162
　vector 56
Electric heating pads 232, 233, 296
　contraindications 233
Electric iron 20
Electric potential 11
Electric power 19
　transmission of 18
Electric shock 59, 60, 163, 193, 297
　causes of 59
　effects of 59
　severe 59, 60
　severity of 59
　treatment of 60
　types of 59
Electrical circuits 10
Electrical current 297
Electrical energy
　and power 19
　storing of 26
Electrical field 297
Electrical impedance 297

Electricity 297
  basics of 1
  conductors of 4
  inertia of 51
  nonconductors of 4
  types of 5
Electrode 21, 26, 96, 135, 154f, 276, 277, 297
  active 293
  coplanar arrangement of 156f
  correct placing of 110, 113, 142, 144
  placement of 106, 107, 111, 130, 171, 173, 175, 181, 184, 188
  types of 126, 277
Electroencephalographs 271
Electrolysis 21, 22, 297
  Faraday's law of 22
  practical application of 23
Electrolyte 21, 297
Electromagnetic induction 44
  Faraday's law of 45
Electromagnetic radiations 62
  laws governing effects of 192
Electromagnetic spectrum 57, 297
  parts of 58t
  uses of 58
Electromagnetic waves 56, 56f, 57
  production of 57
Electromotive force 11, 12, 45f
Electromyogram biofeedback 271
  use of 273
Electromyographic examination 281
Electromyography 45f, 275, 297
  clinical implications of 290
  components of 276
  diagnostic 276
  normalization of 284
  recording system 281f
  types of 276
Electron 4
  charge of 6
Electronic stimulator 77f
Electroplating 23
Electrotherapeutic currents 77
Electrotherapy, modern 2
Electrovalent compounds 4
Encephalin 134
Endocrine myopathies 292
Endogenous opiates, release of 137
Endorphin 134, 137
Energy 220, 297
  conservation 47
  density 220
  law of conservation of 6
  loss
    amount of 262
    transformer 55
  specific amount of 264
Enkephalin 137
Eosine 216
Epicondylitis, lateral 224, 258
Epidermis 204
  thickening of 205

Erb's paralysis 95, 107
Erythema 204
  appears 203
  degree of 209, 209t
  reaction 204
Excitatory cold 263
Exercise 210, 260
Experimental demonstration 48
Exponential current 89
Extracorporeal shock wave therapy 255
Extrinsic semiconductors 16
Exudates, absorption of 137, 145, 199
Eyes 166

F

Facial nerve stimulation 95, 108, 110f
Facioscapulohumeral muscular dystrophy 292
Faintness 163, 194
Faraday's constant 22
Faraday's experiments 44
Faraday's law 22
Faradic current 76, 77f, 93, 94, 106, 297
  modified form of 78f
  unmodified form of 78f
Faradic foot bath 95, 116, 118f
Fibrillation potential 283
Fibroblasts 249
Fibrosis 297
Fibrous tissue, contracture of 93
Filter 297
Fine wire indwelling electrodes 278, 278f
Finger photo transmission 271
Fleming's left hand rule 29, 30f
Fleming's right hand rule 48, 48f, 297
Fluid
  part of 5
  unidirectional movement of 249
Fluorescent tubes 201-203
  arrangement of 203f
Foot drop 114
Force
  effects on magnitude of 28f
  electric lines of 7, 7f, 8, 41
  magnetic line of 31, 33f, 40, 40f, 41, 41f
Forearm muscles 100
Fracture 71
Frequency 246, 297
  band width 280
Frost bite 71
Furadantin 215
Fuse wire 20
Fusion, latent heat of 5, 264
F-wave 288

G

Gallium arsenide 217, 219
Galvanic current 94, 106, 297
Galvanometer 35
Gangrene 194
  precipitation of 163
Gantrisin 215

Gas laser 219
Gases 5
Gauss's law 42
Gauss's theorem 42
Generators, types of 201
Giddiness 163, 194
Goeckerman regimen 206
Gold therapy 216
Golfer's elbow 226, 259
    position of therapist 226
    treatment 226
Gradual reduction 239
Granulation tissues 177
Grid method 220
Griseofulvin 215
Grothus-Drapper law 192, 209, 299
Ground electrode 285
Growth, malignant 143
Guillain-Barre syndrome 288, 289, 291

H

Hairy surface 143
Half-value distance 240
Hand muscles 100
Headache 194
Hearing aids 163, 166
Heat
    transmission of 5
    treatment 248
Heating
    mild 193
    tissues, physiological effects of 159
Heliotherapy 234, 298
Helium-neon laser 219
Hemarthrosis 298
Hematoma 268
Hemiplegia 274
Hemophilic arthritis 184
Hemorrhage 164, 251
Herniated nucleus pulposus 196
Herpes zoster, treatment of 251
High frequency currents 148
High pressure mercury vapor
    lamp 201, 202
    tube 201f
High transcutaneous electrical nerve stimulation 128
Higher energy levels, atoms of 219
High-intensity short duration current 76
Hip joint 177
Histamine-like substance, causes release of 204
Homogeneous medium 62
Hot packs 230, 254, 298
Hot water fomentation 187
Housemaid's knee 261
H-reflex 287
Humerus, fracture shaft of 111
Huygens' principle 65
Hydrocollator 230, 231f
    hot packs 230, 231, 232f
Hydrocortisone 126, 252, 259
Hydrotherapy 298
Hypnotic drugs 215
Hysteresis loss 55

I

Ice massage 262
Impaired skin sensation 233
Implants 251
Incandescent electric lamp 20
Incandescent state 20
Incident ray 63f
Inclusion body myositis 291
Induction
    electrodes 298
    furnace 50
    motor 50
Inductothermy 157
Infectious diseases 196
Inflammation 71, 72
    acute 72, 192
    causes of 71
    chronic 72, 73
    effects on 160
    feature of 72
    phase of 73
    process of 73
Inflammatory exudates 177
Inflammatory muscle disease 290, 291
Infrared lamp 199
    placement of 198, 200
Infrared radiations 58, 71, 189, 298
    contraindications 194
    dangers of 193
    proforma 194
Infrared therapy, applications of 192, 197
Injury
    mechanism of 267
    types of 122
Insertional activity 281, 282, 298
Insulators 21, 298
Intensity 241, 246, 298
Interferential currents, advantages of 136
Interferential therapy 134, 142f, 145f, 298
    basic principles of 134
    physiological effects of 136
    principles of 134
Interpulse interval 298
Interrupted direct current 79, 298
    tests 125
Interrupted galvanic current 80, 93
Intracellular electrode 279
Intrapulse interval 298
Intrinsic semiconductors 16
Inverse square law 192, 208, 298, 299
Iodine 126
Ions 21, 126, 299
    migration of 251
Iontophoresis 125, 298
Iron loss 55
Ischemic tissue 251
Ischemic ulcer 210

J

Joint movement, terminal limitation of 180

K

Kinesiological electromyography 276, 284, 299
Kinetic force produces vibration 4
Knee 182, 183
Kromayer's lamp 201, 202, 202f, 203-205
   construction of 202

L

Lambert-Cosine law 192
Larger radius, current loop of 32f
Laser 299
   beams 218
   physiological effects of 221
   production 218
   properties of 218
   radiations 218
      production of 218
   therapeutic uses of 221
   therapy 217, 217f, 221, 222
      contraindications 222
      dangers 222
      dosage parameters 220
      methods of treatment 222
      techniques of application 220
   types of 219
Latent heat 5
Lateral collateral ligament injuries 183
Lateral ligament injuries 184
Lateral popliteal nerve
   injury 113
   stimulation 95
Lead 97
   acid accumulator 26, 26f
Leclanché cell 24, 25, 25f
   electromotive force of 25
Lenz's law 46, 47, 47f, 299
   experimental verification of 46
Lesion, level of 105
Lewis's hunting reaction 265f, 299
Ligament
   complete rupture of 183
   injuries 178, 181
   partial rupture of 183
   sprain of 182
Light
   interference of 66
   physical principles of 61
   propagation, aspects of 62
   reflection of 63f
   refraction of 63f
   scattering of 65
Limb-girdle muscular dystrophy 292
Lint pad 96, 139
Liquids 5
Local circulation, increase of 231
Long flexor tendons, paralysis of 100
Longitudinal waves 66, 69, 299

Longwave diathermy 148, 167
Lorentz force 34
Low back pain 141
   causes of 196
   etiology 141
Low backache 173, 142f, 194, 196
   etiology 173, 196
   investigations 174, 197
   neurological examination 174, 197
   treatment 174, 197
Low frequency current 76
   apparatus 77f
   indications for 92
   physiological effects of 93
Low intensity lasers 221
Low transcutaneous electrical nerve stimulation 130
Lower limb 289
Low-intensity long duration current 76
Lumbar spondylosis 176
   cause 176
   clinical features 176
   pathology 176
Lumbar vertebra, sacralization of 173, 196
Luminous generators 190
Lymphatic drainage 92

M

Machine circuit 149
Mackintosh 96, 139
Macroelectrode 279
Macroshock 299
Magnesium oxide 126
Magnet
   basic properties of 37
   magnetized 39f
   unmagnetized 39f
Magnetic dipole 42, 42f
   moment 42
Magnetic field 31, 32, 32f, 299
   center 31f
   direction of 33
   lines 43f
Magnetic flux 44
   leakage of 55
Magnetic force 38
Magnetic lines, properties of 40
Magnetic needle 28
Magnetism 42
   molecular theory of 39
Manganese dioxide 24
Maturation, phase of 73
Maxwell's Corkscrew rule 33, 34f, 299
Mechanical wave 67
Medial collateral ligament injuries 182
Medial epicondylitis 226, 259
Medial ligament injuries 185
Median nerve stimulation 94, 99, 101f
Medical galvanism 299
Medium frequency currents 133, 299
Meninges 196
Menstrual cycle 187

Menstruation 164, 167
Mercury
  ionization 201
  vaporization 201
Metabolic diseases 196
Metabolic myopathies 292
Metal
  around area 184
  purification of 23
Metatarsalgia 261
  causes 261
  clinical features 261
  treatment 261
Methoxypsoralens 216
Microbial agents 71
Microcurrent electrical neuromuscular stimulation 131
Micromassage 249
Microshock 299
Microstreaming 249, 249f
Microwave
  diathermy 148, 165, 166f, 299
  production of 165
  radiations 58
Miner's elbow 261
Minor electric shock 59
Modified direct current impulses 82f
Modified faradic current 76, 300
Modulation depth 135
Molecular agitation, amount of 238
Monochromaticity 218, 300
Monophasic current 300
Monoplanar technique 175
Monopolar method 300
Monopolar needle electrode 277
Motor axon, stimulation of 286
Motor nerve 93
  activated, quantity of 84
  conduction
    principles of 285, 285f
    velocity 300
  neuropraxia of 93
  stimulation of 94
Motor neuron disorders 290, 291
Motor point 119f, 120f, 300
Motor stimulation 137
Motor unit action potential 275, 276, 300
  amplitude of 283
  duration of 282
  phase of 283
  rise time of 283
Movement
  pattern of 243
  range of 92
Moving coil galvanometer 34, 35f
Multicolored rainbows 61
Multi-lead electrode 279
Muscle
  Action
    facilitation of 92
    initiation of 92
    re-education of 92
    re-learning of 92
    contraction, effect on 94
  contusion 268
    clinical feature 268
    investigations 268
    treatment 269
  fibers 271
    degeneration of 292
  relaxation of 193
  soreness, delayed onset 252
  strengthening 274
  tissue, effects on 161
  tone 212, 265
Muscular atrophy, progressive 291
Muscular dystrophy 292
  types of 292
Muscular spasm, effect on 231
Muscular tissue, effects of heat on 160
Musculoskeletal conditions 221
Mutual inductance, coefficient of 52
Mutual induction 51, 52f, 300
  coefficient of 52
Myoelectric signal 279
Myofibroblasts 249
Myogenic disorders 290, 291
Myopathy 290, 292
  congenital 292
Myotonic dystrophy 292

N

Neck of femur, fracture in 177
Needle electrode 277
  bipolar 278f
  concentric 278f
  monopolar 278f
  types of 278f
Needle, north pole of 28
Nemec's currents 134
Neoplastic diseases 196
Nerve
  conduction velocity 284, 289, 300
  course of 99, 105, 108
  distal portion of 286
  electrical stimulation of 84
  fibers, conduction of 265
  polarized state of 301
  regeneration of 85, 122
  transmission 83
    resting state 83f
    stimulated state 83f
Nervous system 251
  effects on 265
Nervous tissues, effects of heat on 159
Neural tissues, effects on 265
Neuralgia 178
Neuritis 178
Neurogenic disorders 290
Neurological examination 174, 197
Neuromuscular re-education 273
Neuromuscular system, integrity of 281
Neurons 128
Neuropathy, alcoholic 291
Neuropraxia 85, 93, 103, 106, 290, 300

Neurotmesis 85, 103, 106, 290, 300
Neutron 3
New muscle action, teaching of 92
Nichrome, wire of 20
Non-ohmic conductors 15
Nonsteroidal anti-inflammatory drugs 252
Normal motor unit action potential 282
N-type semiconductor 16, 17*f*
Nucleus 3
Nutritional rickets 214

O

Oculopharyngeal muscular dystrophy 292
Ohm's law 13, 300
   limitations of 13
Olecranon bursitis 261
Open wound 143, 164
Opponens palsy 100
Orthodromic potential, latency of 286
Orthodromic sensory conduction, principles of 287*f*
Oscilloscope 271
Osteoarthritis 177, 196
   knee 144, 145*f*, 178, 179
      classification 144, 179
      clinical features 179
      investigations 180
   secondary 180
   treatment 145
Osteophyte formation 180

P

Pads, correct placing of 100, 113, 142, 144
Pain 74
   acute 74
   chronic 74
   gate control 128
      mechanism of 128, 129*f*
   gate theory 300
   myofascial 300
   relief of 136, 161, 222
   subacute 74
Panmycin 215
Paraffin wax 229
   application of 229
   bath therapy 228, 300
      methods 229
      techniques of application 229
   bath unit 228, 228*f*
      maintenance of 230
Parallel plate capacitor 9, 10*f*
Parasitic myositis 291
Pelvic
   inflammatory disease 187
   pain 187
   tumors 196
   ulcer 175
Periarthritis shoulder 143, 172
   clinical features 172
   contraindications 172
   investigations 172
   placement of electrodes 173

   treatment 172
   types 172
Periodic mechanical disturbance 236
Periodic waves 67
Periosteal pain 248*f*
Peripheral nerve 85
   disorders of 290
   injuries 265, 274
Peripheral neuropathy, diagnostic measure for 287
Peripheral skin temperature 271
Peripheral vascular disease 266
Phenothiazine 216
Phonophoresis 251, 252, 301
   applications 253
   contraindications 253
   effects of 252
   principle 252
Phosphor, type of 202
Photons 62
   reflect 219
Physiologic salpingitis 187
Piezoelectric effect 301
Placebo effect 250
Plane mirrors, applications of 64
Plantar fasciitis 185, 226
   clinical features 186
   incidence 185
   investigation 186, 227
   procedures 186
   treatment 186, 227
Plantar warts 250
Pointing index finger 100
Polarization 66
Polymyositis 291, 292
Polyneuropathy 290
Polyphasic motor unit potentials 291
Population inversions 219
Posteroanterior shoulder 178
Postimmobilization stiffness 198
Potassium citrate 126
Power 220, 301
   density 220
Pregnancy 164, 167, 251
Prepatellar bursitis 261
Pressure 68
   sores 206, 212
      clinical features 212
      treatment 212
   transducers 271
Primary muscle disease 292
Proliferation, phase of 73
Proton 3
   charge of 6
Proximal motor pathways 288
Proximal sensory pathways 288
Psoralens 216
   ultraviolet-A 203
Psoriasis 206, 212
   cause 213
   treatment 213, 214
Psychoneurotic pain 196

Index

P-type semiconductor 16, 17f
Pulse 86, 301
    amplitude 87
    charge 88
    duration 89
    frequency 89
Pulsed electromagnetic energy 210
Pulsed polyphasic current 79f
Pulsed short wave diathermy 164, 301
Pure faradic current 76f, 301
PUVA apparatus 201, 203

Q

Quadriceps
    femoris muscle, wasting of 180
    inhibition 95, 112

R

Radial nerve stimulation 94, 104
Radial shock wave therapy 255
Radiant heat 189
Radiation 5
    extent of penetration of 191f
    laws of 208
    therapy 189, 301
Radiculopathy 289
    diagnostic measure for 287
Radiotherapy 251
Radium poisoning, chronic 196
Rapid information 273
Rarefaction 238f
Rays, depth of penetration of 190
Rebox-type currents 133, 301
Recent fracture 184
Recording 243
    electrode 279, 285, 287
    system 289
Referred pain 74
Reflection 62
    law of 62, 242
Refraction 62
    law of 62, 63
Regeneration, factor influencing rate of 122
Rehabilitation, biofeedback in 272
Renal function 214
Renal rickets 214
Replacing orthosis 93
Resistance 13, 301
    parallel 14, 14f
    series 13, 14f
Rheobase 124, 301
Rheostat 15, 301
    types 15
Rheumatoid arthritis 71, 177, 196
Rickets 206, 214
    type of 214
Right hand
    palm rule 32
    thumb rule 33, 33f
Rigid lattice formation 4
Ruby laser 219
Russian currents 133, 133f, 301

S

Sacral vertebra, lumbarization of 173, 196
Sacroiliac joint infections 196
Sacroiliitis, types of 196
Salicylates 252
Salicylic acid 126, 211
Saline water 97, 139
Salpingitis 178, 187
    local contraindications 187
    placement of electrodes 188
    positioning of patient 188
Sauna bath 235, 302
    phases of 235
    physiological effects of 235
Scalds 163
Scanning method 220
Scar tissue 221, 250
Sciatica 178
    causes 178
    clinical features 178
Sclerosis, subchondral 180
Scoliosis 93
Sebaceous glands 211
Sebum production 211
Seddon's classification 85, 122
Self-induction 51, 51f, 302
    coefficient of 51
Semiconductor 16
    diode laser, invention of 217
    laser 219
    resistance of 16
    types of 16
Semicylindrical framework 202
Sensation, loss of 143, 184
Sensitive galvanometer, conditions for 35
Sensitizers 215
    use of 207
Sensory 105
    feedback mechanism 273
    fibers 264
    loss 102
    nerve 93
        action potential 286, 287f, 288f
        conduction velocity 302
        painful stimulation of 59
        stimulation of 93
    signs 100
Sepsis, acute 251
Shock 59, 302
Shockwave therapy
    apparatus 255f
    dosage parameters 256
    physical principles 255
Shortwave diathermy 148, 148f, 162, 177, 197, 302
    application of 175, 176
    circuit for 149f
    construction 149

contraindications of 164
dangers of 162
methods of applications 150
principles 149
therapeutic effects of 160
working 150
Shoulder arm movements 226
Shunt 35, 36f
uses of 36
Silicon, pure semiconductor of 16
Simian hand 100
Single fiber needle electrodes 278
Sinus 178
crossfire technique for 157f
Sinusoidal current 79, 79f, 302
Skin
and connective tissue 231
conditions, acute 207
conductance activity 271
cross-section of 191f
grafting 207
hypersensitive 143, 162
resistance lowering tray 96, 98f, 140f
preparation of 97, 139
sensation 230
Snell's law 63
Sodium 126
Soft tissue injury 71
Sound
intensity 70
perception of 68
physical principles of 67
pressure 69
propagation of 68
speed of 70
wave 68, 238
characteristics 69
properties 69
Spasticity 274
Spectrum 135
Speedometers 50
Spherical capacitor 9, 10f
Spherical wavefront 65
Spinal cord injury 274
Spinal muscular atrophy 291
Spinal stenosis 196
Spine, pyogenic infections of 196
Spondylolisthesis 173, 196
Spondylosis 196
Spontaneous activity 281, 282, 302
Sprain 302
grades of 268
Stable cavitation 248
Starling's law 72
Static electricity 5, 302
Stelazine 216
Sterile paraffin wax 230
Stimulating electrode 285, 287
Stimulating system 289

Stimulation, effect of frequency of 84
Storage cells 26
Straight conductor carrying current 32, 32f
Strain 302
Strength-duration curve 121, 302
Stress incontinence 137, 146
Strong electromagnets 18
Student's elbow 261
Stylomastoid foramen 109
Subacromial bursitis 261
Subacute injuries, treatment of 262
Subdeltoid bursitis 260, 261
causes 261
clinical features 261
Suberythemal dose 214
Sulfonal 215
Sulfonamides 215
Sulfur-based ointment 211
Sunlight, dispersion of 65f
Superconductivity 17, 18
cause of 18
Superconductors 18
applications of 18
Superficial dermis 193, 204
Superficial epidermis 193
Superficial heating modalities 228
Superficial tissue 237
Super-high frequency electromagnetic waves 59
Supracondylar fracture 100
Suprapatellar bursitis 261
Supraspinatus tendinitis 225, 259
clinical features 225, 259
etiology 259
exercise 260
management 259
physiotherapy 260
treatment 226
Surface electrodes 277, 277f
Sweat glands, effects of heat on 160
Sweating phase 235
Sweep frequency 135
Synovial membrane, inflammation of 177
Synthetic medium 219
Syringomyelia 291

T

Tannic acid 253
Tendinitis 302
Tennis elbow 224, 258
clinical features 225, 258
etiology 224
pathology 224, 258
treatment 225, 258
Tenosynovitis 260
Tensile strength 221
Terramycin 215
Tetracycline 215
Thalazole 215
Theraktin tunnel 201-203, 203f, 204

Therapeutic ultrasound 236*f*
Thermal 71
    effects 248
        uses of 248
        radiation 62
Thermistors 15
Thermistors, applications of 15
Thermostat pilot lamp 229
Thiazide diuretics 215
Thoracic outlet syndrome 289
Thrombophlebitis 164
Thumb, inability of flex interphalangeal of 100
Tibial nerve, submaximal stimulation of 288
Tissues, thermal conductivity of 262
Toweling method 229
Toxic neuropathy 291
Toxicity 196
Tranquilizer 216
Transcutaneous electrical nerve stimulation 127
    apparatus 127*f*
    contraindications 131
    indications for use 130
    methods of treatment 130
    types of 128
Transformer 54, 303
    construction 54
    principle 54
    step-down transformer 54
    step-up transformer 54
    types of 55
    uses of 56
    working 54
Transient cavitation 249
Transverse waves 66, 69
Trauma, treatment of acute 262
Traumatic synovitis 111
Tridymite formation 201
Trigger point 303
Trimethyl psoralens 215
Trolamine salicylate 252
Tuberculosis, extrapulmonary 187
Tuberculous salpingitis 187
Tumors 164, 167, 251
    benign 196
    malignant 196
Two medium frequency currents 134*f*
Two-phase AC generator 53

U

Ulcers 209, 210
    base of 210
    components of 209
    types 209
    venous 209
Ulnar nerve
    injury 103*f*
    stimulation 94, 101, 103*f*
Ultrasonic apparatus, components of 239*f*
Ultrasonic fields 240, 240*f*
Ultrasonic therapy 236, 248
    dosage 246
    methods of application 243
    techniques 243
Ultrasonic waves 239*f*, 303
Ultrasound
    attenuation of 239
    dangers of 250
    frequency of 237
    parameters of 246
    physiological effects of 248
    production of 238
    reflection of 242, 248
    therapeutic uses of 250
    transmission of 239
    treatment heads 237*f*
    uses of 250
    waves, depth of penetration of 237*f*
Ultraviolet irradiations, indications of 205
Ultraviolet radiations 58, 71, 206, 214, 303
    dangers of 206
    dosage, calculation of 209
    physiological effects of 204
    production of 201
    treatment 212
Ultraviolet rays 201, 204
Unconsciousness, stage of 59
Upper limb 289
Uremic neuropathy 291

V

van't Hoff's law 303
Vapocoolant sprays 263
Vaporization, latent heat of 5
Varicose
    ulcers 250
    vein 184, 196
Vascular impairment 181
Vaseline 97, 139
Vasoconstriction 72, 303
Vasodilation 72
Vasospastic disease 266
Venous thrombosis 164
Vertebra, congenital bony malformations of 173, 196
Viral myositis 291
Vitamin D 205
    production of 205
Vitiligo 215
    treatment 215
Volt 11
Voltaic cell 23, 24*f*
Voltameter 21, 36, 36*f*, 303

W

Walk standing 100
Wallerian degeneration 121, 303
Waste products, removal of 94
Water bag method 244, 245, 245*f*, 303
Water-cooled mercury vapor lamp 202

Wave
  longitudinal 69f
  number 69
  phenomenon 67
  properties of 237
  transverse 69f
  types of 66
  velocity of 238
Waveform 86
  asymmetric 89
  biphasic pulse 86f
  monophasic pulse 87f
  shapes 87, 88f
Wavelengths 220
  mixture of 62

Whirlpool bath 233, 233f, 303
Wire mesh guard 190f
Wound 205
  healing 221
Wrist 102
  level of 100, 102

X
Xiphisternum 214

Z
Zinc oxide 126

EU GSPR Authorised Reprsentative
Logos Europe, 9 rue Nicolas Poussin
1700, La Rochelle, France
Phone: +33 (0) 6 67 93 73 78
E-mail: contact@logoseurope.eu